Man-Made Medicine

Duke University Press   Durham and London 1996

MAN-MADE MEDICINE

Women's

Health,

Public Policy,

and Reform

Kary L. Moss, Editor

© *1996 Duke University Press*
All rights reserved
Printed in the United States of America on acid-free paper ∞
Designed by Katy Giebenhain
Typeset in Janson by Keystone Typesetting, Inc.
Library of Congress Cataloging-in-Publication Data appear on the last printed page of this book.

Title page photograph: *Unidentified Model* (83.34) by Thomas Eakins, courtesy of Hirshhorn Museum and Sculpture Garden, Smithsonian Institution. Transferred from the Hirshhorn Museum and Sculpture Garden Archives, 1983. Photograph by Lee Stalsworth.

Contents

Editor's Acknowledgments

. . . .

I would like to thank many people who were essential to the development and execution of this book. First I wish to thank Rachel Toor at Duke University Press, for her support of my initial idea, her skill, and encouragement; she taught me a great deal about effective editing. I also wish to thank Isabelle Katz Pinzler, Joan Bertin, and the American Civil Liberties Union, for providing me, while I was a staff attorney at the Women's Rights Project, with role models and the opportunity and support for working in the area of gender bias in health care.

My thanks especially to the authors of the essays in this book, whose excitement about the project turned an idea into reality. Thank you to the Board of Directors of the Maurice and Jane Sugar Law Center for Economic and Social Justice, and to my secretary, Donna Allen, whose careful attention to detail made the process much easier. Finally, my thanks to my entire family for their loving encouragement and support.

The editor and publisher gratefully acknowledge permission to reprint materials from the following sources: Carol J. Gill, "Cultivating Common Ground: Women with Disabilities," which originally appeared in *Health/Pac Bulletin* (winter 1992); Nancy Krieger and Elizabeth Fee, "Man-Made Medicine and Women's Health: The Biopolitics of Sex/ Gender and Race/Ethnicity," which originally appeared in the *International Journal of Health Services* 24, no. 2 (1994). Both are reprinted by permission of the publishers.

The editor would also like to recognize that the phrase "Man-Made Medicine," used in the title of this book, was borrowed from Nancy Krieger and Elizabeth Fee, who wrote the first essay.

Man-Made Medicine

Introduction

This book examines the effects of tenacious stereotypes upon the delivery of health care to women in the United States, and looks particularly at those factors that shape health care policy. We focus in part upon specific groups of women whose access to the health care system is especially restricted by race and class.

Long after courts determined that it was an impermissible basis for making laws in this country, gender stereotyping has persisted in the health care arena.[1] When women need health care, they enter a system in which institutional biases restrict their access in many different ways. Some of these are obvious: women are excluded from important clinical trials because of their reproductive capacity, thereby precluding the development of safe treatments for them; the medical establishment has not adequately taken up research about certain diseases that are more common to women than men; many programs and services, such as AIDS treatment, for the most part still do not address the needs of women; and pregnant women continue to be excluded from most drug treatment programs. The list goes on.

Bias persists in less obvious ways as well. For instance, the medical and social implications of important differences *among* women remain largely ignored. We know little, for example, about the significance of race on the progression of AIDS in African-American women, who, as of July 1993, comprised over one-half of the nearly 37,000 women diagnosed with AIDS.[2] The notion of women being defined principally through their reproductive capacities remains a driving force in health care research and public policy as well.

The authors — a dedicated group of academics, lawyers, policymakers, and health care activists whose past work has challenged fundamental problems with the system — have been asked here to talk about these issues and discuss the reform measures they believe are essential to generating improvements in the delivery of health care in this country. They draw upon information from various disciplines, demonstrating the close interaction between the legal system, the research and development industry, Congress, academia, and health care professionals, and the necessity for interdisciplinary efforts at reform.

The most common theme in these chapters is that gender stereotyping continues to significantly affect the formation and implementation of public policy. The authors recognize that improvement in the delivery of health care requires work on many fronts: eliminating sex bias in research, testing, and reporting; expanding access to primary care, clinical trials, and research for all women and girls; and working to eradicate the conditions that lead to unwanted pregnancies as well as those, such as poverty, that are at the root of most health problems.

The book does not critique any specific health care plan.[3] The authors do not attempt to articulate a general theory of reform, nor do they discuss every important issue affecting women's health and the health care system. Instead, the book offers an interdisciplinary approach to a complex array of problems that are too often oversimplified by fragmented institutional structures ill-equipped to devise short- and long-range policy solutions.

The book begins with several essays that discuss bias in science, or in its reporting, as it affects the delivery of health care. Nancy Krieger and Elizabeth Fee describe how a "logic of difference" has evolved from the medical community's practice, during the nineteenth and twentieth centuries, of using white men as the "research subject of choice for all health conditions other than women's reproductive health":

> Within medicine, women's health was relegated to obstetrics and gynecology; within public health, women's health needs were seen as being met by maternal and child health programs. Women were perceived as wives and mothers; they were important for childbirth, child care, and domestic nutrition. Although no one denied that some women worked, women's occupational health was essentially ignored because women were, after all, only temporary workers. Outside the specialized realm of reproduction, all other health research concerned men's bodies and men's diseases.
>
> This framework has shaped knowledge and practice to the present. U.S. vital statistics present health information in terms of race and sex and age, conceptualized only as biological variables — ignoring the social dimensions of gender and ethnicity. Data on social class are not collected. At the same time, public health profes-

sionals are unable adequately to explain or to change inequalities in health between men and women and between diverse racial/ethnic groups.

Not enough is known, they argue, about "the many ways that gender as a social reality gets into the body and transforms our biology." That poor women suffer more from cervical cancer while breast cancer is more common among the affluent, for example, is evidence that more than biology is at issue and that the social patterning of disease should not be ignored. They believe the remedy lies in asking what is different and similar across "the social divides of gender, color, and class." To create an alternative understanding, they suggest:

> [W]e must reframe the issues in the context of the social shaping of our human lives — as both biological creatures and historical actors. Otherwise, we will continue to mistake — as many before us have done — what is for what must be, and leave unchallenged the social forces that continue to create vast inequalities in health.

The influence of a distorted view of differences between the sexes, premised on the reproductive abilities of women, is also addressed by Joan E. Bertin, Director of the Program on Gender, Science and Law at the Columbia University School of Public Health, and Laurie R. Beck, Director of Education Policy at the Community Service Society, whose chapter focuses on the role played by the popular press. They begin by recognizing the power of medical and scientific information, which makes it "big news": "It alters individual conduct, shapes social policy, and influences law." The media provide the means by which this information achieves much of its power.

How, they ask, do the media select and communicate this information? To answer that question, they track print media coverage of scientific findings about gender that either confirm or defy gender-role expectations. Specifically, they examine contemporaneous press coverage of seven studies reported in scholarly journals that deal with reproductive risk issues, choosing that topic because it is invested with enormous social importance and because it is an area in which gender roles are socially well defined.

They find that the popular media report more often on studies that find innate gender differences than on those that find little or no sex-based differences. Sometimes the media even report differences where none were found at all. Bertin and Beck explain this occurrence as rest-ing upon journalists' and scientists' urges to buttress social conventions and cultural arrangements with biological data:

> Scientific explanations can be used to "validate a social preference," that is, to legitimize gender-based social norms and the gender-based allocation of roles, privileges, and responsibilities, which are deeply ingrained in our culture. At the same time, rigid sex-based allocations of roles and rights have been recognized as the source of personal, social, and legal wrongs — felt mostly, but not exclusively, by women — and have been legally repudiated. Recognition of these wrongs has stimulated the repudiation of many cultural sex roles and stereotypes, but the process is a tortuous one. This may explain, at least in part, the popular fascination with scientific theories, no matter how poorly derived, that purport to document a biological basis for gender differences and conventional sex-role behaviors. Scientific evidence of gender similarity would not perform the same comforting function, since it would force recognition of the unfairness of some of those traditional arrangements.

Inaccurate reporting has a powerful impact upon public discourse, impeding the capacity for public policy to adequately address women's health needs:

> First . . . the tendency to dichotomize on the basis of sex "generates invidious comparison" and provides "a framework to which cultures can attach a broad range of social differences that in fact have little to do with [anatomical] sex difference." Second, if the goal is to promote accurate science, it is important to determine what differences really exist and what they mean. . . . The focus on the differences between the sexes, moreover, can obscure important similarities and distort scientific inquiry.

The authors note, for example, that "seeing reproductive biology through a 'gendered' lens has prevented important questions from being asked[,] . . . obscured knowledge of the sensitivity of the male reproductive system to toxic insult . . . [and] also has served to rationalize punitive policies toward women."

The efficacy of scientific research for women is also influenced by the nature and degree of consumer involvement in the research process itself. Professor Kay Dickersin and Dr. Lauren Schnaper, of the University of Maryland's School of Medicine, examine how exclusion of consumers from the research process has impacted research about certain diseases and access to certain kinds of treatment for women. They observe, for example, that "[c]ervical, endometrial, ovarian, and breast cancer; endometriosis; conditions related to pregnancy and the menstrual cycle have neither been taken up as special causes by the public nor championed by the 'hidden colleges' in Congress and academe."

They examine the consequences for women, as well as the more general failure to accommodate cultural and economic variations in planning and executing clinical investigations. They look specifically at the role breast cancer activists have played in increasing the amount of money spent on breast cancer research and treatments, and identify generally the benefits to be gained by giving greater attention to issues of concern to women.

The next section of the book, "Moving from the Periphery," examines the impact of bias in research and the impact of gender stereotyping upon specific populations of women. It also looks at the responsiveness of the medical establishment to certain diseases as they affect women and girls. Catherine Teare and attorney Abigail English, of the National Center for Youth Law, describe the various ways in which bias has been manifested in AIDS research and treatment. Exclusion of women from HIV/AIDS research and clinical trials, because of their reproductive capacity and a restrictive definition of the disease itself, has had a profound impact on women individually, as well as on HIV research generally, "by stalling the expansion of knowledge of pharmacokinetics, safety, and efficacy of interventions."

Stereotyping of women as perpetually pregnant in the AIDS context has resulted in the nearly exclusive concern with perinatal transmission, at the expense of studying women's own risk for infection:

> Basic research on the natural history of HIV infection in women — gynecologic manifestations, the effect of pregnancy on disease progression and on treatment, the effects of hormones on the course of the disease, and other topics — has begun in earnest only recently. For some time, however, clinicians have noticed that HIV manifests and progresses differently in women.

The cost of neglect is significant: without an AIDS diagnosis, women cannot qualify for important services, treatment, or benefits. Women's access to HIV testing remains difficult, as does access to reproductive and prenatal care and expensive and specialized treatments. Moreover, the perception that it is still primarily a male disease results in underdiagnosis by physicians who are not alert to its symptoms in women.

Teare and English advocate for a reform agenda that cuts a broad swath across several fields: health care and research, child welfare, and law, among many others. They seek expanded access to primary care for women and girls, especially those with low incomes, funding for clinical trials and research studies, research on the natural history of HIV disease in women and girls, specialized treatment for HIV disease and substance abuse, and appropriate HIV counseling and voluntary testing. They also call for a limitation on mandatory testing of women and girls, and for greater, independent, and confidential access to health care services.

In no other context are the problems resulting from gender bias as apparent as in the context of reproductive health. Controlling the timing and circumstances of motherhood is essential to women's health and well-being as well as to that of their children. The impediments facing women seeking safe and inexpensive reproductive health care are examined by Dr. Wendy Chavkin, an associate professor at Columbia University's School of Public Health, and Professor Ann Scales of the University of New Mexico School of Law.

Dr. Chavkin begins by examining the public health aspects of safe abortions and the ramifications of the provider shortage, restrictions of public funds, and new technological and medical developments, which "herald a new era with profound implications for practice and for public health." She calls for the inclusion of abortion coverage under any health care financing plan as essential to ensure equitable access to this service, removal of financial barriers currently in place, and reintegration of abortion provision into the mainstream of reproductive health services and primary care.

Professor Scales identifies a range of barriers to safe abortions, including recent violence directed at clinics and doctors, lack of public funds to help low-income women obtain abortions, and the legal and social doctrines that operate to impede women's access to this important medical service. She calls upon us to challenge what she calls "liberalist discourse that preconceives each of us as *citizen-blanks:* as equally autonomous vessels of potential self-determination, undetermined and uninfluenced by social context":

> The rhetoric of choice, though valuable in the past, does not nearly encompass the meaning of access to abortion for real women living through real crises.

Scales focuses on four strategies for reform: (1) protection of abortion providers; (2) reinstatement of abortion funding for low-income women;

(3) reduction of the number of unwanted and/or dangerous pregnancies; and (4) redescription of abortion as a constitutional equality right, rather than as a privacy right, so that its role in the lives of women is clarified. The first two agenda items devolve fully on ways to protect women's advances and/or to regain lost ground. The last two involve reconceptualizing strategies about abortion and women's health generally.

The book also focuses on the exclusion of certain populations of women in ways that are not legally remediable (and are in fact legally sanctioned or mandated). Immigrant women, for example, are a special population whose lack of access to quality health care has profound public health implications for them and their families, as well as for the rest of society.

Professor Janet M. Calvo, of City University of New York Law School at Queens College, discusses the ways in which legal definitions of the various types of immigration status (i.e., permanent resident, illegal immigrant, and immigrants allowed to remain in the country pending processing of their applications) impedes access of this group of women to health care. She focuses in particular upon battered women, for example, who have historically avoided health care for fear of jeopardizing their relationships with partners upon whose assistance they depend to gain legal status. Professor Calvo further examines how contagious disease control is impeded by a system that prevents those in need from coming forward for fear of being reported to the Immigration and Naturalization Service. She calls for a redefinition of our current notion of citizenship as the only solution to what has become a public health crisis for this population.

Women living in prison are another special population subject to a "systematic pattern of neglect," as described by Ellen M. Barry, Director of Legal Services for Women with Children:

> While the provision of adequate, responsive, and appropriate medical care is a complex challenge in any context, it is particularly challenging in a correctional setting. Prisons and jails are severely stressful environments — they are often dramatically overcrowded[,] . . . unsanitary and intolerably loud. . . . Nutrition is almost always a low priority.

Barry looks in particular at the experiences of pregnant and parenting women, women with substance abuse problems, and women with HIV/AIDS, and describes the positive changes brought about by litigation. She also finds, however, that reform requires attention to complex social factors, which include change in the attitudes of correctional staff, both medical and nonmedical; an increasingly hostile climate towards prisoners; and an enormous increase in the prison population, particularly among people of color. The needs of women in prison must be included, she argues, in any comprehensive health care agenda. She asks us to remember that "women who are incarcerated today will, in most cases, reenter society in another capacity tomorrow — often as low-income, single mothers with all the same critical health concerns as nonincarcerated, low-income women."

Women in the mental health system are a third population whose health care needs have been sorely neglected. Professor Susan Stefan, of the University of Miami School of Law, examines how treatment of mental illness that excludes consideration of gender and sexuality results in the failure to adequately respond to needs unique to the experiences of many women within the mental health system, such as those involving contraception and reproductive rights. She notes that until now even feminists have failed these women:

> Women's groups whose efforts are devoted specifically to health reform issues rarely include mental health as a principal part of their agenda. Even when these concerns are included, the scope of reform is usually limited to proposals for more funding for research and screening. Yet many of the issues raised by mental health treatment are extremely salient to feminism: unwanted and physically intrusive treatment; coercion into roles of passivity and dependence, and punishment for stepping outside the bounds of those roles; construing "unfeminine" behavior as symptomatic and deviant; and separating women from their children. Although feminists have vocally opposed some forms of forced treatment . . . they have paid little attention to the daily imposition of unwanted electric shock, seclusion and restraint, and forcible medication in institutional settings.

She outlines reforms that would "create a system that recognizes and provides for women's specific gender-related issues, such as reproductive capacity, child custody, and the effects of living with the constant threat of sexual violence." Second, she advocates for a system that would

> replace hierarchy with participation and choice, enforced dependency with enhanced control, isolation with connection, models of pathology with models of recovery and strength, and objectification

and a primarily biological model with an understanding of people as humans interacting with each other and operating in a social context that has a vast influence on their behavior and mental health.

The last specific population singled out in this book is that of women with disabilities. Carol J. Gill, a clinical and research psychologist, describes these women as living in a world of "sexism without the pedestal." She looks at the myriad of obstacles that hinder disabled women's access to health care, including biased attitudes that fail to seriously consider a range of health needs, the isolation of disability within medicine, and the isolation of gender, to the exclusion of women's needs, in social scientific research on disability. Blocked access to health-care facilities, limited consideration of privacy issues by the medical establishment, and treatment without consent are all specific manifestations of this neglect. She calls for eradication of government policies that keep disabled people dependent, national health insurance, and financial support for personal assistance as critical reform measures.

Finally, from a different angle, several authors focus on tools used which have made the health care system more responsive to the needs of women, and ways in which women have been able to remedy harms suffered. For example, grassroots organizing by consumers, lay professionals, and health care workers has been key to improving access to health care, the quality of health services, and the responsiveness of the research establishment to their needs, as fully described by Judy Norsigian, coauthor of the seminal work, *Our Bodies, Ourselves.*

Professor Joyce E. McConnell, a law professor at the University of West Virginia School of Law, examines the potential implications of any reform effort upon the tort system, which women historically have used to remedy injuries, both in the medical malpractice and product liability contexts. In her evaluation of proposals for caps on punitive damages, "loser pay" requirements, enterprise liability, and no-fault liability, she observes that many of these recent proposals may adversely affect the ability of women to obtain compensation and may also fail to accomplish their purported goal of decreasing the cost of health care. Reformers must recognize, she urges, that the tort system has offered the only hope for many women injured by products and doctors. She argues that women's health care advocates and policymakers must not bargain away the only methods available to protect women against negligent health care and defective products.

Each of these chapters represents a significant contribution to the literature. Each author brings her unique experiences — as a woman, an advocate, a scientist, or observer — to a complex set of problems that have profound personal implications.

In order for any of these prescriptions to have any chance of success, leadership at the national level is essential. This was well demonstrated during 1994 when there was much debate about the now failed American Health Security Act (AHSA). There are important lessons to be learned from that particular experience which may guide us in any future efforts.

Unlike the Great War on Poverty, which had an ambitious and defined mission, the goal of the AHSA, at least as articulated by the Clinton administration, was fairly simple: "health security." President Clinton proclaimed, for example, in a speech to a Joint Session of Congress on September 22, 1993: "At long last, after decades of false starts, we must make this our most urgent priority: Giving every American health security — health care that's always there." The principles he defined to "guide our reform": "security, simplicity, and savings; choice, quality, and responsibility."

This discourse was, perhaps not surprisingly, one of free market ideology and cold war rhetoric. Notably absent from his vision were "[t]he traditional liberal themes of doing justice, of attending to the downtrodden, to those on whom society has inflicted much pain and discrimination in the past and whom we have put into dire economic circumstances."[4] He sidestepped the thorny question of health care as a right, and government's role and responsibility to its citizens, to insist upon maintaining the status quo, which treats health care as a matter of contract between private parties. The vision: each employer would provide coverage to its employees. The health security card would ensure that those employees would obtain a comprehensive set of benefits comparable to those offered by Fortune 500 companies.

The incantation of these words — security, simplicity, savings; choice, quality, responsibility — performed a magic trick. Differences in race, income, gender, health, living and working conditions faded away in the public consciousness. All were rendered equal. The government's duty would be done, and health care as a problem resolved.

However, by avoiding a discussion about the values we as a society most cherish, fragmented interest groups were able to focus exclusively on their own narrow and immediate concerns. As observed by Harvard medical economist Rashi Fein: "When debates about money displace those concerned with principles, it is the bookkeeper who dominates the discussion. Such debates, with their focus on the 'practical,' . . . ignore the vision of the kind of society and medical care sector we seek."[5] The public, alienated from its leaders, was left behind.[6] In the absence of a more comprehensive, long-term vision, the chosen vehicle of reform — a law — was doomed.

This result was not all that surprising, while nonetheless disappointing. Historically, laws have proven to be poor vehicles for generating massive social change of the type on everyone's mind at the beginning of the reform effort. The legal and public health systems traditionally come into contact only when something fails. Laws are used to obtain remedies for those injured during the course of medical treatment; they are used by civil rights advocates seeking to increase access to hospitals believed to discriminate against a protected group, or to reform large institutions believed to treat specific groups of people poorly. Sometimes laws, such as those governing the civil commitment process, are used when a person is believed unable to function outside of an institution. And sometimes laws are used punitively, as when pregnant women are prosecuted for drug or alcohol use during pregnancy.[7]

Rarely, however, is the legal system used in a proactive way to empower its users. Legislatures and courts are not the place for enlightened understanding of the meaning of disease. For any law to provide the means for broad-based social change, it must first have the strong and vocal support of consumers themselves. It must take as its inspiration a profound sense of public duty or obligation derived from the existence of a fundamental right.

The inability of the reform effort to do just that meant that few could believe it would make a substantial difference in their own lives. Without the creation of a vested interest, the reform movement lost its energy and base of once strong grassroots support. Those magical words — security, simplicity, and savings; choice, quality, and responsibility — faded away in the face of a more generalized fear of the unknown.

This is not to minimize the influence and power of various industries for whom reform was not in their best interests. Nor is it to minimize the importance of cost containment as a strategy and goal of health care reform. However, leadership in the area of health care policy must operate from the premise of our interdependence as a community and an understanding that the health care system, for many complex reasons, fails a significant section of the population. The sad consequences of our inability to include this failure in the formulation of a vision of reform must become at the very least a part of the public discourse about health care reform. And that public discourse must be translated into particular demands with the weight of energy that drove the civil rights and women's movements. As the chapters in this book demonstrate, anything less is destined to fail because of the complexity and seriousness of the issues.

This book is one contribution to the public debate. It is my hope that the reader will approach this book with the same enthusiasm undertaken by the authors themselves and will close it feeling as enlightened as do I.

Notes

1   See *International Union v. Johnson Controls, Inc.*, 111 S. Ct. 1196 (1991).
2   See chapter 1 at note 73, where Krieger and Fee cite Centers for Disease Control and Prevention, *HIV/AIDS Surveillance Report* 5 (July 1993): 1–19.
3   The authors of the chapters are responsible only for the work contained within their own chapters, and not for each other's work or for the ideas articulated in this introduction.
4   Amitai Etzioni, "How to Transform Society: The Health Care Example," *TIKKUN* 8, no. 6 (1993): 14.
5   Ronald A. Carson, "Reconfiguring Health Care," *TIKKUN* 8, no. 6 (1993): 15.
6   For example, the Health Insurance Association of America (HIAA) spent their time fighting the proposal that would allow purchasing cooperatives to determine what health plans consumers can buy. The American Medical Association spent their time pushing for preservation of patient choice of physicians and for limitations on fees and malpractice protections.
7   See K. Moss, "Recent Update: Substance Abuse During Pregnancy," *Harvard Women's Law Journal* 13 (1990): 278.

The Making and Interpretation of Science

1

MAN-MADE MEDICINE AND WOMEN'S HEALTH

The Biopolitics of
Sex/Gender
and Race/Ethnicity

. . . .

Nancy Krieger and Elizabeth Fee

Introduction

Glance at any collection of national health data for the United States —
whether pertaining to health, disease, or the health care system — and
several features stand out.[1] First, notice that most reports present data
in terms of race, sex, and age. Some races are clearly of more interest
than others. National reports most frequently use racial groups called
"white" and "black" and, increasingly, a group called "Hispanic." Occasionally, we find data on Native Americans and on Asians and Pacific
Islanders. Whatever the specific categories chosen, the reports agree
that white men and women, for the most part, have the best health, at all
ages. They also show that men and women, across all racial groups, have
different patterns of disease. Obviously, men and women differ for conditions related to reproduction (women, for example, do not get testicular cancer), but they differ for many other conditions as well — for
example, men on average have higher blood pressure and develop cardiovascular disease at an earlier age. And, in the health care sector, occupations, just like diseases, are differentially distributed by race and sex.

All this seems obvious. But it isn't. We know about race and sex divisions because this is what our society considers important. This is how
we classify people and collect data. This is how we organize our social
life as a nation. This is therefore how we structure our knowledge about
health and disease. And this is what we find important as a subject of
research.[2]

It seems so routine, so normal, to view the health of women and men as fundamentally different, to consider the root of this difference to be biological sex, and to think about race as an inherent, inherited characteristic that also affects health.[3] The work of looking after sick people follows the same categories. Simply walk into a hospital and observe that most of the doctors are white men, most of the registered nurses are white women, most of the kitchen and laundry workers are black and Hispanic women, and most of the janitorial staff are black and Hispanic men. Among the patients, notice who has appointments with private clinicians and who is getting care in the emergency room; the color line is obvious. Notice who provides health care at home: wives, mothers, and daughters. The gender line at home and in medical institutions is equally obvious.[4]

These contrasting patterns, by race and sex, are longstanding. How do we explain them? What kinds of explanations satisfy us? Some are comfortable with explanations that accept these patterns as natural, as the result of natural law, as part of the natural order of things. Of course, if patterns are that way by nature, they cannot be changed. Others aim to understand these patterns precisely in order to change them. They look for explanations suggesting that these patterns are structured by convention, by discrimination, by the politics of power, and by unreasonable law. These patterns, in other words, reflect the social order of people.

In this essay, we discuss how race and sex became such all-important, self-evident categories in nineteenth- and twentieth-century biomedical thought and practice. We examine the consequences of these categories for our knowledge about health and for the provision of health care. We then consider alternative approaches to studying race/ethnicity, gender, and health. And we address these issues with reference to a typically suppressed and repressed category: that of social class.

The Social Construction of "Race" and "Sex" as Key Biomedical Terms and Their Effect on Knowledge About Health

In the nineteenth century, the construction of "race" and "sex" as key biomedical categories was driven by social struggles over human inequality. Before the Civil War, the dominant understanding of race was as a natural/theological category — black/white differences were innate and reflected God's will.[5] These differences were believed to be manifest in every aspect of the body, in sickness and in health. But when abolitionists began to get the upper hand in moral and theological arguments, proponents of slavery appealed to science as the new arbiter of racial distinction.

In this period, medical men were beginning to claim the mantle of scientific knowledge and assert their right to decide controversial social issues.[6] Recognizing the need for scientific authority, the state of Louisiana, for example, commissioned one prolific proponent of slavery, Dr. Samuel Cartwright, to prove the natural inferiority of blacks, a task that led him to detail every racial difference imaginable — in texture of hair, length of bones, vulnerability to disease, and even color of the internal organs.[7] As the Civil War changed the status of blacks from legal chattel to bona fide citizens, however, medical journals began to question old verities about racial differences and, as importantly, to publish new views of racial similarities.[8] Some authors even attributed black/white differences in health to differences in socioeconomic position. But by the 1870s, with the destruction of Reconstruction, the doctrine of innate racial distinction again triumphed. The scientific community once again deemed "race" a fundamental biological category.[9]

Theories of women's inequality followed a similar pattern.[10] In the early nineteenth century, traditionalists cited scripture to prove women's inferiority. These authorities agreed that Eve had been formed out of Adam's rib and that all women had to pay the price of her sin — disobeying God's order, seeking illicit knowledge from the serpent, and tempting man with the forbidden apple. Women's pain in childbirth was clear proof of God's displeasure.

When these views were challenged in the mid-nineteenth century by advocates of women's rights and proponents of liberal political theory, conservatives likewise turned to the new arbiters of knowledge and sought to buttress their position with scientific facts and medical authority.[11] Biologists busied themselves with measuring the size of women's skulls, the length of their bones, the rate of their breathing, and the number of their blood cells. And considering all the evidence, the biologists concluded that women were indeed the weaker sex.[12]

Agreeing with this stance, medical men energetically took up the issue of women's health and equality.[13] They were convinced that the true woman was by nature sickly, her physiological systems at the mercy of her ovaries and uterus. Because all bodily organs were interconnected, they argued, a woman's monthly cycle irritated her delicate nervous system and her sensitive, small, weak brain. Physicians considered women especially vulnerable to nervous ailments such as neurasthenia and hysteria. This talk of women's delicate constitutions did not apply, of course, to slave women or to working-class women — but it was handy to refute the demands of middle-class women whenever they sought to vote or gain access to education and professional careers. At such moments, many medical men declared the doctrine of separate spheres to be the ineluctable consequence of biology.

At the same time, nineteenth-century medical authorities began to conceptualize class as a natural, biological distinction. Traditional, pre-scientific views held class hierarchies to be divinely ordained; according to the more scientific view that emerged in the early nineteenth century, class position was determined by innate, inherited ability. In both cases, class was perceived as an essentially stable, hierarchical ranking. These discussions of class usually assumed white or Western European populations and often applied only to males within those populations.

With the impact of the industrial revolution, classes took on a clearly dynamic character. As landowners invested in canals and railroads, as merchants became capitalist entrepreneurs, and as agricultural workers were transformed into an industrial proletariat, the turbulent transformation of the social order provoked new understandings of class relationships.[14] The most developed of these theories was that of Karl Marx, who emphasized the system of classes as a social and economic formation and stressed the contradictions between different class interests.[15] From this point onward, the very idea of social classes in many people's minds implied a revolutionary threat to the social order.

In opposition to Marxist analyses of class, the theory of Social Darwinism was formulated to suggest that the new social inequalities of industrial society reflected natural law.[16] This theory was developed in the midst of the economic depression of the 1870s, at a time when labor struggles, trade union organizing, and early socialist movements were challenging the political and economic order. Many scientists and medical men drew upon Darwin's idea of "the struggle for survival," first expressed in the *Origin of the Species* in 1859,[17] to justify social inequality. They argued that those on top, the social elite, must by definition be the "most fit" because they had survived so well. Social hierarchies were therefore built on and reflected real biological differences. Poor health status simultaneously was sign and proof of biological inferiority.

By the late nineteenth century, theories of race, gender, and class inequality were linked together by the theory of Social Darwinism, which promised to provide a scientific basis for social policy.[18] In the realm of race, for example, proponents of Social Darwinism blithely predicted that the "Negro Question" would soon resolve itself — the "Negro" would naturally become extinct, eliminated by the inevitable workings of "natural selection."[19] Many public health officers — particularly in the southern states — agreed that "Negroes" were an inherently degenerate, syphilitic, and tubercular race, for whom public health interventions could do little.[20] Social Darwinists also argued that natural and sexual selection would lead to increasing differentiation between the sexes.[21] With further evolution, men would become ever more masculine and women ever more feminine. As proof, they looked to the upper classes, whose masculine and feminine behavior represented the forefront of evolutionary progress.

Over time, the Social Darwinist view of class gradually merged into general American ideals of progress, meritocracy, and success through individual effort. According to the dominant American ideology, individuals were so mobile that fixed measures of social class were irrelevant. Such measures were also un-American. Since the Paris Commune, and especially since the Bolshevik revolution, discussions of social class in the United States were perceived as politically threatening. Although fierce debates about inequality continued to revolve around the axis of nature versus nurture, the notion of class as a social relationship was effectively banished from respectable discourse and policy debate.[22] Social position was once again equated only with rank, now understood as socioeconomic status.

In the early twentieth century, Social Darwinists had considerable influence in shaping public views and public policy.[23] They perceived two new threats to American superiority: the massive tide of immigration from eastern and southern Europe, and the declining birth rate — or "race suicide" — among American white women of Anglo-Saxon and Germanic descent. Looking to the fast-developing field of genetics, now bolstered by the rediscovery of Gregor Mendel's laws and by T. H. Morgan's fruit fly experiments,[24] biological determinists regrouped under the banner of eugenics. Invoking morbidity and mortality data that showed a high rate of tuberculosis and infectious disease among the immigrant poor,[25] they declared "ethnic" Europeans a naturally inferior and sickly stock and thus helped win passage of the Immigration Restriction Act in 1924.[26] This legislation required the national mix of immigrants to match that entering the United States in the early 1870s, thereby severely curtailing immigration of racial and ethnic groups deemed inferior. "Race/ethnicity," construed as a biological reality, became ever more entrenched as the *explanation* of racial/ethnic differences in disease; social explanations were seen as the province of scientifically illiterate and naive liberals, or worse, socialist and Bolshevik provocateurs.

Other developments in the early twentieth century encouraged biological explanations of sex differences in disease and in social roles. The discovery of the sex chromosomes in 1905[27] reinforced the idea that gender was a fundamental biological trait, built into the genetic constitution of the body. That same year, Ernest Starling coined the term "hormone"[28] to denote the newly characterized chemical messengers that permitted one organ to control — at a distance — the activities of another. By the mid-1920s, researchers had isolated several hormones integral to reproductive physiology and popularized the notion of "sex hormones."[29] The combination of sex chromosomes and sex hormones were imbued with almost magical powers to shape human behavior in gendered terms; women were now at the mercy of their genetic limitations and a changing brew of hormonal imperatives.[30] In the realm of medicine, researchers turned to sex chromosomes and hormones to understand cancers of the uterus and breast and a host of other sex-linked diseases;[31] they no longer saw the need to worry about environmental influences. In the workplace, of course, employers said that sex chromosomes and hormones dictated which jobs women could — and could not — perform.[32] This in turn determined the occupational hazards to which women would be exposed — once again, women's health and ill health were viewed as a matter of their biology.

Within the first few decades of the twentieth century, these views were institutionalized within scientific medicine and the new public health. At this time, the training of physicians and public health practitioners was being recast in modern, scientific terms.[33] Not surprisingly, biological determinist views of racial/ethnic and sex/gender differences became a natural and integral part of the curriculum, the research agenda, and medical and public health practice. Over time, ethnic differences in disease among white European groups were downplayed and instead, the differences between whites and blacks, whites and Mexicans, whites and Asians were emphasized. Color was now believed to define distinct biological groups.

Similarly, the sex divide marked a gulf between two completely disparate groups. Within medicine, women's health was relegated to obstetrics and gynecology; within public health, women's health needs were seen as being met by maternal and child health programs.[34] Women were perceived as wives and mothers; they were important for childbirth, child care, and domestic nutrition. Although no one denied that some women worked, women's occupational health was essentially ignored because women were, after all, only temporary workers. Outside the specialized realm of reproduction, all other health research concerned men's bodies and men's diseases. Reproduction was so central to women's biological existence that women's nonreproductive health was rendered virtually invisible.

Currently, it is popular to argue that the lack of research on white women and on men and women in nonwhite racial/ethnic groups resulted from a perception of white men as the norm.[35] This interpretation, however, is inaccurate. In fact, by the time that researchers began to standardize methods for clinical and epidemiological research, notions of difference were so firmly embedded that whites and nonwhites, women and men, were rarely studied together. Moreover, most researchers and physicians were interested only in the health status of whites and, in the case of women, only in their reproductive health. They therefore used white men as the research subjects of choice for all health conditions other than women's reproductive health and paid attention to the health status of nonwhites only to measure degrees of racial difference. For the most part, the health of women and men of color and the nonreproductive health of white women was simply ignored. It is critical to read these omissions as evidence of a logic of difference rather than as an assumption of similarity.

This framework has shaped knowledge and practice to the present. U.S. vital statistics present health information in terms of race and sex and age, conceptualized only as biological variables — ignoring the social dimensions of gender and ethnicity. Data on social class are not collected. At the same time, public health professionals are unable adequately to explain or to change inequalities in health between men and women and between diverse racial/ethnic groups. We now face the question: is there any alternative way of understanding these population patterns of health and disease?

Alternative Ways of Studying Race, Gender, and Health: Social Measures for Social Categories

The first step in creating an alternative understanding is to recognize that the categories we traditionally treat as simply biological are in fact largely social. The second step is to realize that we need social concepts to understand these social categories. The third step is to develop social measures and appropriate strategies for a new kind of health research.[36]

With regard to race/ethnicity, we need to be clear that "race" is a spurious biological concept.[37] Although historic patterns of geographic isolation and migration account for differences in the distribution of certain genes, genetic variation within so-called racial groups far exceeds that across groups. All humans share approximately 95 percent of their genetic makeup.[38] Racial/ethnic differences in disease thus require something other than a genetic explanation.

Recognizing this problem, some people have tried to substitute the term "ethnicity" for "race."[39] In the public health literature, however, "ethnicity" is rarely defined. For some, it apparently serves as a polite way of referring to what are still conceptualized as "racial"/biological differences. For others, it expresses a new form of "cultural" determinism, in which ethnic differences in ways of living are seen as autonomous "givens" unrelated to the social status of particular ethnic groups within our society.[40] This cultural determinism makes discrimination invisible and can feed into explanations of health status that are as reductionist and individualistic as those of biological determinism.

For a different starting point, consider the diverse ways in which racism operates, at both an institutional and interpersonal level.[41] Racism is a matter of economics, and it is also more than economics. It structures living and working conditions, affects daily interactions, and takes its toll on people's dignity and pride. All of this must be considered when we examine the connection between race/ethnicity and health.

To address the economic aspects of racism, we need to include economic data in all studies of health status.[42] Currently, our national health data do not include economic information—instead, racial differences are often used as indicators of economic differences. To the extent that economics are taken into account, the standard approach assumes that differences are either economic or "genetic." So, for those conditions where racial/ethnic differences persist even within economic strata— hypertension and preterm delivery, for example—the assumption is that something biological, something genetic, is at play. Researchers rarely consider the noneconomic aspects of racism or the ways in which racism continues to work within economic levels.

Some investigators, however, are beginning to consider how racism shapes people's environments. Several studies, for example, document the fact that toxic dumps are most likely to be located in poor neighborhoods and are disproportionately located in poor neighborhoods of color.[43] Other researchers are starting to ask how people's experience of and response to discrimination may influence their health.[44] A recent study of hypertension, for example, found that black women who responded actively to unfair treatment were less likely to report high blood pressure than women who internalized their responses.[45] Interestingly, the black women at highest risk were those who reported *no* experiences of racial discrimination.

Countering the traditional practice of always taking whites as the standard of comparison, some researchers are beginning to focus on other racial/ethnic groups to better understand why, within each of the groups, some are at higher risk than others for particular disease outcomes.[46] They are considering whether people of color may be exposed to specific conditions that whites are not. In addition to living and working conditions, these include cultural practices that may be positive as well as negative in their effects on health. Some studies, for example, point to the importance of black churches in providing social support.[47] These new approaches break with monolithic assumptions about what it means to belong to a given racial/ethnic group and consider diversity *within* each group. To know the color of a person's skin is to know very little.

It is equally true that to know a person's sex is to know very little. Women are often discussed as a single group defined chiefly by biological sex, members of an abstract, universal (and implicitly white) category. In reality, we are a mixed lot, our gender roles and options shaped by history, culture, and deep divisions across class and color lines. Of course, it is true that women, in general, have the capacity to become pregnant, at least at some stages of their lives. Traditionally, women as a group are defined by this reproductive potential. Usually ignored are the many ways that gender as a social reality gets into the body and transforms our biology — differences in childhood expectations about exercise, for example, affect our subsequent body build.[48]

From a health point of view, women's reproductive potential does carry the possibility of specific reproductive ills, ranging from infertility to preterm delivery to cervical and breast cancer. These reproductive ills are not simply associated with the biological category "female," but are differentially experienced according to social class and race/ethnicity. Poor women, for example, are much more likely to suffer from cervical cancer.[49] By contrast, at least among older women, breast cancer is more common among the affluent.[50] These patterns, which at times can become quite complex, illustrate the general point that, even in the case of reproductive health, more than biological sex is at issue. Explanations of women's reproductive health that ignore the social patterning of disease and focus only on endogenous factors are thus inadequate.

If we turn to those conditions that afflict both men and women — the majority of all diseases and health problems — we must keep two things simultaneously in mind. First are the differences and similarities among diverse groups of women; second are the differences and similarities between women and men.

For a glimpse of the complexity of disease patterns, consider the example of hypertension.[51] As we mentioned, working class and poor women are at greater risk than affluent women; black women, within each income level, are more likely to be hypertensive than white women.[52] The risks of Hispanic women vary by national origin: Mexican women are at lowest risk, Central American women at higher risk, and Puerto Rican and Cuban women at the highest risk.[53] In what is called the "Hispanic paradox," Mexican-American women have a higher risk profile than Anglo women, yet experience lower rates of hypertension.[54] To further complicate the picture, the handful of studies of Japanese and Chinese women in the United States show them to have low rates, while Filipina women have high rates, almost equal those of African-Americans.[55] Rates vary across different groups of Native American women; those who live in the Northern plains have higher rates than those in the Southwest.[56] From all this, we can conclude that there is enormous variation in hypertension rates among women.

If we look at the differences between women and men, we find that men in each racial/ethnic group have higher rates of hypertension than women. Even so, the variation among women is sufficiently great that women in some racial/ethnic groups have higher rates than men in other groups.[57] Filipina women, for example, have higher rates of hypertension than white men.[58] Obviously, the standard biomedical categories of race and sex cannot explain these patterns. If we want to understand hypertension, we will have to understand the complex distribution of disease among real women and men; these patterns are not merely distracting details but are the proper test of the plausibility of our hypotheses.

As a second example, consider the well-known phenomenon of women's longer life expectancy. This difference is common to all industrialized countries, and amounts to about seven years in the United States.[59] The higher mortality of men at younger ages is largely due to higher accident rates, and at older ages, to heart disease.

The higher accident rates of younger men are not accidental. They are due to more hazardous occupations, higher rates of illicit drug and alcohol use, firearms injuries, and motor vehicle crashes — hazards related to gender roles and expectations.[60] The fact that men die earlier of heart disease — the single most common cause of death in both sexes — may also be related to gender roles. Men have higher rates of cigarette smoking and fewer sources of social support, suggesting that the masculine ideal of the Marlboro man is not a healthy one. Some contend that women's cardiovascular advantage is mainly biological, due to the protective effect of their hormone levels.[61] Interestingly, however, a study carried out in a kibbutz in Israel, where men and women were engaged in comparable activities, found that the life expectancy gap was only four and a half years — just over half the national average.[62] While biological differences between men and women now receive much of the research attention, it is important to remember that men are gendered beings too.

Clearly, our patterns of health and disease have everything to do with how we live in the world. Nowhere is this more evident than in the strong social-class gradients apparent in almost every form of morbidity and mortality.[63] Yet here the lack of information and the conceptual confusion about the relationship between social class and women's health is a major obstacle. As previously noted, in this country we have no regular method of collecting data on socioeconomic position and health. Even if we had such data, measures of social class generally assume male heads of households and male patterns of employment.[64] This, indeed, is one of the failures of class analyses — that they do not deal adequately with women.[65]

Perhaps the easiest way to understand the problems of class measurements and women's health is to mention briefly the current debates in Britain, a country that has long collected social class data.[66] Men and unmarried women are assigned a social class position according to their employment; married women, however, are assigned a class position according to the employment of their husbands. As British feminist researchers have argued, this traditional approach obscures the magnitude of class differences in women's health.[67] Instead, they are proposing measures of household class that take into account the occupations of both women and their husbands, and also other household assets. Here in the United States, we have hardly any research on the diverse measures of social class in relation to women's health. Preliminary studies suggest we also would do well to distinguish between individual and household class.[68] Other research shows that we can partly overcome the absence of social class information in U.S. medical records by using census data.[69] This method allows us to describe people in terms of the socioeconomic profile of their immediate neighborhood. When coupled with individual measures of social class, this approach reveals, for example, that working-class women who live in working-class neighborhoods are somewhat more likely to have high blood pressure than working-class women who live in more affluent neighborhoods.[70] We thus need to separate conceptually three distinct levels at which class operates — individual, household, and neighborhood.

As a final example of why women's health cannot be understood without reference to issues of sex/gender, race/ethnicity, and social class, consider the case of AIDS.[71] The definition of disease, the understanding of risk, the approach to prevention — all are shaped by our failure to grasp fully the social context of disease. For the first decade, women's unique experiences of AIDS were rendered essentially invisible. The first definition of AIDS was linked to men, because it was perceived to be a disease of gay men and those with a male sex-linked disorder, hemophilia. The very listing of HIV-related diseases taken to characterize AIDS was a listing based on male experience of infection. Only much later, after considerable protest by women activists, were female disorders — such as invasive cervical cancer — made part of the definition of the disease.[72]

Our understanding of risk is still constrained by the standard approaches. AIDS data are still reported only in terms of race, sex, and mode of transmission; there are no data on social class.[73] We know, however, that the women who have AIDS are overwhelmingly women of color. As of July 1993, of the nearly 37,000 women diagnosed with AIDS, over one half were African-American, another 20 percent were Hispanic, 25 percent were white, and about 1 percent were Asian, Pacific Islander, or Native American.[74] What puts these women at risk? It seems clear that one determinant is the missing variable: social class. Notably, the women at highest risk are injection drug users, the sexual partners of injection drug users, and sex workers.[75] The usual listing of behavioral and demographic risk factors, however, fails to capture the social context in which the AIDS epidemic has unfolded. Most of the epidemiological accounts are silent about the blight of inner cities, the decay of the urban infrastructure under the Reagan and Bush administrations, unemployment, the drug trade, prostitution, and the harsh realities of everyday racism.[76] We cannot gain an adequate understanding of risk absent a real understanding of people's lives.

Knowledge of what puts women at risk is of course critical for prevention. Yet, just as the initial definitions of AIDS reflected a male-gendered perspective, so did initial approaches to prevention.[77] The emphasis on condoms assumed that the central issue was knowledge, not male-female power relations. For women to use condoms in heterosexual sex, however, they need more than bits of plastic; they need male assent. The initial educational materials were created without addressing issues of power; they were male-oriented and obviously white — both in the mode and language of presentation. AIDS programs and services, for the most part, still do not address women's needs. Pregnant women and women with children continue to be excluded from most drug treatment programs. And when women become sick and die, we have no remotely adequate social policies for taking care of the families left behind.

In short, our society's approach to AIDS reflects the larger refusal to deal with the ways in which sex/gender, race/ethnicity, and class are inescapably intertwined with health. This refusal affects not only what we know and what we do about AIDS, but also the other issues we have mentioned — hypertension, cancer, life expectancy — and many we have not.[78] As we have tried to argue, the issues of women's health cannot be understood in only biological terms, as simply the ills of the female of the species. Women and men are different, but we are also similar — and we both are divided by the social relations of class and race/ethnicity. To begin to understand how our social constitution affects our health, we must ask, repeatedly, what is different and what is similar across the social divides of gender, color, and class. We cannot assume that biology alone will provide the answers we need; instead, we must reframe the issues in the context of the social shaping of our human lives — as both biological creatures and historical actors. Otherwise, we will continue to mistake — as many before us have done — what is for what must be, and leave unchallenged the social forces that continue to create vast inequalities in health.

Notes

This chapter originally appeared in the *International Journal of Health Services* 24, no. 2 (1994); it is reprinted here by permission of the publisher.

  1 National Center for Health Statistics, *Health, United States, 1991* DHHS Pub. No. (PHS) 92-1232 (Hyattsville, Md.: Public Health Service, 1992); National Center for Health Statistics, *Vital Statistics of the United States — 1988. Vol. I, Natality* DHHS Pub. No. (PHS) 90-1100 (Washington, D.C.: U.S. Government Printing Office, 1990); National Center for Health Statistics, *Vital Statistics of the United States — 1987. Vol. II, Mortality, Part A* DHHS Pub. No. (PHS) 90-1101 (Washington, D.C.: U.S. Govern-

ment Printing Office, 1990); National Center for Health Statistics, *Vital Statistics of the United States—1988. Vol. II, Mortality, Part B* DHHS Pub. No. (PHS) 90-1102 (Washington, D.C.: U.S. Government Printing Office, 1990); U.S. Department of Health and Human Services, *Health Status of Minorities and Low-Income Groups*, 3d ed. (Washington, D.C.: U.S. Government Printing Office, 1991).

2   N. Krieger, "The Making of Public Health Data: Paradigms, Politics, and Policy," *Journal of Public Health Policy* 13 (1992): 412–427; V. Navarro, "Work, Ideology, and Science: The Case of Medicine," in *Crisis, Health, and Medicine: A Social Critique*, ed. V. Navarro (New York: Tavistock, 1986), 142–182; E. Fee, ed., *Women and Health: The Politics of Sex in Medicine* (Amityville, New York: Baywood, 1983); S. Tesh, *Hidden Arguments: Political Ideology and Disease Prevention Policy* (New Brunswick, N.J.: Rutgers, 1988).

3   N. Krieger, D. Rowley, A. A. Herman, B. Avery, and M. T. Phillips, "Racism, Sexism, and Social Class: Implications for Studies of Health, Disease, and Well-being" American Journal of Preventative Medicine (in press).

4   I. Butter, E. Carpenter, B. Kay, and R. Simmons, *Sex and Status: Hierarchies in the Health Workforce* (Washington, D.C.: American Public Health Association, 1985); P. C. Sexton, *The New Nightingales: Hospital Workers, Unions, New Women's Issues* (New York: Enquiry, 1982); B. Melosh, *The Physician's Hand: Work, Culture and Conflict in American Nursing* (Philadelphia: Temple University Press, 1982); S. Wolfe, ed., *Organization of Health Workers and Labor Conflict* (New York: Baywood, 1978); P. H. Feldman, A. M. Sapienza, and N. M. Kane, *Who Cares for Them? Workers in the Home Care Industry* (New York: Greenwood, 1990).

5   N. Krieger, "Shades of Difference: Theoretical Underpinnings of the Medical Controversy on Black/White Differences in the United States, 1830–1870," *International Journal of Health Services* 17 (1987): 256–278; W. Stanton, *The Leopard's Spots: Scientific Attitudes Towards Race in America, 1815–59* (Chicago: University of Chicago Press, 1960); N. Stepan, *The Idea of Race in Science, Great Britain, 1800–1860* (Hamden, Conn.: Archon, 1982); W. D. Jordan, *White Over Black: American Attitudes toward the Negro, 1550–1812* (Chapel Hill: University of North Carolina Press, 1968).

6   C. E. Rosenberg, *No Other Gods: On Science and American Social Thought* (Baltimore, Md.: Johns Hopkins University Press, 1976); G. H. Daniels, "The Process of Professionalization in American Science: The Emergent Period, 1820–1860," *Isis* 58 (1967): 151–166; W. G. Rothstein, *American Physicians in the 19th Century: From Sects to Science* (Baltimore, Md.: Johns Hopkins University Press, 1972).

7   S. A. Cartwright, "Report on the Diseases and Physical Peculiarities of the Negro Race," *New Orleans Medical Surgery Journal* 7 (1850): 691–715; S. A. Cartwright, "Alcohol and the Ethiopian: Or, the Moral and Physical Effects of Ardent Spirits on the Negro Race, and Some Accounts of the Peculiarities of That People," *New Orleans Medical Surgery Journal* 10 (1853): 150–165; S. A. Cartwright, "Ethnology of the Negro or Prognathous Race—A Lecture Delivered November 30, 1857, before the New Orleans Academy of Science," *New Orleans Medical Surgery Journal* 15 (1858): 149–163.

8   R. Reyburn, "Remarks Concerning Some of the Diseases Prevailing among the Freedpeople in the District of Columbia (Bureau of Refugees, Freedmen and Abandoned Lands)," *American Journal of Medical Science* n.s. 51 (1866): 364–369; J. Byron,

"Negro Regiments — Department of Tennessee," *Boston Medical and Surgical Journal* 69 (1863): 43–44.

9   E. Foner, *Reconstruction: America's Unfinished Revolution, 1863–1877* (New York: Harper & Row, 1988); J. S. Haller Jr., *Outcasts from Evolution: Scientific Attitudes of Racial Inferiority, 1859–1900* (Urbana: University of Illinois Press, 1971); G. W. Stocking, *Race, Culture, and Evolution: Essays in the History of Anthropology* (New York: Free Press, 1968); D. Lorimer, *Colour, Class and the Victorians* (New York: Holmes & Meier, 1978); V. N. Gamble, ed., *Germs Have No Color Line: Blacks and American Medicine, 1900–1940* (New York: Garland, 1989).

10 G. J. Barker-Benfield, *The Horrors of the Half-Known Life: Male Attitudes toward Women and Sexuality in Nineteenth-Century America* (New York: Harper & Row, 1976); E. Fee, "Science and the Woman Problem: Historical Perspectives," in *Sex Differences: Social and Biological Perspectives*, ed. M. S. Teitelbaum (New York: Anchor/ Doubleday, 1976), 175–223; L. Jordanova, *Sexual Visions: Images of Gender in Science and Medicine between the Eighteenth and Twentieth Centuries* (Madison: University of Wisconsin Press, 1989); B. Ehrenreich and D. English, *Complaints and Disorders: The Sexual Politics of Sickness* (New York: Feminist Press, 1973).

11 C. E. Russett, *Sexual Science: The Victorian Construction of Womanhood* (Cambridge: Harvard University Press, 1989); R. Hubbard, *The Politics of Women's Biology* (New Brunswick, N.J.: Rutgers University Press, 1990).

12 E. Fee, "Nineteenth-Century Craniology: The Study of the Female Skull," *Bulletin of the History of Medicine* 53 (1979): 415–433; C. Smith-Rosenberg and C. E. Rosenberg, "The Female Animal: Medical and Biological Views of Woman and Her Role in 19th Century America," *Journal of American History* 60 (1973): 332–356; S. J. Gould, *The Mismeasure of Man* (New York: W. W. Norton, 1981).

13 C. Smith-Rosenberg, "Puberty to Menopause: The Cycle of Femininity in Nine- teenth-Century America," *Feminist Studies* 1 (1973): 58–72; C. Smith-Rosenberg, *Disorderly Conduct: Visions of Gender in Victorian America* (New York: Knopf, 1985); J. S. Haller and R. M. Haller, *The Physician and Sexuality in Victorian America* (Urbana: University of Illinois Press, 1974); R. D. Apple, ed., *Women, Health, and Medicine in America: A Historical Handbook* (New Brunswick, N.J.: Rutgers University Press, 1990).

14 R. Williams, *Culture & Society: 1780–1950* (New York: Columbia University Press, 1958, rev. ed. 1983).

15 K. Marx, *Capital*, Vol. 1 (New York: International Publishers, 1967, orig. 1867).

16 R. Hofstadter, *Social Darwinism in American Thought* (Boston: Beacon, 1955); R. M. Young, *Darwin's Metaphor: Nature's Place in Victorian Culture* (Cambridge: Cambridge University Press, 1985); D. J. Kevles, *In the Name of Eugenics: Genetics and the Uses of Human Heredity* (New York: Knopf, 1985); A. Chase, *The Legacy of Malthus: The Social Costs of the New Scientific Racism* (New York: Knopf, 1977).

17 C. Darwin, *On the Origin of Species by Means of Natural Selection, or the Preservation of Favoured Races in the Struggle for Life* (London: Murray, 1859).

18 Hofstadter, *Social Darwinism in American Thought*; Young, *Darwin's Metaphor*; Kevles, *In the Name of Eugenics*; Chase, *The Legacy of Malthus*; all sources *supra* note 16.

19 Haller, *Outcasts from Evolution*, *supra* note 9; M. J. Anderson, *The American Census: A Social History* (New Haven: Yale University Press, 1988).

20 F. L. Hoffman, *Race Traits and Tendencies of the American Negro* (New York: American Economic Association, 1896); S. Harris, "Tuberculosis in the Negro," *Journal of the American Medical Association* 41 (1903): 827; L. C. Allen, "The Negro Health Problem," *American Journal of Public Health* 5 (1915): 194; E. H. Beardsley, *A History of Neglect: Health Care for Blacks and Mill Workers in the Twentieth-Century South* (Knoxville: University of Tennessee Press, 1987).

21 Fee, "Science and the Woman Problem," *supra* note 10; Hofstadter, *Social Darwinism in American Thought, supra* note 16; P. Geddes and J. A. Thompson, *The Evolution of Sex* (London: Walter Scott, 1889).

22 K. M. Ludmerer, *Genetics and American Society: A Historical Appraisal* (Baltimore, Md.: Johns Hopkins University Press, 1972).

23 Hofstadter, *Social Darwinism in American Thought, supra* note 16; Ludmerer, *Genetics and American Society, supra* note 22; J. Higham, *Strangers in the Land: Patterns of American Nativism, 1860–1925* (New Brunswick, N.J.: Rutgers University Press, 1955); M. H. Haller, *Eugenics: Hereditarian Attitudes in American Thought* (New Brunswick, N.J.: Rutgers University Press, 1963); D. K. Pickens, *Eugenics and the Progressives* (Nashville, Tenn.: Vanderbilt University Press, 1968); M. King and S. Ruggles, "American Immigration, Fertility, and Race Suicide at the Turn of the Century," *Journal of Interdisciplinary History* 20 (1990): 347–369; C. N. Degler, *In Search of Human Nature: The Decline and Revival of Darwinism in American Social Thought* (Oxford: Oxford University Press, 1991).

24 G. E. Allen, *Life Science in the Twentieth Century* (Cambridge: Cambridge University Press, 1978); W. E. Castle, "The Beginnings of Mendelism in America," in *Genetics in the Twentieth Century*, ed. L. C. Dunn (New York: Macmillan, 1951), 59–76; J. S. Wilkie, "Some Reasons for the Rediscovery and Appreciation of Mendel's Work in the First Years of the Present Century," *British Journal of the History of Science* 1 (1962): 5–18; T. H. Morgan, *The Theory of the Gene* (New Haven: Yale University Press, 1926).

25 A. M. Kraut, *The Huddled Masses: The Immigrant in American Society, 1800–1921* (Arlington Heights: Harlan Davison, 1982); G. W. Stoner, "Insane and Mentally Defective Aliens Arriving at the Port of New York," *New York Medical Journal* 97 (1913): 957–960; S. T. Solis-Cohen, "The Exclusion of Aliens from the United States for Physical Defects," *Bulletin of the History of Medicine* 21 (1947): 33–50.

26 K. Ludmerer, "Genetics, Eugenics, and the Immigration Restriction Act of 1924," *Bulletin of the History of Medicine* 46 (1972): 59–81; E. Barkan, "Reevaluating Progressive Eugenics: Herbert Spencer Jennings and the 1924 Immigration Legislation," *Journal of the History of Biology* 24 (1991): 91–112; A. M. Kraut, "Silent Travelers: Germs, Genes, and American Efficiency, 1890–1924," *Social Science History* 12 (1988): 377–393.

27 J. Farley, *Gametes & Spores: Ideas About Sexual Reproduction, 1750–1914* (Baltimore, Md.: Johns Hopkins University Press, 1982); G. Allen, "Thomas Hunt Morgan and the Problem of Sex Determination," *Proceedings of the American Philosophical Society* 110 (1966): 48–57; S. Brush, "Nettie M. Stevens and the Discovery of Sex Determination by Chromosomes," *Isis* 69 (1978): 163–172.

28 E. Starling, "The Croonian Lectures on the Chemical Correlation of the Functions of the Body," *Lancet* 2 (1905): 339–341, 423–425, 501–503, 579–583.

29 J. E. Lane-Claypon and E. H. Starling, "An Experimental Enquiry into the Factors Which Determine the Growth and Activity of the Mammary Glands," *Proceedings of*

the Royal Society of London, Series B: Biological Sciences 77 (1906): 505–522; F. A. Marshall, *The Physiology of Reproduction* (New York: Longmans, Green, 1910); N. Oudshoorn, "Endocrinologists and the Conceptualization of Sex," *Journal of the History of Biology* 23 (1990): 163–187; N. Oudshoorn, "On Measuring Sex Hormones: The Role of Biological Assays in Sexualizing Chemical Substances," *Bulletin of the History of Medicine* 64 (1990): 243–261; M. Borrell, "Organotherapy and the Emergence of Reproductive Endocrinology," *Journal of the History of Biology* 18 (1985): 1–30.

30 D. L. Long, "Biology, Sex Hormones and Sexism in the 1920s," *Philosophical Forum* 5 (1974): 81–96; I. G. Cobb, *The Glands of Destiny (A Study of the Personality)* (New York: Macmillan, 1928).

31 E. Allen, ed., *Sex and Internal Secretions: A Survey of Recent Research* (Baltimore, Md.: Williams and Wilkins, 1939); R. Frank, *The Female Sex Hormone* (Springfield, Ill.: Charles C. Thomas, 1929); A. E. C. Lathrop and L. Loeb, "Further Investigations of the Origin of Tumors in Mice. III. On the Part Played by Internal Secretions in the Spontaneous Development of Tumors," *Journal of Cancer Research* 1 (1916): 1–19; J. E. Lane-Claypon, *A Further Report on Cancer of the Breast, With Special Reference to its Associated Antecedent Conditions. Reports on Public Health and Medical Subjects, No. 32* (London: His Majesty's Stationary Office, 1926); J. M. Wainwright, "A Comparison of Conditions Associated with Breast Cancer in Great Britain and America," *American Journal of Cancer* 15 (1931): 2610–2645.

32 Apple, *Women, Health, and Medicine in America, supra* note 13; W. Chavkin, ed., *Double Exposure: Women's Health Hazards on the Job and at Home* (New York: Monthly Review Press, 1984); B. Ehrenreich and D. English, *For Her Own Good: 150 Years of the Experts' Advice to Women* (New York: Anchor, 1979).

33 P. Starr, *The Social Transformation of American Medicine* (New York: Basic, 1982); E. Fee, *Disease and Discovery: A History of the Johns Hopkins School of Hygiene and Public Health* (Baltimore, Md.: Johns Hopkins University Press, 1987); E. Fee and R. M. Acheson, eds., *A History of Education in Public Health: Health that Mocks the Doctors' Rules* (Oxford: Oxford University Press, 1991).

34 Fee, *Women and Health, supra* note 2; Apple, *Women, Health, and Medicine in America, supra* note 13; R. Meckel, *Save the Babies: American Public Health Reform and the Prevention of Infant Mortality, 1850–1920* (Baltimore, Md.: Johns Hopkins University Press, 1990).

35 J. Rodin and J. R. Ickovics, "Women's Health: Review and Research Agenda as We Approach the 21st Century," *American Psychologist* 45 (1990): 1018–1034; B. Healy, "Women's Health, Public Welfare," *Journal of the American Medical Association* 266 (1991): 566–568; R. L. Kirchstein, "Research on Women's Health," *American Journal of Public Health* 81 (1991): 291–293.

36 Krieger et al., "Racism, Sexism, and Social Class," *supra* note 3.

37 R. Lewontin, *Human Diversity* (New York: Scientific American Books, 1982); J. C. King, *The Biology of Race* (Berkeley: University of California Press, 1981); R. Cooper and R. David, "The Biological Concept of Race and Its Application to Epidemiology," *Journal of Health Politics Policy Law* 11 (1986): 97–116.

38 Lewontin, *Human Diversity, supra* note 37.

39 R. Cooper, "Celebrate Diversity — Or Should We?" *Ethnicity and Disease* 1 (1991): 3–7; D. E. Crews and J. R. Bindon, "Ethnicity as a Taxonomic Tool in Biomedical and Biosocial Research," *Ethnicity and Disease* 1 (1991): 42–49.

40   L. Mullings, "Ethnicity and Stratification in the Urban United States," *Annals of the New York Academy of Sciences* 318 (1978): 10–22; J. R. Feagin, *Racial and Ethnic Relations*, 3d ed. (Englewood Cliffs, N.J.: Prentice-Hall, 1989).

41   J. R. Feagin, "The Continuing Significance of Race: Anti-Black Discrimination in Public Places," *American Sociology Review* 56 (1991): 101–116; P. Essed, *Understanding Everyday Racism: An Interdisciplinary Theory* (Newbury Park, Calif.: Sage, 1991); N. Krieger and M. Bassett, "The Health of Black Folk: Disease, Class and Ideology in Science," *Monthly Review* 38 (1986): 74–85.

42   V. Navarro, "Race or Class versus Race and Class: Mortality Differentials in the United States," *Lancet* ii (1990): 1238–1240; N. Krieger and E. Fee, "What's Class Got to Do with It? The State of Health Data in the United States Today," *Socialist Review* 23 (1993): 59–82.

43   S. Polack and J. Grozuczak, *Reagan, Toxics and Minorities: A Policy Report* (Washington, D.C.: Urban Environment Conference, 1984); Commission for Racial Justice, United Church of Christ, *Toxic Wastes and Race in the United States: A National Report on the Racial and Socioeconomic Characteristics of Communities with Hazardous Waste Sites* (New York: United Church of Christ, 1987); E. Mann, *L.A.'s Lethal Air: New Strategies for Policy, Organizing, and Action* (Los Angeles: Labor/Community Strategy Center, 1991).

44   N. Krieger, "Racial and Gender Discrimination: Risk Factors for High Blood Pressure?" *Social Science and Medicine* 30 (1990): 1273–1281; C. A. Armstead, K. A. Lawler, G. Gordon, J. Cross, and J. Gibbons, "Relationship of Racial Stressors to Blood Pressure and Anger Expression in Black College Students," *Health Psychology* 8 (1989): 541–556; S. A. James, A. Z. LaCroix, D. G. Kleinbaum, and D. S. Strogatz, "John Henryism and Blood Pressure Differences among Black Men. II. The Role of Occupational Stressors," *Journal of Behavioral Medicine* 7 (1984): 259–275; W. W. Dressler, "Social Class, Skin Color, and Arterial Blood Pressure in Two Societies," *Ethnicity and Disease* 1 (1991): 60–77.

45   Krieger, "Racial and Gender Discrimination," *supra* note 44.

46   R. G. Fruchter, K. Nayeri, J. C. Remy, C. Wright, J. G. Feldman, J. G. Boyce, and W. S. Burnett, "Cervix and Breast Cancer Incidence in Immigrant Caribbean Women," *American Journal of Public Health* 80 (1990): 722–724; J. C. Kleinman, L. A. Fingerhut, and K. Prager, "Differences in Infant Mortality by Race, Nativity, and Other Maternal Characteristics," *American Journal of Diseases of Children* 145 (1991): 194–199; H. Cabral, L. E. Fried, S. Levenson, H. Amaro, and B. Zuckerman, "Foreign-born and US-born Black Women: Differences in Health Behaviors and Birth Outcomes," *American Journal of Public Health* 80 (1990): 70–72.

47   R. J. Taylor and L. M. Chatters, "Religious Life," in *Life in Black America*, ed. J. S. Jackson (Newbury Park, Calif.: Sage, 1991), 105–123; I. L. Livingston, D. M. Levine, and R. D. Moore, "Social Integration and Black Intraracial Variation in Blood Pressure," *Ethnicity and Disease* 1 (1991): 135–149; E. Eng, J. Hatch, and A. Callan, "Institutionalizing Social Support through the Church and into the Community," *Health Education Quarterly* 12 (1985): 81–92.

48   R. Hubbard, *The Politics of Women's Biology* (New Brunswick, N.J.: Rutgers University Press, 1990); M. Lowe, "Social Bodies: The Interaction of Culture and Women's Biology," in *Biological Woman — The Convenient Myth*, ed. R. Hubbard, M. S. Henefin, and B. Fried (Cambridge, Mass.: Schenkman, 1982), 91–116.

49 Fruchter et al., "Cervix and Breast Cancer Incidence in Immigrant Caribbean Women," *supra* note 46; S. S. Devesa and E. L. Diamond, "Association of Breast Cancer and Cervical Cancer Incidence with Income and Education among Whites and Blacks," *Journal of the National Cancer Institute* 65 (1980): 515–528.

50 N. Krieger, "Social Class and the Black/White Crossover in the Age-specific Incidence of Breast Cancer: A Study Linking Census-derived Data to Population-based Registry Records," *American Journal of Epidemiology* 131 (1990): 804–814; N. Krieger, "The Influence of Social Class, Race and Gender on the Etiology of Hypertension Among Women in the United States," in proceedings of the conference *Women, Behavior, and Cardiovascular Disease*, sponsored by the National Heart, Lung, and Blood Institute, Chevy Chase, Md., September 25–27, 1991 (in press).

51 Krieger, "The Influence of Social Class, Race and Gender on the Etiology of Hypertension," *supra* note 50; *Report of the Secretary's Task Force on Black & Minority Health, Volume IV: Cardiovascular and Cerebrovascular Disease, Part 2* (Washington, D.C.: U.S. Department of Health and Human Services, 1986).

52 U.S. Department of Health and Human Services, *Health Status of Minorities and Low-Income Groups*, 3d ed. (Washington, D.C.: U.S. Government Printing Office, 1991).

53 M. Martinez-Maldonado, "Hypertension in Hispanics, Asians and Pacific Islanders, and Native Americans," *Circulation* 83 (1991): 1467–1469; P. U. Caralis, "Hypertension in the Hispanic-American Population," *American Journal of Medicine* 88, suppl. 3b (1990): 9s–16s.

54 S. M. Haffner, B. D. Mitchell, M. P. Stern, H. P. Hazuda, and J. K. Patterson, "Decreased Prevalence of Hypertension in Mexican-Americans," *Hypertension* 16 (1990): 225–232.

55 Martinez-Maldonado, "Hypertension in Hispanics," *supra* note 53; G. R. Stavig, A. Igra, and A. R. Leonard, "Hypertension and Related Health Issues among Asians and Pacific Islanders in California," *Public Health Reports* 103 (1988): 28–37; A. Angel, M. A. Armstrong, and A. L. Klatsky, "Blood Pressure among Asian Americans Living in Northern California," *American Journal of Cardiology* 54 (1987): 237–240.

56 J. S. Alpert, R. Goldberg, I. S. Ockene, and P. Taylor, "Heart Disease in Native Americans," *Cardiology* 78 (1991): 3–12; Martinez-Maldonado, "Hypertension in Hispanics, Asians and Pacific Islanders, and Native Americans."

57 *Report of the Secretary's Task Force on Black & Minority Health*, *supra* note 51.

58 U.S. Department of Health and Human Services, *Health Status of Minorities and Low-Income Groups*, *supra* note 52; Stavig et al., "Hypertension and Related Health Issues among Asians and Pacific Islanders in California," *supra* note 55.

59 I. Waldron, "Sex Differences in Illness, Incidence, Prognosis and Mortality: Issues and Evidence," *Social Science and Medicine* 17 (1983): 1107–1123; D. L. Wingard, "The Sex Differential in Morbidity, Mortality, and Lifestyle," *Annual Review of Public Health* 5 (1984): 433–458.

60 Ibid.

61 E. Gold, ed., *Changing Risk of Disease in Women: An Epidemiological Approach* (Lexington, Mass.: Colbamore, 1984).

62 V. Leviatan and J. Cohen, "Gender Differences in Life Expectancy among Kibbutz Members," *Social Science and Medicine* 21 (1985): 545–551.

63 S. L. Syme and L. Berkman, "Social Class, Susceptibility and Sickness," *American Journal of Epidemiology* 104 (1976): 1–8; A. Antonovsky, "Social Class, Life Expec-

tancy and Overall Mortality," *Milbank Memorial Fund Quarterly* 45 (1967): 31–73; P. Townsend, N. Davidson, and M. Whitehead, *Inequalities in Health: The Black Report and The Health Divide* (Harmondsworth, England: Penguin, 1988); M. G. Marmot, M. Kogevinas, and M. A. Elston, "Social/economic Status and Disease," *Annual Review of Public Health* 8 (1987): 111–135; V. Navarro, "Race or Class versus Race and Class," *supra* note 42.

64   Krieger and Fee, "What's Class Got to Do with It?" *supra* note 42; H. Roberts, ed., *Women's Health Counts* (London: Routledge, 1990).

65   A. Dale, G. N. Gilbert, and S. Arber, "Integrating Women into Class Theory," *Sociology* 19 (1985): 384–409; V. Duke and S. Edgell, "The Operationalisation of Class in British Sociology: Theoretical and Empirical Considerations," *British Journal of Sociology* 8 (1987): 445–463; N. Charles, "Women and Class — A Problematic Relationship," *Sociology Review* 38 (1990): 43–89.

66   M. Morgan, "Measuring Social Inequality: Occupational Classifications and Their Alternatives," *Community Medicine* 5 (1983): 116–124; K. A. Moser, H. Pugh, and P. Goldblatt, "Mortality and the Social Classification of Women," in *Longitudinal Study: Mortality and Social Organization. Series LS, No. 6*, ed. P. Goldblatt (London: His Majesty's Stationary Office, 1990), 146–162.

67   Roberts, *Women's Health Counts, supra* note 64.

68   N. Krieger, "Women and Social Class: A Methodological Study Comparing Individual, Household, and Census Measures as Predictors of Black/White Differences in Reproductive History," *Journal of Epidemiology and Community Health* 45 (1991): 35–42; P. Ries, "Health Characteristics According to Family and Personal Income, United States," *Vital Health Statistics*, ser. 10, no. 147 (1985), National Center for Health Statistics, DHHS Pub. No. (PHS) 85-1575.

69   Devesa and Diamond, "Association of Breast Cancer and Cervical Cancer Incidence with Income and Education among Whites and Blacks," *supra* note 49; N. Krieger, "Overcoming the Absence of Socioeconomic Data in Medical Records: Validation and Application of a Census-based Methodology," *American Journal of Public Health* 82 (1992): 703–710.

70   Krieger, "Overcoming the Absence of Socioeconomic Data in Medical Records," *supra* note 69.

71   K. Carovano, "More than Mothers and Whores: Redefining the AIDS Prevention Needs of Women," *International Journal of Health Services* 21 (1991): 131–142; PANOS Institute, *Triple Jeopardy: Women & AIDS* (London: Panos, 1990); K. Anastos and C. Marte, "Women — The Missing Persons in the AIDS Epidemic," *HealthPAC* (winter 1989): 6–13.

72   Centers for Disease Control, "1993 Revised Classification System for HIV Infection and Expanded Surveillance Case Definition for AIDS among Adolescents and Adults," *Morbidity and Mortality Weekly Report* 41 (1992): 961–962; R. Kanigel, "U.S. Broadens AIDS Definition: Activists Spur Change by Centers for Disease Control," *Oakland Tribune*, January 1, 1993, A1.

73   Centers for Disease Control and Prevention, *HIV/AIDS Surveillance Report* 5 (July 1993): 1–19.

74   Ibid.

75   PANOS Institute, *Triple Jeopardy, supra* note 71.

76   E. Drucker, "Epidemic in the War Zone: AIDS and Community Survival in New

York City," *International Journal of Health Services* 20 (1990): 601–616; N. Freudenberg, "AIDS Prevention in the United States: Lessons from the First Decade," *International Journal of Health Services* 20 (1990): 589–600.

77 E. Fee and N. Krieger, "Thinking and Rethinking AIDS: Implications for Health Policy," *International Journal of Health Services* 23 (1993): 323–346.

78 E. Fee and N. Krieger, "Understanding AIDS: Historical Interpretations and the Limits of Biomedical Individualism," *American Journal of Public Health* (in press).

2

OF HEADLINES AND HYPOTHESES

*The Role of Gender in Popular
Press Coverage of Women's Health
and Biology*

Joan E. Bertin and Laurie R. Beck

Introduction

Medical and scientific information wields enormous power, and this makes it big news. It alters individual conduct, shapes social policy, and influences law:

> [M]edicine is becoming a major institution of social control, nudging aside, if not incorporating, the more traditional institutions of religion and law. It is becoming the new repository of truth, the place where absolute and often final judgments are made by supposedly morally neutral and objective experts. And these judgments are made, not in the name of virtue or legitimacy, but in the name of health. . . . [T]oday the prestige of *any* proposal is immensely enhanced, if not justified, when it is expressed in the idiom of medical science.[1]

The need for accurate information about women's health, in both the research lab and the pressroom, is especially important in light of the current focus on health care reform and on women's health. In the effort to address deficiencies in the health care system and to define the needs of women within that system, press coverage of medical and scientific research on women and gender is likely to influence public perceptions and affect policy proposals that address public concerns. If either the research or the public understanding of the state of scientific knowledge about women's health is incomplete or inaccurate, policies intended to address women's health needs may fail to achieve their beneficial goals. The need for accurate reporting and unbiased biomedical data about women's health has always existed. If anything, the stakes may now be higher.

A recent headline reads, "Women Smokers Appear to Run Higher Risk."[2] The article reports on a study finding that the risk of lung cancer for women is double that for men at the same levels of exposure. Is this a new breakthrough in women's health, signifying that women are more vulnerable than men to the effects of tobacco smoke? This is what the headline and lead paragraphs suggest, but at the end of the article the reader learns that other studies report that the risk for male smokers is higher. So are women more vulnerable to the effects of tobacco smoke? That is unclear. It is well recognized that lung cancer is an equal opportunity disease and that smoking cigarettes is risky behavior for both sexes. Even if there is a differential risk, it is unlikely that medical advice will change, since both sexes are strenuously counseled against cigarette use.

This report, like many discussed below, confirms certain common assumptions — that women and men are biologically different, that women are physically and biologically more vulnerable, and that women engage in "masculine" activities at their peril. Are these assumptions valid, or does this story invoke biological and scientific explanations to reinforce culturally preferred roles and behaviors? Did the underlying research evaluate other subgroup differences in susceptibility, or did it examine only gender-based differences? Did it consider intra-sex, as well as inter-sex, variation? How does the increased risk associated with gender, if it exists, compare with other known risk factors? Is the study valid? Useful? Newsworthy?

In this chapter, we consider these kinds of questions and evaluate some of the factors that influence reporting on women's health and biology. We address the print media only, and focus our attention on reports from major national newspapers or news services. Through computer searches of major newspaper files, we tracked coverage of specific scientific findings about gender reported in scholarly journals, in an attempt to discern patterns and raise questions about how information is selected and communicated. Although we read hundreds of articles, this was not intended to be a comprehensive study or a systematic review of the literature. Our research indicates that gender does influence some press reports of women's health issues in ways that can be misleading, and we present here some representative examples to illustrate the point; however, we draw no inference about how often this occurs. The patterns that emerge from our review do suggest areas of particular concern and avenues for future research.

Science as a Culturally Embedded Activity

Any evaluation of the possible influence of gender on press reports of women's health issues is hampered by the fact that scientific inquiry itself may be influenced by gender in ways that may not be readily apparent. We begin, therefore, with a brief historical discussion of the effects of culture on science, the difficulty of creating bias-free science, and the implications of these observations for press coverage of scientific studies about women.

> Science, since people must do it, is a socially embedded activity. . . . Facts are not pure and unsullied bits of information; culture also influences what we see and how we see it. . . . [S]ome topics are invested with enormous social importance but blessed with very little reliable information. When the ratio of data to social impact is so low, a history of scientific attitudes may be little more than an oblique record of social change. . . . [M]any questions are formulated by scientists in such a restricted way that any legitimate answer can only validate a social preference.[3]

Women's health and biology is one of those topics that is "invested with enormous social importance" but often "blessed with very little reliable information." The risk that science will be used to "validate a social preference" is consequently great, as has been the case historically.

In his classic study *The Mismeasure of Man*, Stephen Jay Gould studied the science of intelligence testing and quantification and found that it was used "invariably to find that oppressed and disadvantaged groups — races, classes, or sexes — are innately inferior and deserve their status."[4] The craniology movement of the nineteenth century sought to prove that intelligence was a function of brain size and thereby to establish male intellectual preeminence over women.[5] Darwin used a different "scientific" theory to achieve the same result:

> The chief distinction in the intellectual powers of the two sexes is shown in man's attaining to a higher eminence, in whatever he takes

up, than can woman. . . . [I]f men are capable of a decided pre-eminence over women in many subjects, the average mental power in man must be above that of woman.[6]

Consistent with this logic, at the end of the nineteenth century the Surgeon General of the United States asserted as a "scientific fact" that "the brain of a woman is inferior in at least nineteen different ways to the brain of a man."[7]

The claim that women were inherently intellectually inferior to men justified women's exclusion from intellectual endeavors, so that they could devote themselves to domestic activities. It was postulated, again as a "scientific fact," that education and intellectual activities undermined women's reproductive capacities.[8] Popular medical advice reflected these assumptions:

> At puberty, girls were advised to take a great deal of bed rest in order to help focus their strength on regulating their periods — though this might take years. Too much reading or intellectual stimulation in the fragile stage of adolescence could result in permanent damage to the reproductive organs, and sickly, irritable babies. . . . Every mental effort of the mother-to-be could deprive the unborn child of [phosphates, a] vital nutrient, or would so overtax the woman's own system that she would be driven to insanity.[9]

One Harvard professor declared that "higher education would cause women's uteruses to atrophy."[10]

As these examples indicate, gender-based roles and expectations can and do influence scientific inquiry and the interpretation of data. Science is sometimes used to reinforce cultural arrangements, by suggesting that they are "natural," if not inevitable. Cultural arrangements and expectations may preclude certain questions from being asked, or may cause discordant but accurate information to be disregarded. During a period in which traditional allocation of gender roles and responsibilities are challenged and social tensions intensify as a result,[11] biological theories buttressing culturally preferred behavior may become even more appealing. The historical record of complex and subtle interactions between science and culture thus suggests the need for caution in interpreting and applying scientific information about women's biology and gender difference. As Gould asks, "By what right, other than our own biases, can we . . . hold that science now operates independently of culture and class?"[12]

Translating Science: Science as News

Even trained professionals often find it hard to interpret and apply research data.[13] Translating such information so that it can be properly understood by a lay audience adds another layer of complexity. The popular press faces both these challenges and moreover adds its own gloss on the information, reflecting its own agenda: selling news.

The very idea of science as "news" is antithetical to the nature of scientific knowledge. Treating scientific developments as news stories in and of itself invites distortion. Science is a process by which hypotheses are formulated, tested, and replicated under various circumstances, and placed in context with other relevant information.[14] Individual studies usually can be interpreted correctly only in the context of the whole body of data on a particular subject. The failure to contextualize bits of information leads to widespread confusion over how one study can be reported to "prove" that caffeine causes miscarriage, while another "proves" the opposite. Similarly, one year a study made headlines reporting that exercise disrupts menstruation; another year the hypothesis was disproved. Readers buffeted by such reports hardly know what to think.

These studies are not necessarily contradictory. Studies are often reported as if they conclusively "prove" a proposition, when they only tend to show that a particular explanation is more or less likely. Sometimes, studies on animals are offered to support a conclusion in humans, when the extrapolation may be inappropriate. Often, limitations noted by scientists in their studies are not conveyed in press reports. Reporters themselves may have little training in discerning limitations or flaws in studies that make their conclusions limited or unreliable. Conversely, scientists are sometimes insufficiently cautious when describing their findings to reporters, and are quoted for propositions that a study does not support. One pattern that is all too apparent is that studies that confirm what is expected are often accepted uncritically, by reporters and readers alike.

The stylistic format imposed by many newspapers and magazines also presents a challenge to accurate science reporting. Stories often begin with a "human interest" anecdote about an individual, who is supposed to exemplify the issues in the story. This journalistic device may "hook" readers, but it is deceptive unless there is evidence that the information about the individual can be generalized. For example, one report on pregnant women at work began with an anecdote about a woman who said that she could not concentrate on her job when she felt fetal movement.[15] The article gave no indication of whether this experience was common, how it compared with workers' reports of concentration difficulties from other causes, whether there was any objectively measurable effect on work performance, or the like. In sum, this tells us nothing from a scientific perspective about the impact of pregnancy on work performance.

If the report presented credible evidence that the "average" pregnant woman experiences problems with work performance, this would indicate a more general phenomenon, but it still would provide only limited information. Reporting the average alone reveals nothing about the extent of variation, or the proportion of subjects who do not conform to the average. We know, for example, that the "average" ever-married woman in the United States has two children, but this does not indicate how many ever-married women have no children, or have one, three, four, etc. Furthermore, the average does not define or represent what is "normal," although this is a common misunderstanding. For example, if the average height for women is five feet four inches, a woman who is five feet eight inches tall is not abnormal, even though she is not "average." As these examples indicate, scientific methods and terms do not always translate easily to other contexts, and the limitations of data collection, analysis, and reporting are often overlooked or misunderstood. An appreciation of the precise meaning of certain common scientific terms and conventions is essential to accurate presentation and understanding of scientific findings, posing a challenge to reporters and readers alike.

Selection and Placement of News: Confirming the Expected

Out of the hundreds of thousands of stories reported in scientific journals, which ones are selected? And what makes front-page news? To try to find out, we tracked contemporaneous press coverage of seven scientific studies that focused on reproductive risk issues. We picked studies that concerned reproductive risks because it is a topic that is invested with the type of "enormous social importance" to which Gould refers and because it is an area in which gender roles are socially well defined. We selected studies that confirm gender-role expectations and studies that defy such expectations. Some studies focus on male reproductive health and others focus on female risk factors in reproduction. As noted previously, we did not attempt either to select a representative sample or to perform a comprehensive review, but rather undertook a series of case studies.

Three of our case studies (Category A) evaluated women's prenatal use of alcohol or drugs and concluded, contrary to prevailing social messages, that the effect on fetal health or pregnancy outcome (at certain exposure levels) was not consequential or had been overstated. One study (Category B) reported that drug use had a negative effect on fetal growth. Three studies (Category C) looked at the effects of paternal exposures to drugs on pregnancy and birth.

Category A: Counterintuitive Studies
The first study in this category appeared in a prestigious medical journal, *The Lancet*, and addressed the effects of prenatal cocaine usage, a topic then (as now) much in the news.[16] It demonstrated that the deleterious effects of prenatal exposure to cocaine may have been overstated. This study, however, received no press coverage whatsoever in major national newspapers.[17] The study evaluated all abstracts relating to the effects of cocaine use on pregnancy that were submitted to a scientific journal for publication over a nine-year period and reported: "Of the negative (showing no adverse effect) only 1 (11%) was accepted, whereas 28 of the 49 positive abstracts were accepted (57%)." The authors evaluated the quality of the research reflected in the abstracts to determine if that might explain the selections and concluded it did not; indeed, they reported that "the negative studies [were] superior in almost every variable studied." As a result, they concluded that

> most scientific studies were not rejected because of scientific flaws, but rather because of bias against their nonadverse message. The subconscious message may be that if a study did not detect an adverse effect of cocaine, when the common knowledge is that this is a "bad drug," then the study must be flawed.

They concluded that the bias in publication "may lead to distorted estimation of the teratogenic risk [risk of birth defects] of cocaine."

On its merits, this study should have been front-page news. The social importance of the issue can hardly be overstated: at the time the study was published, numerous women around the country were being prosecuted for prenatal "child" abuse or a similar charge, based on drug toxicology tests on newborns. Yet it received no mention.

The second item in this category, a commentary published in the *Journal of the American Medical Association* (*JAMA*) that also questions whether the effects of cocaine use on pregnancy have been overstated, met virtually the same fate. Only one regional newspaper picked it up, and the report was buried deep in the paper.[18] Finally, the third article in this category, a review article entitled "Alcohol Use in Pregnancy: What is the Risk?"[19] reviewed the medical literature on prenatal alcohol use and concluded that the risk from low to moderate consumption had not been documented. The article criticized the standard advice that pregnant women should abstain completely from drinking alcoholic beverages during pregnancy. Like the cocaine article, this article was not reported at all in major national newspapers.[20]

Category B: Confirming the Expected
In contrast, a study demonstrating some adverse effects of prenatal cocaine and marijuana use[21] was mentioned in nine major news stories, some of which were syndicated and therefore widely reported. In fact, while the study observed impaired fetal growth associated with drug use, it explicitly noted that no "cause and effect relationship" could be demonstrated. Furthermore, the study also demonstrated that cigarette smoking had a more deleterious effect on fetal growth than either cocaine or marijuana use. None of these limitations was recognized in the press reports. One front-page story that reported on this among other studies referred in the headline to a "growing army of damaged children" and began with the statement: "A growing body of scientific data indicates that children whose mothers used cocaine during pregnancy may face long-term developmental problems more serious than the much publicized irritability and lethargy many of these babies exhibit in the days and weeks following birth."[22] Another report said that the "largest and most conclusive study of drug use in pregnancy had found that the use of cocaine or marijuana impairs fetal development."[23]

Only one newspaper article, written by a pediatrician,[24] tempered the message and observed what the researchers themselves had published in one of the Category A articles that received no press coverage: that the effects of drugs on fetal and child development are poorly understood and that it is difficult, if not impossible, to separate out the risk factors in some pregnancies in which drugs, alcohol, poverty, malnutrition, violence, illness, and homelessness may all play a role in undermining the pregnant woman's health and that of her future child.[25]

Category C: What's That Again?
The final group of articles documented risks to male reproduction and to the children of men exposed to drugs and alcohol. Unlike the first group, these studies received some press attention, although not as much as did the Category B study on fetal risks. What is striking about these articles is their content. One study that reported an association between

father's drinking and reduced infant birthweight[26] was consistently described as "surprising," "preliminary," and "unexpected." This characterization appeared in almost all reports, even though the researcher herself noted that reports associating alcohol consumption with damage to the male reproductive system have existed for a hundred years. Similarly, a study documenting an increased risk of certain cancers in the children of men who smoke[27] was consistently depicted as "speculative."

A second study, published in *JAMA*, reported that cocaine binds to sperm,[28] and received heavy coverage and generally serious treatment. Most news articles explored the potential significance of the study as well as other literature on male-mediated reproductive risk, and many sought opinions from several experts.[29] Only one paper ran the story on the front page.

It is difficult to generalize from this small sample, but some interesting patterns do emerge. First, certain counterintuitive data were virtually ignored, while others were not. In this group, the distinguishing feature seems to relate to the content of the message: the press was simply unwilling to print a story suggesting that maternal drug use may not produce the dire fetal health effects commonly attributed to it, even if that is true. In contrast, stories suggesting that drugs may be as bad for men as they are for women received some press attention, some of it admirable in its thoroughness, some of it unnecessarily tentative. The articles that confirmed social expectations more often appeared on the front page and stated their conclusions more definitively, even if the proof was inconclusive. In contrast, evidence that is not consistent with social expectations (e.g., that male alcohol use is associated with reduced infant birthweight) was accorded substantially less credibility, and was often represented as interesting and peculiar. The difference in selection and placement of articles was not apparently related to the quality of the science; even in studies by the same authors, studies that confirmed expectations and conventional social behavior norms were featured, while studies that challenged the "prevailing wisdom" were not. Nor do we believe that these observations can be explained entirely by the source of the scientific data; counterintuitive messages were often ignored, even when published in prestigious journals such as *JAMA* and *The Lancet*.

To Generalize or Not to Generalize: On Rats, Voles, and Moms

Questions of credibility are central to reporters and experts alike. Since scientific information is always evolving, it is often difficult to determine when a particular conclusion can be reached, and with what degree of certainty. In other words, how much evidence is sufficient to justify a particular conclusion? What constitutes proof? To evaluate how these questions are handled in media reports, and to assess the role of extraneous social factors, we looked at some examples of how the press treats experimental, or animal, data.

Experimental data provide important information in many health-related contexts. Such data can be critical to fill in gaps in research on humans, to explain biological processes that are poorly understood in humans, and to provide information when research cannot be performed on humans as a practical or ethical matter, or, if done on humans, would inevitably be inconclusive. It is a particularly important tool for assessing the potential health effects of toxic agents.

In our review, reliance on animal data and the willingness to extrapolate from animals to humans closely followed the themes noted above: such data are reported and believed when they confirm the expected, but not otherwise. The likelihood of extrapolating (i.e., generalizing) the findings of animal studies to humans increases considerably when the findings support socially approved gender roles for humans. Consider the following case studies.

A feature article carried the following headline: "What Makes a Parent Put Up with It All?"[30] The headline on the continuation of the story read: "Studying the Role of Hormones in Motivating Parental Behavior." The reader would never know from these headlines that the article is based on data about *prairie voles*. Moreover, the story itself freely extrapolates the findings to humans. It states that this study of prairie voles has finally shed light on "the biochemical basis of parental behavior":

> After long groping about in the dark, scientists are at last gaining clues to the biochemical basis of parental behavior. They are learning precisely what hormonal signals impel males and females to pair up into cooperative units and assume the demands of rearing and protecting young.

The story reports that "two hormones . . . appear to be essential to family and other social relationships among *mammals*. . . . the same peptides that are important for things like uterine contractions and feeding an infant are also important for monogamous social bonds and *parental* behavior" (emphasis added). Thus, the hormone oxytocin in females "arouse[s] an urge to cuddle, a zeal for mating, and a willingness to care for the young," while vasopressin is responsible in males "for transforming a naive young male into an affectionate and aggressively protective partner and father." Aggression, we are told, "is one way of expressing attachment." Buried in the article is the warning that "the role of vasopressin in human behavior remains in the realm of speculation."

The fact that this study was reported at all is curious, given its arcane title: "A Role for Central Vasopressin in Pair Bonding in Monogamous Prairie Voles."[31] This topic hardly appears newsworthy or relevant to the general public. Moreover, the study itself plainly announces that its findings are limited to *prairie voles*, a significant point obscured in the press reports.

Compare this article's willingness to extrapolate from animal data with another front-page science article about aggressive behavior in female hyenas. The headline reads "Hyenas' Hormone Flow Puts Females in Charge,"[32] and plainly announces that these data cannot be applied to humans. In reporting a study of hormones that cause *female* animals to be aggressive, the data are reported as pertaining only to animals, not to humans. The article states that the hyenas' behavior results from "a bizarre balance of hormones." The study is described as "using a *strange* animal to test ideas that can be applied to more conventional cases" (emphasis added). The hyena is "strange" because both male and female fetuses are exposed to high levels of "male" hormones. But in this case, the hormones that allegedly induce aggressive behavior are not "male" and the resulting behavior is not "strange." Rather, it is apparently normal for the hyena.

Now consider coverage of experimental data confirming a male contribution to birth anomalies. The story was brief, introduced by the headline "Defective Offspring of 'Alcoholic' Rats." It states:

> Male rats that consumed large amounts of alcohol before breeding sired male offspring that suffered from learning disabilities and low levels of the male sex hormone testosterone, scientists have reported.[33]

The article quotes one of the study's investigators as saying "I would be hesitant to extrapolate our findings to the human alcoholic." Contrast this with the following article, reprinted here in its entirety:

> Fetus Gets 'Taste' for Alcohol?
> A pregnant women [*sic*] who drinks, even though not enough to cause birth defects, may be predisposing their [*sic*] unborn children to a life of alcohol abuse, a new experiment suggests.

"The implication here is that [if] a woman drinks during pregnancy, even at levels not high enough to cause birth defects, she may be influencing her child's drinking behavior in later life," said Dr. Jan Johnson, who led the research at the University of North Carolina.

The experiments, conducted on laboratory animals at the university School of Medicine, showed that dogs whose mothers were fed alcohol before giving birth chose to consume more alcohol and did it faster than dogs whose mothers were not given alcohol.

Dr. Johnson said the evidence could not be considered conclusive until more tests were made.

Dr. Johnson said many animals, including monkeys and rats, apparently find drinking alcohol pleasurable and will administer it to themselves if given the chance.[34]

The manner of interpretation and application of these animal data reflect and perpetuate the values, norms, and beliefs of our culture. The behavior of both the male and female prairie vole was credited and generalized because it is consistent with conventional human behavior; in contrast, the female hyenas' behavior and biology were characterized as "strange" and "bizarre," because aggressive behavior in women and girls, which plainly exists, is not culturally valued. Experimental evidence of male-mediated birth defects is presumed to be irrelevant to humans, because it defies social norms assigning women principal if not exclusive responsibility for healthy pregnancy and birth. Studies that demonstrate a biological basis for women's singular responsibility for the production of healthy offspring, in contrast, are well received and easily extrapolated to humans, as the final article demonstrates.

Gender Difference as News

The lack of consistency in the approach to similar kinds of data reveals the urge to buttress social conventions and cultural arrangements with biological data.[35] Scientific explanations can be used to "validate a social preference," that is, to legitimize gender-based social norms and the gender-based allocation of roles, privileges, and responsibilities, which are deeply ingrained in our culture.[36] At the same time, rigid sex-based allocations of roles and rights have been recognized as the source of personal, social, and legal wrongs — felt mostly, but not exclusively, by women — and have been legally repudiated.[37] Recognition of these wrongs has stimulated the repudiation of many cultural sex roles and stereotypes, but the process is a tortuous one.[38] This may explain, at least in part, the popular fascination with scientific theories, no matter how poorly derived, that purport to document a biological basis for gender differences and conventional sex-role behaviors. Scientific evidence of gender similarity would not perform the same comforting function, since it would force recognition of the unfairness of some of those traditional arrangements.

Predictably, then, the popular press more often and more prominently reports studies that find innate gender difference than studies that show little or no sex-based difference. For example, a recent front-page article, "He-Men in Training; Dolls or Trucks — The Play's the Thing," began:

> Truck? Check. Helicopter? Check. Barbie Doll? Uh . . . nope. UCLA psychologist Melissa Hines watches 3- to 8-year-old girls and boys play with toys. The noted neuroscientist's quest: To find out how females and males are different and why. . . . The ongoing study is part of a growing body of gender-difference research indicating that males and females do indeed differ in some areas of behavior and cognition — and at least some of those differences may be rooted in *biology*.[39]

According to the story, "*the prenatal androgen exposure tends to be associated with choices like cars and trucks*" (emphasis added).

This story made it to the front page not because readers have a particular interest in trucks or Barbie but because the story uses science to confirm that boys and girls really are inherently different. We are led to believe that all boys are influenced by prenatal androgen but that girls are not. All fetuses, however, are exposed to some levels of androgen, and exposure levels vary within each sex. In sum, the story proceeds from a hypothesis that is not openly stated and certainly not proved — that the gender differences observed in toy selection are the result of biology. The story does not ask about the children's three to eight years of socialization — whether that may have contributed to the selections and been a better predictor of children's toy choices than prenatal androgen. To know whether toy selection is related in some way to gender, the research would have to rule out alternative explanations for the behavior, explain the role of androgen in both sexes, and account for the fact that some children do not conform to the generalization.

Dichotomizing on the basis of sex invites comparison and ranking, and studies purporting to document sex-based differences often assign a higher value to the characteristics attributed to men than to those attributed to women. For example, one article that reported alleged sex-based differences in coping with stress said that girls focus more on their feelings, while boys pursue "diverting activities."[40] The girls, who behave "just like their moms," are said to be *"less skilled than males* at shrugging off hassles" (emphasis added). This study, a self-report of personal stress, could just as easily have been interpreted as indicating that girls are more willing than boys to confront stress, deal with it, and admit to it. The reporter could also have described the findings without characterizing one group as more or less skilled than the other.

The fascination with gender difference sometimes leads to the reporting of differences where none exist. Here, too, in the comparison of purported differences, girls lose out. A recent front-page story began with the headline: "To Help Girls Keep Up: Math Class without Boys."[41] One would expect the article to demonstrate that girls' math skills are inferior to boys'. If not, why the need to help girls keep up? The story begins with the anecdotal experiences of Amber, Cara, and Laura who couldn't make it in math and sciences class. (Remember the pregnant woman who couldn't concentrate when she felt fetal movement?) There's also a graph showing a fifty-point difference between male and female math scores on the Scholastic Aptitude Test (SAT) over the past twenty years. The story contains some data from the United States Department of Education in a table entitled "As Girls Grow, Math Skills Decline" (table 1). The text accompanying the table states: "Although girls and boys enter 8th grade with about the same . . . achievement level, girls soon fall behind."

However, the data do not really support this conclusion. Both boys and girls lose ground and the differences between them are really quite small. Which is more salient: the difference between boys and girls or the difference between eighth graders and twelfth graders? Do these data indicate that there is a gender difference in math ability, or do they suggest that math achievement of boys and girls is fairly comparable? Given room for measurement error and bias in testing, the only accurate conclusion is that the difference, if any, is minor.

Not all reporters got this particular story wrong. Another article on sex-based differences in math ability concluded that gender-based differences in math achievement have narrowed to the point that they are now insignificant.[42] This story also explained that scores on standardized aptitude tests do not always correlate with math achievement, especially for girls.[43] While this example demonstrates that some press reports are attentive to the issues that matter in reporting scientific data and are

Table 1. As Girls Grow, Math Skills Decline (percentage
of students in grade at each math achievement level)

	Advanced	Proficient	Basic skill	Below basic
8th grade				
Boys	4	21	37	38
Girls	4	20	38	37
12th grade				
Boys	3	15	47	35
Girls	1	13	49	37

more accurate as a result, it also shows that the myth of female inferiority
dies hard. One story confirmed it, the other refuted it, but the myth itself
is a palpable presence in both.

Such myths resurface, sometimes in more subtle ways. For example,
one article, headlined "Subtle but Intriguing Differences Found in the
Brain Anatomy of Men and Women," began: "Researchers who study
the brain have discovered that it differs anatomically in men and women
in ways that may underlie differences in mental abilities."[44] The article
reviewed other studies purporting to show that the size of different parts
of the brain is causally related to different abilities in men and women
and concluded that "new research is producing a complex picture of the
brain in which differences in anatomical structure seem to lead to advantages on certain mental tasks." The story acknowledged that these findings are based on preliminary and small-scale studies. It further observes
that "the brains of men and women are far more similar than different."
If so, why wasn't that the focus of the story? Why instead were tentative
findings highlighted and their limitations underemphasized? And why
are differences, even if they exist, used to rank the sexes (one gaining an "advantage" over the other), rather than to describe individual
characteristics?

What is the problem with the focus on gender difference, some may
wonder. Why not celebrate the differences between the sexes?

Characterizing an attribute as gender-based has important consequences. First, as noted above, the tendency to dichotomize on the basis
of sex "generates invidious comparison" and provides "a framework to
which cultures can attach a broad range of social differences that in fact
have little to do with [anatomical] sex difference."[45] Second, if the goal is
to promote accurate science, it is important to determine what differences really exist and what they mean. Assume, for example, that an ele-

phant's brain is larger than a human's. That would not necessarily signify that elephants are smarter than humans.[46] As this suggests, merely observing a physiological difference is not enough. If differences do exist, either on average or across the board, are they meaningful? Do the larger brains of elephants (or men) mean that they are "smarter" than humans (or women)? In addition, it is necessary to know whether the difference exists for all members of each group, or only for some. If some women have brains that are as large or larger than some men, brain size, by definition, cannot be a gender-based characteristic.

The focus on the differences between the sexes, moreover, can obscure important similarities and distort scientific inquiry. In the area of reproductive biology, for example, sex-based physiological and biological differences are well documented. The focus on those differences, and the cultural values attached to the female role in reproduction, have had anomalous results. Concentrating on reproductive success as a function of women's biology, few scientists have thought to inquire about males. Seeing reproductive biology through a "gendered" lens has prevented important questions from being asked and obscured knowledge of the sensitivity of the male reproductive system to toxic insult (consistent with the male myth of strength and invulnerability). It also has served to rationalize punitive policies toward women. Some employers, rather than improving workplace conditions, have denied fertile women access to lucrative jobs to preclude the possibility of fetal harm; as a result, some women have become sterilized to keep their jobs.[47] Women have been labeled neglectful or even abusive for engaging in conduct even arguably harmful to the fetus, and some have gone to jail.

Recent research provides evidence that male exposure to toxic chemicals, radiation, drugs, alcohol, and cigarettes can reduce fertility, interfere with conception, affect the course of pregnancy, and potentially affect the health of a future child.[48] If the vulnerability of both sexes to reproductive injury were better recognized, employment policies that exclude fertile women and prosecutions of pregnant women for prenatal "child" abuse would more easily have been recognized as unscientific and irrational.

Conclusion

The media can serve many useful functions in reporting on women's health issues. They can generate public attention for important issues, stimulate needed debate, and encourage legislative, regulatory, and other public policy responses. Press coverage can also help women assess the extent of particular health risks, weigh the benefits and disadvantages of various treatment options, make health-enhancing lifestyle choices, and the like. A great deal of scientific information cannot be adequately understood, however, without knowledge of the scientific method and an appreciation for the fact that scientific inquiry can be influenced by cultural biases and that press reports reflect and sometimes magnify this problem. We have used reporting on scientific issues generally to illustrate how the process works, with the ultimate goal of identifying the factors that increase the possibility of bias and diminish the reliability of information. The discerning reader can then make judgments about the likelihood that a particular study, or the popular report of it, contains trustworthy information.

Our preliminary review reveals some disquieting examples of distortion in the popular interpretation of scientific theories and research about women's biology. We have observed the reporting of "scientific" rationales to support conventional sex-role behavior, which is particularly marked in reports of studies relating in some way to childbearing and mothering. It is often impossible to determine from reading a press report whether the bias or distortion derives from the underlying data or was added by the translation into the vernacular. In either case, the issues most susceptible to distortion are those that are "invested with enormous social importance," to use Gould's phrase — issues in which there is a cultural investment in a particular result.

We do not suggest that scientific research is so tainted as to be useless. A great deal of important and useful information exists in medical journals and newspapers. However, it is important to recognize the point at which scientific knowledge leaves off and social preferences or values begin. This is especially critical in the effort to construct a health care system that will meet the needs of women for accurate information and beneficial services.

Notes

Thanks to Jeanne Mager Stellman, Isabelle Katz Pinzler, Mary S. Henifin, and Patricia Campbell for sharing their insights on many of the topics addressed in this chapter; to Susan Cott Watkins for her helpful comments on an earlier draft; and to Robin Finn, graduate student in the School of Public Health at Columbia University, for her indispensable research assistance. The Herman Goldman Foundation, the General Service Foundation, the Moriah Fund, and the Jessie Smith Noyes Foundation provided support of Ms. Bertin's research and the Program on Gender, Science and Law at Columbia University.

As this article neared completion, the authors learned of the sudden and untimely death of Professor Irving Kenneth Zola, who is quoted in the opening paragraph. His work offers a unique perspective and critical insights, for which we are very grateful. His work was an inspiration; he will be missed by many.

1   I. K. Zola, "Medicine as an Institution of Social Control," *Social Review* 20 (1972): 487.

2   "Women Smokers Appear to Run Higher Risk," *New York Times*, January 4, 1993, sec. C, p. 3.

3   S. J. Gould, *The Mismeasure of Man* (New York: W. W. Norton, 1981), 22–23. For a more recent exploration of the influence of culture and gender on a specific discipline, see S. C. Watkins, "If All We Knew About Women Was What We Read in *Demography*, What Would We Know?" *Demography* 30 (1993): 551–577. Watkins's comprehensive analysis is notable, among other things, for its careful methodology, which focused on the potential for bias in the creation and interpretation of data. Other studies have evaluated the potential for bias in reporting of data; see, e.g., G. Koren et al., "Bias Against the Null Hypothesis: The Reproductive Hazards of Cocaine," *Lancet* 2 (1989): 1440–1442, discussed *infra*.

4   Gould, *Mismeasure of Man*, 25.

5   M. Lowe, "Social Bodies: The Interaction of Culture and Women's Biology," in *Biological Woman: The Convenient Myth*, ed. R. Hubbard, M. S. Henifin, and B. Fried (Cambridge: Schenkman, 1982), 91–116.

6   Quoted in Hubbard et al., *Biological Woman*, 29.

7   Quoted in W. Kaminer, *A Fearful Freedom: Women's Flight from Equality* (New York: Pergamon, 1990), xiv.

8   L. M. Newman, *Men's Ideas/Women's Realities: Popular Science, 1870–1915* (New York: Pergamon, 1985).

9   B. Ehrenreich and D. English, *For Her Own Good: 150 Years of the Experts' Advice to Women* (Garden City, N.J.: Doubleday, 1979), 127.

10   Ibid., 128.

11   S. Faludi, *Backlash: The Undeclared War Against American Women* (New York: Crown, 1991).

12   Gould, *Mismeasure of Man*, 74.

13   See, e.g., G. H. Guyatt et al., "Users Guide to the Medical Literature: How to Use an Article about Therapy of Prevention — A. Are the Results Valid?," *Journal of the American Medical Association* 270 (1993): 2598–2601.

14   National Academy of Sciences et al., *Responsible Science: Ensuring the Integrity of the Research Process* (Washington, D.C.: National Academy Press, 1992).

15   A. L. Cowan, "Trend in Pregnancies Challenges Employers," *New York Times*, April 17, 1989, sec. A, p. 1.

16   Koren et al., "Bias Against the Null Hypothesis," *supra* note 3. Canadian newspapers, however, have reported on similar research by this author and colleagues. See, e.g., C. Maloney, "Cocaine and Pregnancy: Study Shows Users Who Quit Drug Have Normal Babies," *The Ottawa Citizen*, August 10, 1991, E12.

17   We searched "Major Newspapers Files" in The Nexis Service (online database of Mead Data Central, Inc.).

18   L. C. Mayes et al., "Commentary: The Problem of Prenatal Cocaine Exposure: A Rush to Judgment," *Journal of the American Medical Association* 267 (1992): 406–408. This commentary was featured in a story in *New York Newsday*, June 28, 1992, 51.

19 J. Alpert and B. Zuckerman, "Alcohol Use in Pregnancy: What is the Risk?" *Pediatrics in Review* 12 (1992): 375–379.

20 In contrast, the *New York Times* has featured numerous articles emphasizing the risks of even moderate alcohol consumption during pregnancy. See E. Rosenthal, "When a Pregnant Women Drinks," *New York Times Magazine*, February 4, 1990, 30; and D. Goleman, "Lasting Costs for a Child from Mother's Early Drinks," *New York Times*, February 16, 1989, sec. B, p. 10. See also C. Leerhsen and E. Schaefer, "Pregnancy + Drinking = Problems: Even Moderate Drinking Can Cause Fetal Damage," *Newsweek*, July 31, 1989, 57.

21 B. Zuckerman et al., "Effects of Maternal Marijuana and Cocaine Use on Fetal Growth," *New England Journal of Medicine* 320 (1989): 762–768. Zuckerman coauthored the commentary by Mayes et al., "The Problem of Prenatal Cocaine Exposure," *supra* note 18.

22 B. D. Colen, "Cocaine Babies: Doctors Are Becoming Increasingly Alarmed about the Long-Term Prospects for a Growing Army of Damaged Children," *New York Newsday*, March 27, 1990, 1.

23 G. Kolata, "Study Ties Drugs to Impaired Fetuses," *New York Times*, March 23, 1989, sec. B, p. 13.

24 P. Klass, "Tackling Problems We Thought We Solved," *New York Times*, December 13, 1992, sec. 6, p. 55.

25 See Mayes et al., "The Problem of Prenatal Cocaine Exposure," *supra* note 18.

26 R. Little and C. Sing, "Father's Drinking and Infant Birthweight: Report of an Association," *Teratology* 36 (1987): 59–65.

27 E. M. John, D. A. Savitz, and D. P. Sandler, "Prenatal Exposure to Parent's Smoking and Childhood Cancer," *American Journal of Epidemiology* 133 (1991): 123–132.

28 R. A. Yazigi et al., "Demonstration of Specific Binding of Cocaine to Human Spermatozoa," *Journal of the American Medical Association* 266 (1991): 1956–1959.

29 E.g., K. F. Schmidt, "The Dark Legacy of Fatherhood," *U.S. News and World Report*, December 14, 1992, 94, 96.

30 N. Angier, "What Makes a Parent Put Up with It All?" *New York Times*, November 2, 1993, sec. C, p. 1.

31 J. T. Winslow et al., "A Role for Central Vasopressin in Pair Bonding in Monogamous Prairie Voles," *Nature* 365 (1993): 545–547.

32 N. Angier, "Hyena's Hormone Flow Puts Females in Charge," *New York Times*, September 1, 1992, sec. C, p. 1.

33 "Defective Offspring of 'Alcoholic' Rats," *New York Times*, January 2, 1990, sec. C, p. 6.

34 "Fetus Gets 'Taste' for Alcohol?" United Press International, June 13, 1984, Wednesday, A.M. Cycle, Domestic News, dateline Chapel Hill, N.C.

35 Reportage on how surrogate care affects infants and young children provides another good example of this phenomenon. See, e.g., E. Eckholm, "Learning If Infants Are Hurt When Mothers Go to Work," *New York Times*, October 6, 1992, sec. A, p. 1. The question is whether children in families where both parents work outside the home, or where the only parent present works outside the home, suffer as a result of the fact that a parent does not care for them during the day. The way in which this article was framed, however, reveals a bias in favor of assigning the role of child care to women, along with the responsibility for insuring the well-being of children.

36   Kaminer, *Fearful Freedom, supra* note 7.

37   See, e.g., *Orr v. Orr,* 440 U.S. 268 (1979) and *Mississippi University for Women v. Hogan,* 458 U.S. 718 (1982).

38   Faludi, *Backlash, supra* note 11.

39   M. A. Hogan, "He-Men in Training: Dolls or Trucks — The Play's the Thing," *Los Angeles Times,* April 28, 1993, sec. E, p. 1.

40   M. Elias, "Shedding Light on Human Behavior," *USA Today,* March 16, 1993, 6D.

41   J. Gross, "To Help Girls Keep Up: Math Class Without Boys," *New York Times,* November 24, 1993, sec. A, p. 1.

42   M. Gladwell, "Pythagorean Sexism: Who Says Men Are Better at Math? Not the Numbers," *Washington Post,* March 14, 1993.

43   This fact, among others, led a federal judge to conclude that the Scholastic Aptitude Test (SAT) discriminates against girls and could not be used as the basis for state-awarded scholarships. See *Sharif v. New York State Dep't of Education,* 709 F. Supp. 345 (S.D.N.Y. 1989).

44   D. Goleman, "Subtle but Intriguing Differences Found in the Brain Anatomy of Men and Women," *New York Times,* April 11, 1989, sec. C, p. 1.

45   C. F. Epstein, *Deceptive Distinctions: Sex, Gender, and the Social Order* (New Haven: Yale University Press, 1988).

46   The craniologists' arguments were defeated by this logic, pressed persuasively by Helen Hamilton Gardener, who observed that if intelligence were a function of brain weight " 'Almost any elephant is . . . perhaps an entire medical faculty.' " Kaminer, *Fearful Freedom, supra* note 7, xiv.

47   *International Union, UAW v. Johnson Controls,* 499 U.S. 187 (1991).

48   See, e.g., B. Robaire and B. F. Hales, "Paternal Exposure to Chemicals Before Conception: Some Children May Be at Risk," *British Medical Journal* 307 (1993): 341–342.

3

REINVENTING MEDICAL RESEARCH

Kay Dickersin and
Lauren Schnaper, M.D.

Introduction

In 1995, an estimated 185,000 women in the United States developed breast cancer and approximately 46,000 women died from the disease. It is estimated that approximately 2.6 million women in the U.S. are living with breast cancer: 1.6 million who have been diagnosed and 1 million who have not yet been diagnosed but have the disease. Incidence has been increasing steadily over the past fifty years, and the mortality rate has remained essentially unchanged. Although African-American women have a lower incidence of the disease than white women, their mortality rate is higher.

Public attention to the importance of breast cancer has increased over the past several years, largely because of the prominent activities of a number of grassroots and other organizations who joined together in 1991 to form the National Breast Cancer Coalition (NBCC). The primary objective of the NBCC is to facilitate the eradication of breast cancer, and one of its specific goals is to increase research into the causes, prevention, and cure of the disease. Its members seek more funding for breast cancer research and also wish to see the money spent wisely. The NBCC believes that consumer involvement in every step of the research process is necessary to achieve eradication of the disease. We propose in this article that the way all research is conducted should be "reinvented"; that is, consumers should be more involved in the research process: designing, implementing, interpreting, and disseminating research findings. We use the work of the NBCC as a case study in our discussion.

A wide variety of groups formed the first NBCC Board of Directors. These groups included small breast cancer support groups, such as Arm-in-Arm in Baltimore; local groups oriented toward providing both support and access to care for women without sufficient financial means, such as the Linda Creed Foundation in Philadelphia; cancer groups oriented toward special populations, such as the Mary Helen Mautner Project for Lesbians with Cancer; larger grassroots advocacy groups, such as Breast Cancer Action in California; coalitions such as the Massachusetts Breast Cancer Coalition and California Association of Breast Cancer Organizations; and professional and nonprofit organizations, such as the Faulkner Hospital Breast Center, the National Alliance of Breast Cancer Organizations, and the American Cancer Society.

Only months after its first meeting, the NBCC held its first national rally in Washington, D.C. Its purpose was to deliver over 600,000 letters from citizens around the country to members of Congress and President Bush, demanding an increase in funding for breast cancer research. This initial effort was the cornerstone for a series of stunning successes, including increases in funding for breast cancer research from $90 million in 1991 to $410 million in 1993. In an unusual move, Congress reappropriated $210 million of the "star wars" defense plan to breast cancer research, deciding to house the research program under the U.S. Department of Defense, rather than move the funds to an agency on the domestic side.

The NBCC next demanded a national action plan for breast cancer, including research, that would put in place a system for planning and accountability. On May 2, 1993, a second national breast cancer rally was held on the Mall in Washington, D.C., to kick off the NBCC's campaign to deliver 2.6 million signatures to President Clinton requesting this plan. On October 18, 1993, the coalition delivered the signatures to President Clinton; this ceremony held on the Ellipse in front of the White House, was marked by a concomitant march and rally that drew busloads of citizens from all over the United States.

At the White House meeting, President Clinton pledged support for a National Action Plan; work toward that goal was begun in December of the same year under the leadership of Secretary of Health and Human Services Donna Shalala. Proceedings setting the stage for the plan were released in April 1994. Action points include research, health care policy, health care delivery, and education of consumers,[1] providers, and scientists. A common thread in all four areas is the need for consumer involvement at every level. In the next step efforts have been focused on six priority areas: consumer involvement at every level of research; ensuring access by women to clinical trials; providing information about breast cancer to women, providers, and others, using the "information superhighway"; development of a national breast cancer tissue bank as a research resource; development of a plan regarding testing and follow-up of women at risk for carrying the breast cancer susceptibility gene; and determination of the etiology of breast cancer. Six working groups comprised of consumers, scientists, and representatives of government and industry now coordinate activities related to these priorities.

Despite making impressive strides in directing more medical and scientific attention to breast cancer and contributing successfully to setting priorities, women consumers need more involvement in the planning, conduct, and oversight of research. It is not enough to demand that women and women's health be the "subject" of more research. Where it has existed, consumer involvement in guiding the design and conduct of research has largely been indirect and men have had considerably more input than women. For example, men have had the vast majority of seats in Congress, and some claim that this has resulted in more funding for clinical research on men.[2] Perhaps even more important, men have dominated positions of power in medical schools and major research institutions, such as the National Institutes of Health. As members of study sections and advisory boards, as directors of institutes, chairs of departments, and presidents of institutions, they have had the ability to direct funds per their recommendations. Thus, men, as both scientists and nonscientists, have had a disproportionate ability to influence the selection of research questions and to award funding that makes research possible, while women have been largely excluded.

This lack of influence may be a large part of the reason that a number of major trials in the 1970s and 1980s relating to prevention of cardiovascular mortality (funded by the National Institutes of Health) excluded women, despite the fact that about the same number of deaths from heart disease occur in women and men each year in the United States. These trials included the Physicians' Health Study, testing the efficacy of aspirin; the Coronary Drug Project, testing various drug regimens; and MRFIT (Multiple Risk Factor Intervention Trial), testing smoking and dietary counseling interventions in men at high risk of coronary heart disease. Despite the enormous cost of these trials to the U.S. taxpayer, their results provided no information on the effect of these preventive interventions in women.

As the women's movement has matured, there has been a growing collective interest in issues relating to women's health. The publication of *Our Bodies, Ourselves*[3] in 1973 was perhaps the first formal response by women to increasing sentiment that women's health needs had been ignored. At about the same time, the enrollment of women in medical school began increasing dramatically across the United States. In 1985, the U.S. Public Health Service issued a report from its Task Force on Women's Issues, which concluded that there had been a historical lack of focus on women's health research. In response, the NIH in 1986 instituted a policy of greater inclusion of women in clinical research, although a 1990 report by the Government Accounting Office (GAO) found that they had failed to fully implement it.[4] This led to inclusion of language in the 1993 NIH Revitalization Act requiring NIH clinical studies to include sufficient populations of women and minority populations to allow a valid analysis of these subgroups. The Institute of Medicine Committee on the Ethical and Legal Issues Relating to the Inclusion of Women in Clinical Studies issued its report the following year, stating that it was unable to draw conclusions about women's participation in clinical research from available data. They recommended that the NIH establish a registry of clinical studies to allow investigation of gender issues in the future.[5]

Although the U.S. government has now taken steps to increase participation of women in research and to monitor that participation, these do not guarantee that the research undertaken or the questions asked will be relevant to health issues that are important to women. Consumers have demanded more research, but rarely have they demanded that they themselves play a direct role in guiding the research.

The Current Research Paradigm in the United States

Consumers must understand the current paradigm for conducting research in the United States to be able to understand the many places where their voices are needed. Traditionally, consumers have not been part of the review, critique, and approval of research, nor have they been part of planning or executing research projects. However, they are integral to research — as the volunteers who make it possible, as the consumers or "users" of medical care services to whom any results will be applied, and as the individuals raising or contributing funding. It can be argued that consumers are, in fact, research "subjects" unless they have a meaningful voice at every level where decisions are made.

The current system of research involves semiautonomous groups of clinicians and investigators planning, carrying out, monitoring, and disseminating the work. In recent years, however, there has been a tendency for government agencies to exert more influence over the direction of research by limiting funding to specific questions they determine to be important. In other words, ideas for research that start with investigators' questions may be less likely to be funded than proposals that respond to a government agency's specific request. Scientists do not like this approach, because they feel it sets unnatural boundaries on areas ripe for research, stifles creativity, discourages risk taking that may lead to important advances, and limits opportunities to follow unexpected leads.

Scientists and providers interested in a common area of investigation typically design a study together. Rarely, if ever, are consumers part of the study planning team, although they may be brought in for several hours as part of a "focus group" that discusses issues related to the topic being studied, to help with generating hypotheses.[6]

If outside funding is sought, scientific "peers" review the proposed work for merit and approval in a "study section." An advisory council at the funding agency approves funding for meritorious proposals that meet programmatic goals. Institutional review boards review proposals at the institution(s) where the research will be carried out, and recommend changes to the protocol and patient consent process where they feel it is warranted. In a clinical trial of a new or existing intervention, a data and safety monitoring committee may exist to advise on ethical issues and to examine the data for beneficial or harmful trends as the study proceeds. Research results are presented in journal articles and reports to the medical and scientific community. Prior to publication, a manuscript is reviewed by "peers" and editors; if it is found to meet minimum standards, it will be accepted as is, or the author may be asked to revise it, in an effort to limit the publication of poor research and to improve acceptable work.

Consumers and lay people[7] may sit on the "advisory councils" of funding agencies — as they do, for example, at the National Institutes of Health (NIH), where they contribute to setting programmatic goals for an institute and giving final approval to funding decisions. Lay people are also likely to sit on institutional review boards of medical institutions; however, they are more likely to be lawyers than patients. Sometimes data and safety monitoring boards include lay people — most often members of the clergy or, again, lawyers. Even when they are included as part of these processes, however, consumers may not represent any constituency. They may owe their inclusion simply to being an acquaintance of the person who made the appointments to the committee. The advantages of consumer affiliation with a constituency are numerous and will be discussed later; suffice it to say that this concept is not limited to

consumers serving on committees: scientists and others involved in research are considered to represent both a "common" voice (e.g., the
current state of medical knowledge in a field, adherence to scientific
principles) and an individual voice.

Formal exclusion of consumers from the research process has probably resulted from both the isolation of biomedical research from its
practical applications and the autonomy that we as a society have granted
health care providers in administering interventions to patients. Historically, scientists have claimed a right to pose their own research questions and to proceed in directions of their own choosing. The argument
is that science is an endeavor best driven by intellectual and creative
spark, not by practical needs specified by others. Where practical needs
are included in the motivation to conduct scientific research, typically
they have been defined by the scientists themselves without input from
the public. Similarly, health care providers, most often physicians, have
claimed and been granted the right to make decisions regarding patient
care based on their personal knowledge and best judgment. Indeed,
physicians may try out a new type of surgery they have read about in a
journal article without asking anybody's permission; yet if they wish to
do formal testing on how well the surgery actually works, they must
receive permission from their institutional review board or ethics committee. This situation provides a disincentive to doctors to be part of
research efforts investigating the efficacy of health care interventions
and an incentive to practice medicine based on training, experience, and
hunch.

Consumers have also been willing to grant relative autonomy to both
scientists and health care providers, because they do not understand
complex scientific/medical language and processes. Public trust in the
medical community exists because it has seemed as if there is no alternative. As is true for other professions, the length, specialty, and hands-on
nature of a doctor's formal education cannot be readily duplicated by a
consumer who wishes to understand fully his or her condition. With
improved science education and broad dissemination of findings from
medical research, however, consumers know a lot more than they once
did, and there is a greater desire for input. For example, the Internet has
numerous user groups devoted to medical conditions such as breast
cancer and AIDS. Patients exchange information about their own experiences as well as ask and answer questions. Patients can obtain research
citations related to their interests and even engage in on-line critiques of
the latest findings with relative ease. With increasing recognition that

relatively little progress has been made in curing and preventing diseases such as breast cancer and that the traditional research model focusing on mortality does not address many of the questions important to women, consumers have demanded more input into the research and health care processes.

Barriers to Consumer Involvement

Consumer involvement can be perceived by providers and scientists as an obstacle to research. From the provider's perspective, the process of obtaining consent for participation in a research study is more time-consuming than delivery of standard medical care. Yet it is also possible that establishment of a mutually informed provider-patient relationship in the context of a trial takes less provider time, overall, because of increased patient satisfaction. Many scientists feel that consumers may not understand the scientific complexity of a problem and will therefore slow down the research design and approval process. This reasoning implies that the best decisions in planning and carrying out research are made by individuals with identical viewpoints. The point of consumer involvement is to bring new ideas to the table, which will almost certainly slow the process.

While some argue that consumers may be unscientific, and this might be correct, it does not follow that they will be unintelligent or irrational. Just as there is a selection process for any scientific collaborator in a research project, there should be a similar process for choosing consumer collaborators, involving comparable selection criteria that include the ability to work in a group, knowledge about the area that he or she represents, and the existence of positive recommendations from others, including the support of the people they represent. For example, the Army Medical Command for 1993–94, with the help of its contracting agency, identified appropriate consumers for its Integration Panel, the advisory board responsible for making the final funding decisions regarding disbursement of $235 million allocated for breast cancer research. In 1995, the Army will expand consumer participation to its study selections, the groups that review the research proposals for scientific merit. Identification and selection of consumers will involve a process similar to the one used to identify scientist candidates for study sections.

Finally, scientists are concerned that consumers may be "biased." Individual consumers are indeed likely to have a bias, as is any individual, including a scientist. Consumers representing a constituency, however, have a responsibility to represent more than just their personal point of view. They bring their own experience and the understanding of others' needs and experiences. In addition, a consumer representative who is accountable to a constituency will be told when or if she or he has become locked into a single position or has failed to represent adequately the group's views.

The consumer brings to the table concerns different from those of a doctor treating women with breast cancer or a researcher who has studied women with breast cancer. For example, a clinical trial of a given chemotherapy for cancer may examine laboratory test results and mortality as its major outcomes, but not proportion of time spent nauseated, days hospitalized or separated from one's family, cessation of fertility, compromise of sexual function, number of months of life gained and the quality of those months, and so forth.

Setting the Stage for Advocacy

Since Victorian times, health care decision making in the United States has been largely within the purview of physicians. Additional players have been other health care professionals; the government, acting for the uninsured, underinsured, and elderly; and third-party payers. The role of the average consumer traditionally has been limited to choosing a physician, and this ability to choose has been limited by other factors, such as the system of financing. In addition, patients often grant physicians a level of autonomy that allows them to assume a paternalistic role. Nevertheless, assumptions on the physicians' part that their greater knowledge of medicine translates automatically into knowledge of what is best for patients has drawn increasing skepticism from the public. With greater mass communication, consumers have become more aware of medical knowledge and on an individual basis have demanded new or existing interventions (for example, tamoxifen treatment or mastectomy for women at high risk of breast cancer).

Patients can be quite powerful in terms of setting health care policy when they band together to insist that a treatment be made widely available. For example, in the case of third-party payment for autologous bone marrow transplants (ABMT) in women with breast cancer, many states have responded to public demand by instituting laws requiring reimbursement for this procedure, despite a price tag estimated to be in excess of $200,000. At the time legislation was passed in these states, there was no reliable evidence that this treatment cured breast cancer or even prolonged life. Lobbying efforts by grassroots breast cancer groups in Virginia and Massachusetts, for example, effected legislation mandating payment for this procedure.

In terms of health research, consumers are less likely to have an impact when they work as individuals than when they work as a group. Their influence, both on medical professionals and on other consumers, is necessarily limited because of their lack of a constituency. After the initial thrust of an individual's argument is heard, she may tend to be marginalized or adopt the view of the medical profession. Furthermore, individual activists who do not represent a consumer group may not be knowledgeable regarding current consumer issues that differ from their own. Nor are they necessarily able to communicate their experiences to other consumers.

Individuals can have an important pioneering role, however. In her book *Why Me?* (later titled *Alternatives*) and in other writings, Rose Kushner[8] urged doctors to recognize the evidence that lumpectomy was as effective as mastectomy, in terms of survival, for women with breast cancer. "She is probably the single most important person in leading to this major change in breast surgery," said Dr. Bruce Chabner, former director of the Division of Cancer Treatment at the National Cancer Institute. While her early writings were cautious in terms of counseling women to participate in clinical trials, she modified her views with increased experience. As a consumer representative, she was a member of the Advisory Board of the National Cancer Institute from 1980 to 1986 and served until her death in 1990 as president of BreastPac, a fund created to support the election of legislators who favor increased funding for breast cancer research.

Women consumers have long been involved with lobbying for increased research funding — as mothers of children with cancer and polio, as daughters of women with Huntington's Disease, as uninfected women working as part of the AIDS advocacy movement. However, until recently, women have not lobbied en masse for research related specifically to their own diseases and conditions. Cervical, endometrial, ovarian, and breast cancers; endometriosis; conditions related to pregnancy and the menstrual cycle have neither been taken up as special causes by the public nor championed by the "hidden colleges" in Congress and academe.

The most successful medical advocacy movements in the United States have utilized preexisting political structures[9] and have reached the general public through celebrity example. When the AIDS movement began, it was based on the already well-organized gay rights movement, and was advanced through the journalistic talents of Randy Shiltz and others as well as through the efforts of many members of the performing arts who were victims of the disease. The Right to Life movement, using its strong religious and political base, successfully banned the anti-progestin Mifepristone (RU 486) in the United States, despite the fact that it not only can be used for abortions but has other actions that may hold promise (e.g., in the treatment of Cushing's disease and breast cancer).[10] The Grey Panthers, a strong health-advocacy group for the elderly, has been successful in their campaign for increased funding in Alzheimer's disease research, which was boosted by the poignant 1994 revelation of the decline of the artist Willem de Kooning.[11]

The stunning success of the National Breast Cancer Coalition in its first few years of operation can be attributed in part to a confluence of political and newsworthy events. The year the Coalition was formed, 1991, was the Year of the Woman. In that year, the Congressional Caucus for Women's Issues submitted the Breast Cancer Challenge to the medical research community and the National Cancer Institute, naming five goals related to prevention and cure of breast cancer, to be achieved by the year 2000. Also in 1991, in a report picked up by the media, the United States General Accounting Office called attention to the increasing incidence, and unchanged mortality, of breast cancer.[12] The diagnoses and treatment of Presidents' wives (e.g., Betty Ford, Nancy Reagan), as well as movie and television stars, were highlighted in the media internationally. Thus breast cancer attracted the attention of women who had been sensitized to women's health issues through the media as well as those who were part of the established feminist network (for example, as part of the National Women's Health Network or The Feminist Majority).

Community Activism Related to Medical Research

Community "walks" and "runs" to raise money for various areas of health research are legion. Most occur on a local or statewide basis, such as the AIDS Walk and the Race for the Cure (for breast cancer). Few are nationwide in scope, although the National Breast Cancer Coalition has coordinated local rallies, such as Mother's Day rallies against breast cancer that highlight the genetic and family nature of the disease. These efforts are useful for raising public awareness about a disease but are too general to have much of an impact on the quantity or quality of research in specific areas.

Community activists have also demanded that research be performed specifically to address local health problems. The involvement of community groups in helping discover the adverse effects of chemical dumping at Love Canal is one of the best-known examples.[13] In 1985, the Kendall Lakes Women Against Cancer was formed in southern Florida when three women under the age of 45 on a single tennis team were diagnosed with breast cancer. They surveyed their neighbors and found that others also had the disease. Suspecting an abnormally high incidence, they attempted to discover if the incidence was indeed high and, if so, the possible etiologies. They received considerable media attention and were able to raise enough money to conduct an epidemiologic study investigating environmental contamination as a possible cause of the apparent increase of breast cancer in the community.[14]

Training Consumers for a Seat at the Research Table

To accommodate the new paradigm of including consumers in the research process, the NBCC has instituted an educational program. The pilot phase of the program has been tested on the Board of Directors of the NBCC and has involved a series of one-day workshops on various scientific and research topics: basic science (including DNA replication, transcription, translation, cell cycle, cell signaling, genetic linkage, mutation, and other areas); research methods (including the principles of biostatistics, descriptive epidemiology, observational studies, clinical trials, screening tests, and meta-analysis); current knowledge from breast cancer clinical research; and the epidemiology of breast cancer. Members of the Board and others have also undergone formal advocacy training to learn how the legislative and research funding systems work, the role of advocacy in these domains, and the goals and policies of the NBCC.

This program has been funded for widespread application to breast-cancer consumer activists who wish to be included in the research process. In 1995, the NBCC has launched Project LEAD (Leadership, Advocacy, and Education Development), a four-day training program for grassroots activists around the United States. Courses covering research and leadership topics similar to those tested in the pilot project will be offered in four cities during the year. Faculty include prominent investigators from the research community as well as NBCC Board members.

The major aim of the course is to prepare breast cancer consumers for positions on the various advisory boards and study teams. The course does not aim to create scientist-consumers, because this would mitigate the independent views a consumer can offer; rather it aims to help women be comfortable with the process of research and with presenting their points of view in research settings.

As noted earlier, the Army Medical Command, as part of its own breast cancer research program, has decided to include consumers in its study sections. Consumers will not be primary reviewers of research applications but are expected to contribute to discussion of the proposals and to vote on a priority score. As part of the new endeavor, the Army plans to study the effect of consumers on the study section process. In another example, the University of California, San Francisco and California Pacific Medical Center breast cancer SPORE (Specialized Programs of Research Excellence), a joint research group funded by the National Cancer Institute, has had consumers as part of its project review process since 1993.

Dividends of Consumer Involvement in the Research Process

Participating as a Volunteer in Clinical Trials

Every patient wants to receive the best available care. What most patients do not know is that the vast majority of medical and surgical interventions have never been properly tested in the context of a randomized trial, but are phased in by consensus after having been used routinely by practitioners. For example, the modified radical mastectomy replaced the Halsted radical mastectomy without benefit of scientific testing regarding its effect on survival. More recently, laparoscopy rapidly replaced open exploration for many types of abdominal surgeries, also without first being subjected to randomized trials. Tamoxifen, an anti-estrogen oral medication used to prevent second primary breast cancers, has been advocated by many clinicians for short-term use in the treatment of fibrocystic changes of the breast — without evidence that it is safe or effective.[15] Thus, participation in a clinical trial has indirect benefits, in that all of society will gain from the knowledge obtained, as well as possible direct benefits, in that the patient herself will benefit if she is allocated to the superior treatment (assuming there is one). Yet some patients still believe that the newest treatment is likely to be the best and that participating in a randomized clinical trial is being a "guinea pig." Part of the problem is that randomization, whereby a patient is assigned to treatment by a random process similar to flipping a coin, is not well understood. Not even all doctors recognize that randomized clinical trials are the best method for demonstrating efficacy and safety of new treatments when compared with standard therapies or no treatment.[16] Randomization tends to ensure that the two or more treatment groups are similar in all respects related to the potential success of the treatment (e.g., age of the patient, stage of the disease). Studying a treatment's efficacy using groups that were not assigned randomly, such as comparing one doctor's practice to another, may be biased. For example, one doctor may tend to be referred the healthiest patients in town because she is known to have access to the latest treatment and doctors want their patients with the best chances of recovery to receive the new intervention. Another doctor may be referred older patients because she is known to accept Medicare payment.

The reasons behind consumers' decisions to participate in clinical trials may be practical, personal, altruistic, or all three. In some instances, enrollment in a clinical trial may be the only way a patient can gain access to a new type of treatment that has already been popularized in the press. Originally, this was the case with AZT, in which the only way to have a 50 percent chance of gaining access to the drug was via the clinical trial.[17] Patients may also enroll in clinical trials because they believe that institutions participating in clinical research are on the forefront of scientific discovery, have state-of-the-art equipment, and more knowledgeable medical staffs.[18] Others simply want to be a part of the fight against their illness.

The number of patients with cancer who entered into clinical trials each year has been estimated to be approximately 2 percent of those considered eligible.[19] Physician investigators repeatedly fail to accrue the number of subjects needed in the time originally allocated for recruitment, presumably because they overestimate the actual numbers of eligible patients they see each year. It is widely believed, and there is some evidence, that the majority of patients will follow the advice of their doctor to enter a randomized trial. There have always been practical objections, both by physicians and patients, regarding participation in clinical trials: inconvenience, cost when not funded by an outside source, concern about being treated like a "guinea pig," and a "hunch," usually on the part of the primary treating physician, that one treatment is superior to another.

Lack of access to health care in general has limited participation by the poor and minorities in clinical trials. Dr. Harold Freeman, chief of the Department of Surgery at Harlem Hospital Center and chair of the President's Cancer Panel, has stated that researchers do not accommodate cultural and economic variations in planning and executing clinical investigations.[20] In response to this and other similar criticism, the National Cancer Institute (NCI) began a pilot program to help minority women become their own advocates. Through Save Our Sisters, black women between the ages of 50 and 74 in rural North Carolina have been recruited and trained as lay "advisors" to help their peers obtain screening mammography. Through networking and ingenuity, this group has branched into other activities. In addition to pursuing their stated purpose of mammography education, they have formed a committee that helps women understand and use the health care system and a training committee to recruit additional advisors. They also participate in the administration of breast cancer support groups and distribute community educational materials.[21]

Developing and Asking Relevant Research Questions

Women consumers can help develop research questions specifically aimed at and relevant to women. Providers traditionally have been interested in preventing "serious" adverse outcomes (e.g., death) and thus clinical research questions have focused on these. In the case of breast cancer, for example, most research has centered on methods for prolonging survival and has neglected quality-of-life issues. For example, research has shown that giving "adjuvant" chemotherapy (medical therapy given in addition to the primary surgical treatment) to premenopausal women diagnosed with early breast cancer is associated with increased survival.[22] Given this information, most newly diagnosed women would agree to receive adjuvant treatment. Many might also ask, "What is the chance that I will have nausea and lose my hair?" Some might ask, "Should I expect to gain weight? What is weight gain due to, and what can I do to prevent it?" And a few might ask, "Will I experience menopause? What are my chances of conceiving a child after treatment? How will my sex life be affected?" Data have not been consistently collected, analyzed, and presented for these outcomes, despite the fact that this information is important to many women.

There are numerous examples where consumers have helped to develop new hypotheses and guide important research. A mother suggested that her daughter's exposure to diethylstilbestrol in utero might have caused her daughter's adenocarcinoma of the vagina; a mother of a child with Lyme disease drew a spot map of the homes of children with similar symptoms, leading to an understanding of the origins of the condition; and a mother of a child with Down's syndrome first hypothesized that a low level of alphafetoprotein might serve as a marker that could be tested prenatally for the chromosomal abnormality associated with the disease.

The NIH-funded Breast Cancer Prevention Trial, a multicenter trial in which either tamoxifen or a placebo is given to women at risk for breast cancer, has received tremendous scrutiny, much of it initiated by consumers, with regard to aspects of its design and other issues. However, there are other important issues, related to study outcomes and data collected, that should also be addressed as part of the trial. For example, had women with breast cancer or women taking tamoxifen been formally involved in the trial's design, trial participants might have been asked additional questions at follow-up. Tamoxifen, a "hormonal" adjuvant therapy frequently prescribed for women with breast cancer, may cause younger women to enter menopause. Hypotheses relating to the proportion of women who enter menopause, the reversibility of that phenomenon, and the effects of the treatment on sexual enjoyment, cognitive function, and overall sense of well-being, might have been suggested and data collected to allow testing had women consumers been involved at the outset.

Consumers can make sure that important risks are explored in a study and, where they are known, included in the consent form and monitored closely. Hazel Cunningham, an individual whose mother had breast cancer and died of complications possibly related to her tamoxifen treatment, has mounted a one-woman battle to see that the Breast Cancer Prevention Trial addresses ethical issues appropriately.[23] For many years she has warned of the potential side effects of tamoxifen, and only recently has one of them, the increased risk of endometrial cancer, been generally recognized and accepted. The consent form of the Breast Cancer Prevention Trial has been modified to reflect this and other risks, and regular endometrial biopsies are now recommended for participants. However, the monitoring guidelines have not been applied consistently across trials of tamoxifen. Even trials funded by the same institute (i.e., the National Cancer Institute) vary by whether routine endometrial biopsies or just routine pelvic examinations are recommended. While women in the Breast Cancer Prevention Trial are recommended to have routine biopsies, women in treatment trials are not. This inconsistency implies that active surveillance for endometrial cancer of women taking tamoxifen is more important for women without breast cancer than for women with breast cancer. Women's groups, such as the NBCC and the National Women's Health Network, are currently active in raising the issue of this disparity in the lay press and with the funding agency, but future resolution of this type of problem is no substitute for proper design from the start.

There is no question that breast cancer activists have been responsible for increasing attention to the role of environmental agents in the development of breast cancer. For example, community activist groups One in Nine and the Adelphi Breast Cancer Support Project in Long Island, New York, have been instrumental in securing congressional funding for a research investigation into the high local rate of breast cancer. This study, the Long Island Breast Cancer Study Project, aims to examine the contribution of various environmental and occupational factors in the etiology of breast cancer.

Until recently, women over the age of 70 have been excluded from breast cancer clinical trials. Consequently, little is known about the biological activity of tumors and women's response to treatment in this age group. Although there are few data, it is a commonly held belief that breast cancer behaves in a more indolent fashion in postmenopausal women. In 1992, M. E. Costanza, Professor of Medicine at the University of Massachusetts School of Medicine, and well known for her work in breast cancer clinical trials, put forth a research agenda that specifically addresses screening, prevention, the effect of comorbidity, education, and treatment in this population.[24] Thus, clinical trials involving older women have begun as a result of pressure by their advocacy groups.

Ethical Issues

Consumer involvement in decisions regarding research design and operation is of special importance where ethical issues are concerned. Currently, most if not all federally funded, multicenter clinical trials have data and safety monitoring boards as part of their structure. As noted earlier, there is typically a lay person on the board and this person is often a representative of the clergy or a lawyer, not a consumer representative. Less often it is a person with the condition being studied, that is, a consumer. While a single person cannot speak to all points of view held by others with the condition, she or he is perhaps more likely to bring up a point of view specific to the situation. For example, it was learned recently that the trials within the National Surgical Adjuvant Breast Project (NSABP) of the NCI Cancer Cooperative Studies program had not had data and safety monitoring boards. The National Breast Cancer Coalition has taken the position that if consumers had been involved on steering, executive, and data and safety monitoring committees, the discovery and disclosure of fraudulent reporting of data associated with the NSABP trials might have been better handled. Although no one can say for sure, consumer involvement might have resulted in the introduction of new ideas and commitments.

Physicians need to reevaluate dogma and be willing to admit uncertainty. It is because so few treatments have been scientifically investigated that the range of treatments in clinical practice is broad. For example, for women with lobular neoplasia (lobular carcinoma in situ) of the breast, some surgeons suggest observation and follow-up and others suggest bilateral mastectomy. Too little is known about the efficacy of either approach to make evidence-based treatment decisions, yet for reasons noted earlier, most clinicians recommend to their patients that they accept a given treatment rather than that they participate in research. Yet many people feel that when a treatment has not yet been properly or fully evaluated for efficacy, it is more ethical for it to be administered in the context of a randomized trial than in the context of routine care, where there is no acknowledgement of the experimental nature of the intervention. Either approach means that some patients may receive less than optimal care. In the clinical trial setting, however, data theoretically are properly collected, analyzed, and disseminated.

The need to test interventions for efficacy goes well beyond new treatments. Members of breast cancer families have become involved in discussions regarding future interventions since identification of a family of genes for inherited breast cancer. While scientists have emphasized ensuring the validity and reliability of any new genetic test prior to its marketing, breast cancer survivors have suggested the need to study the effectiveness of "preventive" measures such as prophylactic mastectomy and earlier mammography prior to their widespread recommendation. Survivors have also emphasized the need to test the utility of genetic counseling prior to its generalized acceptance.

Health Care Reform as an Opportunity for Consumer Involvement

Health care reform, whether implemented by an act of Congress or by third-party payers de facto, provides an opportunity to bridge the gap between delivering the most up-to-date health care and advancing research. Under our current system, most health care interventions applied have not been rigorously tested as to their efficacy. Even when there has been adequate testing and an intervention has been found to be beneficial, there is often no incentive to implement the findings; practice often has lagged decades behind what is known from research.[25] Two examples of problems related to the research/practice gap follow:

–Prior to the outcome of randomized trials now under way that investigate the efficacy of autologous bone marrow transplant (ABMT) for late-stage breast cancer, a jury awarded $89 million to the family of a woman who was denied coverage of ABMT by her HMO.[26] The cost of ABMT for the woman was estimated to be about $212,000. The problem is that many doctors recommend ABMT as possibly beneficial, without sufficient evidence. Some insurance companies will pay for the treatment, others will not. The proper approach is to pay for an unproven treatment only in the context of a randomized clinical trial.

–Guidelines for mammography of women under 50 have recently come under fire. At the present time, there is not sufficient evidence that mammography in women aged 40 to 49 confers a significant survival advantage. It is not clear whether mammography is useful in the younger age group or whether the survival advantage is smaller than that seen in the older group. Additional data are needed to demonstrate this advantage. Randomly assigning all women aged 40 to 49 to some form of screening — for example, mammography (or another imaging technique) plus clinical breast exam versus clinical breast exam alone — and paying for health care for women assigned to both groups will address this controversy and arrive at a conclusion sooner than any other approach.

Our health care system must allow payment for diagnostic, preventive, and treatment services when a clear benefit has been shown. Health care must also be covered if it is administered in the context of an "approved" clinical trial. For example, ABMT is a tremendously expensive therapy and has not yet been shown to be efficacious for breast cancer treatment. The best way to pay for this therapy is in the context of a randomized controlled trial: women would be randomly assigned to receive ABMT or the standard treatment, and regardless of the assignment, treatment would be covered by payors. Paying for ABMT administered outside a trial setting will result in a failure to determine the efficacy of ABMT, since recruitment to ongoing trials will be impacted.[27]

Currently, reimbursement for untested procedures may actually be better than for new procedures administered in the context of a trial, even when physicians are reimbursed for both trial and regular-practice patient care. If only half of a doctor's patients in a trial get the test treatment (e.g., ABMT), compared to all patients in a practice setting, then payment for services in the trial setting would be decreased — even halved — compared to payment in the practice setting, assuming the test treatment is more expensive and all treatments are reimbursed. The NBCC has taken a position supporting reimbursement for treatments for which efficacy has not been established when they are received in the context of a randomized trial. If and when it is made, a consumer-driven provision such as this may well be the most significant advance made so far to speed the applications of medical research.

The situation is complex: whether we move to health care reform or not, a smaller proportion of dollars will be available for health care than was so in the past. Research will increasingly affect access to treatment. For this reason and others, it is essential that consumers are involved in helping to establish and implement the research agenda.

Notes

Ms. Hilda Bastian and Ms. Sharon Batt provided critical readings of chapter drafts and made numerous helpful comments. Dr. Iain Chalmers has outlined a number of areas where public involvement would improve health care research, and many of these are included in this chapter.

1 "Consumers" in this context are defined as individuals who have the medical condition or use the health care system under study. Typically, consumers are rarely included in the process of research except as subjects. The term "subjects" — although widely used, even by so-called ethics committees — implies passivity on the part of those who are volunteering their lives and well-being to research. The term is also dehumanizing, in that the "subject" under study is also the "topic" being examined.

2 S. Rosser, "Gender Bias in Clinical Research: The Difference It Makes," in *Reframing Women's Health: Multidisciplinary Research and Practice*, ed. A. J. Dan (Thousand Oaks, Calif.: Sage, 1994).

3 Boston Women's Health Collective, *Our Bodies, Ourselves* (New York: Simon and Schuster, 1973).

4 Summary of Mark V. Nadel on problems in implementing the National Institutes of Health Policy on Women in Study Populations, given in testimony before the Subcommittee on Health and the Environment, Committee on Energy and Commerce, House of Representatives, June 18, 1990, Washington, D.C.: GAO.

5 A. C. Mastroianni, R. Faden, and D. Federman, eds., *Women and Health Research: Ethical and Legal Issues of Including Women in Clinical Studies*, Report of the Committee on Ethical and Legal Issues Relating to the Inclusion of Women in Clinical Studies, Division of Health Sciences Policy, Institute of Medicine (Washington, D.C.: National Academy Press, 1994).

6 R. A. Krueger, *Focus Groups: A Practical Guide for Applied Research*, 2d ed. (Thousand Oaks, Calif.: Sage, 1994).

7 As noted earlier, we use the term "consumer" to refer to a person who has a condition

or experience relevant to the research under question. We use "lay person" to refer to a person without scientific or medical training. The terms are not mutually exclusive.

8 G. Kolata, "Rose Kushner, 60, Leader in Breast Cancer Fight," *New York Times*, January 10, 1990, p. B5.

9 R. M. Wachter, "AIDS, Activism, and the Politics of Health," *New England Journal of Medicine* 236 (1992): 128–133.

10 W. Regelson, "RU 486: How Abortion Politics Have Impacted on a Potentially Useful Drug of Broad Medical Application," *Perspectives in Biology and Medicine* 35 (1992): 330–338.

11 P. Plagens, "The Twilight of a God," *Newsweek*, March 7, 1994, 64–66.

12 U.S. General Accounting Office, *Breast Cancer, 1971–1991: Prevention, Treatment and Research*, GAO/PEMD92-12 (Washington, D.C.: U.S. GAO, December 1991).

13 S. Schwartz, P. White, and R. Highes, "Environmental Threats, Communities, and Hysteria," *Journal of Public Health Politics* (1985): 58–77.

14 H. V. McCoy, E. J. Trapido, C. B. McCoy, N. Strickman-Stein, S. Engel, and I. Brown, "Community Activism Relating to a Cluster of Breast Cancer," *Journal of Community Health* 17 (1992): 27–36.

15 *A Practical Approach to Breast Disease*, ed. L. F. O'Grady, K. K. Lindfors, L. P. Howell, and M. B. Rippon (Boston: Little, Brown, 1995), ch. 8, p. 125.

16 S. Hellman and D. S. Hellman, "Of Mice But Not Men: Problems of the Randomized Clinical Trial," *New England Journal of Medicine* 324 (1991): 1585–1589.

17 C. Levin, N. N. Dubler, and R. J. Levine, "Building a New Consensus: Ethical Principles and Politics for Clinical Research on HIV/AIDS," *IRB: Rev. Hum. Subjects Res.* 13 (1991): 1–17.

18 B. R. Cassileth, E. J. Lusk, D. S. Miller, and S. Hurwitz, "Attitudes Toward Clinical Trials Among Patients and the Public," *Journal of the American Medical Association* 248 (1982): 968–970.

19 W. Lawrence, "The Impact of Clinical Trial Protocols on Patient Care Systems," *Cancer* 72, suppl. (1993): 2839–2841.

20 H. P. Freeman, "The Impact of Clinical Trial Protocols on Patient Care Systems in a Large City Hospital," *Cancer* 72, suppl. (1993): 2834–2838.

21 E. Eng, "Save Our Sisters Project," *Cancer* 72, suppl. (1993): 1071–1075.

22 Early Breast Cancer Trialists' Collaborative Group, "Systemic Treatment of Early Breast Cancer by Hormonal, Cytotoxic, or Immune Therapy," *Lancet* 339 (1992): 71–85.

23 H. Cunningham, *Re: Tamoxifen. Citizen Petition to FDA*, Doc. No. 93P-0356/CP1, 1993 (filed Sept. 18, 1993).

24 M. E. Costanza, ed., "Breast Cancer Screening in Older Women," *Journal of Gerontology* (1992): 47.

25 E. M. Antman, J. Lau, B. Kupelnick, F. Mosteller, and T. C. Chalmers, "A Comparison of Results of Meta-analyses of Randomized Control Trials and Recommendations of Clinical Experts," *Journal of the American Medical Association* 268 (1992): 240–248.

26 E. Eckholm, "$89 Million Awarded Family Who Sued HMO," *New York Times*, December 30, 1993, p. A1, A12.

27 G. Kolata, "Women Resist Trials to Test Marrow Transplants," *New York Times*, February 15, 1995, p. C8.

Moving from the Periphery

4

THE WOMEN'S HEALTH MOVEMENT IN THE UNITED STATES

Judy Norsigian

Introduction

The Women's Health Movement (WHM) in the United States had its origins in the late 1960s when women's groups, health and medical providers, and others organized a nationwide effort to legalize abortion. Many of these groups subsequently took up other health issues. Some established women-controlled health centers, some produced women's health publications[1] and educational materials, and others carried out a number of women's health advocacy projects, often with the goal of changing public policies affecting women's health.[2]

Nationally, the WHM found a unified voice with the establishment of the Washington, D.C.–based National Women's Health Network in 1976. The Network emphasized federal health policy, which, up to that point, had had little or no feminist consumer input; collaborated with progressive health and medical professionals; and increased contact with members of the media. The Network is now a powerful and credible presence among members of Congress, administrators in key federal agencies, and other important policymakers and has had, for example, major input in the decisions by the Food and Drug Administration to label various drugs and devices used by women.

Early groups in the WHM were primarily white and middle-class in their composition and orientation, although they sometimes addressed the concerns of poorer women and women of color. During the 1980s, many women of color created both local and national organizations[3] to focus more intensively on their priority issues. Women with disabilities, older women, overweight women, and lesbians also organized to form new groups,[4] as well as to raise specific issues within existing women's health groups. This growing diversity of individuals and organizations generated new tensions and conflicting analyses of the same problems, although the general environment has been one where many values and goals are held in common. Differential access to financial resources has at times caused resentment, making it more difficult for many to participate in cooperative ventures.

During the last decade the WHM has been trying to influence the national health care reform debate. Whether *all* women's health and medical needs will be better met under a new national health plan remains to be seen.

The Need for a Women's Health Movement

Health and medical care has been an area of great importance to women in the United States for many reasons. First, women are the major users of health and medical services, seeking care for themselves even when essentially healthy (for example, for birth control, pregnancy and childbearing, and menopausal discomforts). Because women live longer than men, they have more problems with chronic diseases and functional impairment, and thus require more home-based services as well.[5]

Second, women are frequently the "health brokers" for the family, arranging care for children, spouses, or relatives; they are also the major caregivers for those around them. Third, women represent the great majority of health workers; 85 percent in the hospital setting and 75 percent overall. Also, 69 percent of all health care workers are people of color. However, only 20 percent of physicians are women — up from about 10 percent two decades ago[6] — and women still have a relatively small role in policy setting in all arenas.[7] This is especially true in medical schools, where women represent less than 10 percent of all tenured faculty.[8]

Fourth, in most medical institutions women have faced discrimination on the basis of sex, class, race, age, and disability, and have experienced condescending, paternalistic, and culturally insensitive treatment.[9] Certain groups of women (older women, women of color, fat women, women with disabilities, and lesbians) routinely confront discriminatory attitudes and practices and even outright abuse.[10]

Fifth, it is usually difficult for women to obtain good health and medical information, especially for nonconventional forms of treatment, to ensure informed decision making.[11] This problem is intensified for low-income women and those who do not speak English, in part because their class, race, and culture are often markedly different from those of their health care providers.

Sixth, women have been subjected to inappropriate medical interventions such as unnecessary cesarean sections, unnecessary hysterectomies, and overmedication with psychotropic drugs (especially tranquilizers and antidepressants).[12] Inadequate technology assessment is partially responsible for this inappropriate and sometimes dangerous use of medical technologies.

And finally, the health and medical care system has failed to recognize the importance of preventive and routine care and has been generally unwilling to evaluate and incorporate effective nonallopathic treatments. For women, many of whose unique health and medical problems do respond to preventive and nonallopathic approaches, this failure has special consequences.

The Women's Health Movement during the 1970s and 1980s

Much of the activity of the early WHM focused on basic education and sharing of information and experiences about health and sexuality, often in a small group setting. *Our Bodies, Ourselves,* for example, which became one of the most popular books about women's health, emerged out of an unmet need to demystify medical care and redefine and reclaim female sexuality. The first edition, a 112-page, newsprint book published by the New England Free Press in late 1970, resulted from meetings and informal "courses" organized by women who met at a women's liberation conference in the spring of 1969. The phenomenal success of this "underground" publication (over 250,000 copies were sold, mainly by word of mouth, until commercial publication in 1973) demonstrated women's profound need for clear, comprehensive information about their bodies as well as about health and medical care.

Collective ignorance about the most elemental aspects of anatomy, physiology, and reproduction, coupled with the growing anger of many women about frequent mistreatment by a mostly white, privileged, and male medical profession, helped to spark numerous initiatives, from self-help groups to women-controlled health centers. Women taught one another how to perform cervical self-examinations, shared information about self-help treatments for vaginal infections, established advocacy groups that sought to make medical institutions and professionals more responsive to their needs, joined local health planning boards, and even became involved in the training of medical students (for example, the teaching of pelvic exams).[13]

Critiques of medicine as an institution of social control over women[14] emerged alongside analyses exposing problems such as racism, classism, sexism, ageism, ableism, and homophobia. Women also protested the emphasis on pathology and treatment versus prevention. Some argued that this led to the overmedicalization of women's lives, which turned normal events such as childbearing and menopause into necessarily disabling conditions requiring routine medical intervention.

As part of the solution to these myriad problems, women's health advocates sought to increase the decision-making power of women at all levels by working to place women in policy-making positions in medical institutions, educational settings, legislatures and local governing bodies, and relevant governmental agencies. Medical schools have seen little improvement over the past two decades, but there have been more female legislators and hospital administrators, two female Surgeons General,[15] and the first female director at the National Institutes of Health.[16] Even President Clinton's major effort to bring about health care reform in the early 1990s was headed by a woman — Hillary Rodham Clinton. Having women in influential positions does not necessarily change health and medical institutions, especially when powerful corporate interests are at stake, but it has lent legitimacy to raising the special concerns of women.

Many women's health activists have argued that the language of the WHM has been co-opted by larger institutions that remain generally unresponsive to women's needs. They argue that most women directly affected by particular problems still do not have an adequate voice in the organizations and institutions dealing with those problems.

Activists urge that initiatives and programs designed to address particular problems — such as high infant mortality rates or high rates of HIV infection among women in a given community — involve women from that community, including women experiencing these very problems. At a conference on women's health research, sponsored by the National Institutes of Health, activists succeeded in garnering support for a recommendation that committees reviewing breast cancer research proposals include lay women who themselves have or have had breast cancer.[17] Programs or policies that foster "empowerment," a term often used to describe this kind of involvement in problem solving, are still few and far between, especially in low-income communities and communities of color.

In addition to particular health issues such as contraception, abortion, cancer, gynecological problems, childbearing, and menopause, the WHM has recognized other factors central to overall health and well-being: safer, cleaner, less stressful living and working environments; adequate food and housing for all; reduced violence against women, recognizing that such violence contributes substantially to women's health and medical problems; and a national health program that would guarantee everyone access to needed care.[18] Making sure that the many links among these issues are repeatedly articulated remains a high priority.

Accomplishments of the Women's Health Movement

The successes have been many and varied. In the early 1970s, lack of information about birth control pills[19] and a growing awareness among women about problems associated with their use, led to organized protests, including disruption of special hearings in Congress conducted by Senator Gaylord Nelson. Fortuitously, Barbara Seaman, author of *The Doctor's Case Against the Pill*, and Alice Wolfson met at the Nelson hearings; several years later they cofounded the National Women's Health Network with Dr. Mary Howell, Belita Cowan, and Phyllis Chesler.

One important result of women's efforts to obtain more and better information about oral contraceptives (as well as other drugs) was the introduction of the Patient Package Insert (PPI) program by the Food and Drug Administration (FDA). The PPI, a very detailed summary of known problems and contraindications associated with a particular drug, provided women with important information, albeit in a dense, difficult-to-read format. Although a planned expansion of this program to other widely used drugs was subsequently eliminated during the Reagan administration, the Clinton administration resumed the program.[20]

A related struggle involved the provision of PPIs for so-called estrogen-replacement-therapy hormones. Not long after PPIs appeared for estrogen products, the Pharmaceutical Manufacturers Association (PMA), joined by the American College of Obstetricians and Gynecologists (ACOG), sued the FDA in an effort to block the distribution of PPIs for estrogen products. In response, four women's and consumer organizations, led by the National Women's Health Network (NWHN), entered the case as codefendants and filed an amicus brief cogently arguing for the right to such basic information. And we won. PPIs for estrogen products were retained.

Although difficult to prove, it is likely that pressure from the WHM played a significant role in increasing the number of nurse practitioners who provide primary care services for women. Many women's health activists believe that the greater likelihood of being cared for by a nurse practitioner or nurse-midwife often has improved the quality of care experienced by many women.[21]

Sterilization abuse, a long-standing problem for poor women in the United States, became the focus of a government inquiry after activists, journalists, and community organizations documented and publicized the degree to which certain women, especially women of color and Native American women, were sterilized without informed consent.[22] This happened in a variety of ways: some women agreed to be sterilized without fully understanding what it meant, especially when information was given in terminology they did not understand; others were told that their public welfare benefits would be denied unless they agreed to sterilization; and some were told that the procedure was reversible, when, of course, that was not true.

Special hearings[23] resulted in regulations designed to curb the incidence of abuse among federally funded sterilizations. These regulations included a thirty-day waiting period, the provision of information in a language clearly understood by the woman, and prohibition of the use of hysterectomy solely for the purpose of sterilization. Though far from a perfect solution, these regulations have been somewhat effective.

Ironically, with the exception of a handful of states in the United States, low-income women who are on Medicaid can obtain a federally funded sterilization but *not* a federally funded abortion. This limitation has led some women to "choose" sterilization because they have so few options. As the WHM continues to emphasize, without access to *all* reproductive health services, there can be no real choice in matters of childbearing.

During the 1970s, women-controlled health centers emerged as an alternative to the conventional delivery of health and medical care. Many were organized in a nonhierarchical fashion, with physicians having little or no policy-making roles. Most offered self-help groups that taught cervical self-exams, abortion services that were often the only ones in the region, and support groups for dealing with experiences such as premenstrual problems, infertility, and menopause. They also pioneered a more thorough, client-centered approach to informed consent. Because of these women-controlled health centers, abortion services became firmly entrenched as outpatient health services. In 1992 only 7 percent of abortions were performed in hospitals, whereas in 1973 more than half of all abortions had been performed in hospitals.[24] This assured that first-trimester abortions in this country would be appropriately demedicalized. (In contrast, European countries have adhered to a more medical, hospital-based approach.)

Unfortunately, relatively few of these centers have survived, especially in the face of competition from imitative facilities run by hospitals.[25] Some continue to offer an important model of how to provide responsive care in a politically conscious fashion. Several produce outstanding newsletters that are distributed nationally.

As early as the mid-1970s the WHM addressed controversies surrounding breast cancer. For many years the standard practice of American doctors, upon doing a breast biopsy and finding malignant tissue, was to proceed immediately with a mastectomy. Several years of hard work during the 1970s, especially on the part of activist and journalist Rose Kushner, who has since died from the disease, resulted in a landmark recommendation by the National Cancer Institute that in most cases breast biopsies should be performed as part of a two-step procedure. The panel advised that a diagnostic biopsy specimen be studied with permanent histologic sections before various treatment options are discussed. This represented an important step forward in the treatment of breast cancer, and also increased general awareness of the importance of nonsurgical treatments.

In the early 1980s, the WHM publicized the early results of clinical trials as, for example, in instances where lumpectomies represented an improved approach over more radical forms of surgery. Activists also challenged the overuse and misuse of chemotherapy.[26] By the late 1980s, WHM activists and other women with breast cancer founded the first of many grassroots women's cancer groups that challenged the failure of the breast cancer establishment to adequately address causation and prevention of breast cancer.[27] In the early 1990s, many of these groups formed the National Breast Cancer Coalition, which has continued to press for laywomen's involvement in breast cancer policy setting at all levels.[28]

Challenges for the 1990s and Beyond

If one protests long and loudly enough, even the United States Congress will eventually take note. Starting several years ago, a package of bills known as the Women's Health Equity Act has been introduced in Congress due to the leadership of several senior female members of

Congress, including Barbara Mikulski, Patricia Schroeder, Mary Rose Oakar, and Olympia Snowe. The current package of twenty-five bills addresses research, services, and prevention in such areas as breast and ovarian cancer, sexually transmitted diseases (STDs), contraceptive research, infertility, osteoporosis, and adolescent pregnancy. Many activists hope to see more positive action in prevention and early intervention.

However, congressional attention can result in federal action even without legislation. For example, in 1993 Senator Barbara Mikulski chaired a hearing on the continued problem of unnecessary hysterectomies. This has led to federal funding for studies of the effectiveness of, and alternative approaches to, hysterectomy. In addition to these legislative efforts, the National Institutes of Health launched an ambitious new Women's Health Initiative, which will result in the allocation of $600 million during the next decade to research on heart disease, osteoporosis, and breast cancer.[29] Most women's health activists are pleased with the Initiative because it will address pressing questions unanswered by currently available data: Does the regular and prolonged use of hormones beginning at menopause increase the risk of breast cancer? Does combined hormone therapy (progestins *plus* estrogen) reduce the loss of bone mass, as estrogen alone does? Does hormone therapy prevent heart disease, especially in women for whom no special risk factors are apparent?

However, many activists remain frustrated by the underfunding of key areas of research. For example, the National Cancer Institute has not adequately funded any studies of environmental factors that affect breast cancer risk, especially organochlorines. This is despite mounting evidence implicating environmental carcinogens as a cause of several cancers, including breast cancer.[30] Ironically, the National Cancer Institute's major recent contribution to breast cancer prevention research was a study of tamoxifen, a fairly potent drug with some significant risks and side effects.[31] Activists have criticized this clinical trial as a study in "disease substitution" rather than disease prevention.[32]

On the positive side, consumer health activists now have a slightly greater role in discussions at the National Institutes of Health. Whether we will be able to influence the NIH research agenda will be one of the major challenges during the coming years.

Contraceptive vaccine research represents another thorny issue for the WHM. Many women's health advocates believe that the potential problems associated with vaccine research[33] do not justify forging ahead in this area. They point to the potential for abuse, because there exists no antidote or means of short-term reversibility. Even where fully informed women choose the vaccine, there is the possibility that they can develop autoimmune disorders *after* getting the vaccine.

Instead of more vaccine research, many women's health activists urge that contraceptive research priorities be reordered. They advocate placing greater emphasis upon female-controlled barrier methods of contraception, especially in an era where STDs (especially AIDS and HIV infection) are epidemic. They have welcomed, for example, the development of the female condom, improved male condoms, and new types of diaphragms and cervical caps.[34] Beginning in 1989, health activists campaigned successfully to convince the FDA to eliminate unnecessary testing requirements for barrier methods of contraception.[35]

Over the past decade several organizations — including the World Health Organization, the Population Council, and the International Women's Health Coalition — have attempted to foster greater mutual understanding among women's health advocates, scientists, and funders by setting up opportunities for discussion in relatively informal settings.[36] Whether the WHM will sway funders and researchers sufficiently to alter current trends in contraceptive development remains to be seen.

Norplant, in the United States, has generated more controversy than any other birth control method during the past few years. The National Black Women's Health Project, one of several national women's health organizations that has opposed the FDA approval of Norplant, has characterized "Norplant and Teens" as a "Dangerous Combination."[37] Although many women have welcomed this long-acting method, others have emphasized its problems.[38] In 1994 a coalition of groups, including women-of-color, reproductive rights groups, asked the FDA to require manufacturers of long-acting contraceptives to include written consent forms with these products.[39]

A recent concern of the global women's health movement has been the growing trend, especially among environmental groups, to label population growth as a primary cause of environmental degradation. Activists fear that this trend could lead to more overzealous family-planning programs,[40] driven by demographic goals rather than women's reproductive health needs. The result might well be more cases of sterilization abuse or systematic disregard for women's decisions to discontinue long-acting contraceptive methods, like Norplant, that require provider assistance for removal.

Recently, activists have protested the unethical and growing use of quinacrine, a sclerosing agent, as a means of nonsurgical sterilization in countries such as Indonesia, India, Pakistan, and Vietnam.[41] Many women's health advocates point out that provider-dependent methods, such as injectables and implants offer special opportunities for misuse, as when a provider will not remove an implant upon a woman's request. These methods are inappropriate where women's rights to decent treatment are not recognized.

To ensure that women's voices would be a significant presence at the 1994 World Conference on Population held in Cairo, Egypt, numerous coalitions and meetings organized to articulate a women-centered position on the subject of population.[42] Some feminists believe that a "feminist population policy" is an oxymoron, while others argue that population policies might strengthen women's reproductive rights, if such policies emphasize good-quality family-planning services that respect women's rights.

Childbirth represents a continuing problematic area for the WHM. In general, childbirth remains a highly medicalized experience for most women, when it could and should be an essentially normal event requiring little or no intervention beyond basic forms of human support and caregiving. Although there certainly has been progress over the last twenty to thirty years, attempts to expand midwifery options or to increase the number of out-of-hospital birthing centers remain quite controversial. The cesarean section rates in the United States, averaging one in four births nationwide, remain inexcusably high.

For a number of reasons, including the litigious climate in the United States, there has been very little change in the nature of obstetrical training. In some areas we have lost ground. For example, access to home and birth center alternatives has been curtailed or limited through restrictions in health insurance or HMO coverage, withdrawal of malpractice insurance for providers, or lack of trained personnel.

One important effort to shape the future debate about childbirth in the United States, and to establish the central importance of the midwifery model of care, is a landmark document entitled *Childbearing Policy Within a National Health Program: An Evolving Consensus for New Directions*.[43] This document, a collaborative effort of the Boston Women's Health Book Collective, National Black Women's Health Project, National Women's Health Network, and the Women's Institute for Childbearing Policy, provides a complete discussion of the benefits of midwifery care in a primary care model. It stands as an outstanding recent contribution of the Women's Health Movement.

Abortion and reproductive rights remain centerpiece WHM concerns. Pro-choice groups are extremely well-organized and are attracting young women and men to their ranks. Advocates for reproductive rights have learned that a multifaceted approach is crucial to securing accomplishments and making further progress. Political pressure must be maintained on elected officials; the courts must be used as an arena for setting policy and to educate the public about the real consequences of both proposed and actual public policies; and advocates must be able to participate more fully in the regulatory process. Possibly most important of all, we need to ensure adequate numbers of trained abortion providers, so that a legal right does not become meaningless in the face of dwindling abortion services.[44] The increasing violence and lethal attacks on abortion clinics will make it all the harder to attract clinic staff in many communities.

The current AIDS epidemic has raised a new set of difficult issues. What happens to a woman's right to anonymous Human Immunodeficiency Virus (HIV) testing as HIV infection rates soar and increasing numbers of babies are born with HIV infection? If women seek treatment through government-funded entitlement programs, must we then risk the discriminatory treatment that seems inevitably to accompany disclosure of HIV infection and AIDS?

Other difficult questions remain with us as well. As fetal rights continue to be juxtaposed in opposition to women's rights, what will happen to women who use legal and illegal drugs during pregnancy, or who refuse the advice of doctor-recommended C-sections, or who want to work in settings that may involve exposure to reproductive health hazards? There are already cases of court-ordered cesarean sections, discriminatory workplace policies that have been upheld in some of our courtrooms, and child-abuse convictions of women who were substance-dependent and became pregnant.[45]

One might see all these punitive measures as the inevitable corollary to advances in reproductive technology. Or they might be viewed as a backlash to the gains of the women's movement over the past two decades. Increased participation of women in the public policy arena has aided efforts to hold back this tide. There is still a long way to go to ensure that less privileged women, women without degrees and professional backgrounds, have access to information, education, and the decision-making arenas that profoundly affect their lives.

Another area of difficulty involves determining when a technology or treatment in its research phases ought to gain legitimacy as bona fide "safe and effective" treatment warranting widespread use.[46] Some advocates argue that these technologies, especially those affecting reproduction, expand women's choices, while others emphasize their potential for exploitation and their tendency to elevate the rights and status of men and fetuses while reducing women to baby carriers with fewer and fewer rights.[47]

The WHM must also acknowledge the difficulties they have had in forging a truly multiracial and multicultural effort. While coalition efforts among groups predominantly comprised of women of color and those predominantly comprised of white women have often resulted in comprehensive, coordinated efforts on certain issues, most of these organizations do not work together on a daily basis.

In order to enhance diversity within and between organizations, many white women with long histories of working on particular issues or with particular organizations have had to give up some power. This has often been difficult. While both the Board and staff of the National Women's Health Network, for example, are much more diverse (half of the Board are women of color), it took a long time and generated substantial conflict.

In addition, priority issues for some women-of-color groups have on occasion come in conflict with priority issues of more mainstream organizations. Thus, in the late 1970s, a collaborative effort among several grassroots and women's health organizations led to the development of sterilization abuse regulations, but that effort drew initial opposition from the National Organization for Women, which opposed the thirty-day waiting period contained within the regulations as violative of the rights of those women seeking immediate sterilization.

As part of the larger women's movement, which has yet to find better ways of sharing power and resources among the many women's organizations that claim to hold values and goals in common, the WHM faces an extraordinary challenge to strengthen ties among the various organizations working under its umbrella. Leadership exercised by women-of-color organizations, such as the National Black Women's Health Project, has offered a unique opportunity for larger, white-dominated women's groups to demonstrate their support and commitment to broader causes not initially defined by white women.

Women's organizations frequently have difficulty achieving greater ethnic and racial diversity. Some of these problems result from the inevitable growing pains that face all organizations as they evolve and mature. Stephanie Riger has described, for example, a "founders trap," which is the "reluctance of founders to institutionalize leadership by establishing procedures and policies which do not require their personal judgment."[48] In cases where founders have been primarily white women, this resistance serves to reinforce elements of structural racism. Conflicts between staff and boards, often dominated by those who founded a particular organization, frequently develop because of varying expectations or levels of commitment to a particular issue or set of issues.

Issues such as an adequate salary schedule or accommodation to the realities of single motherhood may become as important or more important than the particular mission of an organization. These issues, along with differences due to age or experience levels, may reflect or appear to reflect racial and cultural differences. Women's health organizations must be prepared to deal with these concerns; failure to address them adequately may prevent many women's health groups from achieving or maintaining diversity within their organizations.

Understanding how race and class affect the organizational development process is a central challenge facing the WHM. Many WHM groups have relied to a great extent upon a "self-help" model as a principal organizing vehicle. This approach involves organizing around issues that are closest to one's own experience. Thus, women whose mothers have died of breast cancer might take on the issue of funding for breast cancer research over some other causes, such as women in prison or the mental health system or women immigrants. Unfortunately, women in these latter groups usually lack the resources needed to initiate and sustain a self-help project without considerable outside assistance.

This problem is exacerbated by the media's distortion of women's health concerns. The mainstream media are increasingly controlled by a very small monopoly, and many pressing concerns, as described by Ben Bagdikian in *Media Monopoly*, simply do not get a platform. Thus, stories about breast self-exam or mammography abound, while the role of the environment in breast cancer causation is rarely mentioned. These distortions make it harder for women's health advocates to forge solutions and to obtain public support and appreciation for the full complexity of the issues facing women.

The Health Care Reform Debate and Women

For many activists, the health care reform debate, prompted by the election of President Clinton, poses the most significant challenges facing women. Not until the early 1990s were women's voices given even minimal consideration. Now at least a dozen women's groups and coalitions have developed principles against which they measure any health care reform proposals.

Some groups, like the Washington, D.C.–based Campaign for Women's Health, have developed a "model benefits package," which includes services frequently excluded from conventional insurance policies and HMOs. In March 1994 the Massachusetts Women's Health Care Coalition issued a statement, supported by more than fifty organizations, that included a set of basic principles as well as a specific critique of President Clinton's Health Plan.[49] The Coalition will measure any future reform effort based on the following principles:[50]

Universality: Health care should be everyone's right. It should go beyond medical coverage to include outreach and education that will ensure that all people know how to obtain care.

Equality: Benefits should be standard and broad, offering the same quality of care to all. Low-income people should not experience barriers that limit access (such as unaffordable premiums and payments at the doctor's office). It is essential to eliminate the current multitiered system.

Diversity: People should be able to choose culturally and linguistically appropriate care, non-Western methods of treatment, and community-based providers. Governing bodies should reflect the diversity of the population served.

Social responsibility: Health is not just an individual, personal problem but the responsibility of the community and the government. Health services are more similar to fire or police services than to restaurants or car dealerships.

Many elements of President Clinton's proposal, which foundered in late 1994, represented positive and important advances for women. These included the promise of universal coverage; an expanded standard benefits package, which included free prenatal care and regularly scheduled preventive and early detection services for women, including mammography, prescription drugs, birth control and abortion; and broader mental health and substance abuse benefits.

However, Clinton's plan was inadequate in several key respects. For example, its reliance upon a premium-based payment system was inherently regressive. A woman with children earning $20,000 a year as a secretary would have paid the same 20 percent share of the family premium as her $55,000-a-year boss. It is critical that any national health program include a percent-of-income cap on premiums and all out-of-pocket expenses. Also, several million undocumented women and their families would have lost coverage and had no access to anything other than emergency care. The lack of a sliding scale in subsidies was another deficiency of the plan.

Additionally, required co-payments and deductibles in the Clinton plan would have actively impaired women's access to health care. A well-respected study by the Rand Corporation has shown that while co-payments do discourage provider visits, they do not distinguish between necessary and unnecessary care. The inclusion of co-payments in any reform proposal ignores the reality of many women's lives and the true driving forces behind spiraling costs. What really drives up costs are unnecessary procedures ordered by doctors (worth an estimated $200 billion per year in excess medical costs); inappropriate distribution of high-technology; out-of-control capital spending; and expensive marketing and administration. Lastly, the Clinton plan — like other proposals — offered no plan for adequate consumer control over services.

Women's health advocates must continue to address these types of concerns in their critiques of future health care reform effort.

Conclusion

As the WHM moves into the next century, the ability to build broad coalitions will, to a large extent, determine the political effectiveness of women's health care advocates. The emergence of "single-issue" organizations, such as the Endometriosis Association and the Interstitial Cystitis Association, may make it harder to keep the broader feminist context in focus. The WHM's success in influencing national health care reform during the 1990s and beyond will depend upon effective collaboration and networking among many diverse organizations.

Although the WHM has had a significant impact on the consciousness of many, most medical institutions remain largely unchanged. Many of the inequities that stirred feminists to action in the early 1970s continue to exist. Poverty, the single most important factor affecting health and well-being, continues to affect a growing percentage of the population. Violence persists as a major cause of disability and death among women. Amidst worsening statistics, it will take patience, stubborn persistence, and a good sense of humor to sustain a movement that has had much to be proud of.

Notes

1   For example, see *HealthRight* (New York: Women's Health Forum, 1974–1979), *WomenWise* (Concord, N.H.: New Hampshire Feminist Health Center), and the *Santa Cruz [Calif.] Women's Health Center Newsletter* (Santa Cruz: Santa Cruz Women's Health Center).

2   For an extended discussion of what has happened to many of these groups, see "Women's Health Movement Organizations: Two Decades of Struggle and Change," a report by Sandra Morgen and Alice Julier, 1991. Copies available from Sandra Morgen, Center for the Study of Women in Society, Prince Lucien Campbell Hall, University of Oregon, Eugene, OR 97403.

3   For example, these organizations include the National Black Women's Health Project (Atlanta, Ga.), the National Latina Health Organization (Oakland, Calif.), the Native American Health Education Resource Center (Lake Andes, S.D.), and the National Women of Color Reproductive Health Coalition.

4   For example, the Project on Women and Disability (Boston, Mass.), Lyon-Martin Women's Health Center (San Francisco, Calif.), and *Radiance: A Publication for Large Women* (Oakland, Calif.: Radiance Enterprises).

5   See Jo-Ann Lamphere Thorpe and Robert J. Blendon, *The Impact of Population Aging on Women* (Southport, Conn.: Southport Institute for Policy Analysis, 1991).

6   Teresa M. Rackauckas, "Women in Medicine: Numbers Growing, Roles Changing," *American Medical News*, November 9, 1992, 40–41.

7   Ibid.; *Empowering Women in Medicine*, Report of the Feminist Majority Foundation and American Women's Medical Association (AMWA) (Washington, D.C.: AMWA, 1991); Kim Painter, "Female M.D.'s Lack Fair Share of Power," *USA Today*, September 10, 1991.

8   American Women's Medical Association, Testimony before the Office of Research on Women's Health, National Institutes of Health, March 23, 1992.

9   Sue Fisher, *In the Patient's Best Interest* (New Brunswick, N.J.: Rutgers University Press, 1986); Ellen Lewin and Virginia Olesen, eds., *Women's Health and Healing: Towards a New Perspective* (New York: Tavistock, 1985).

10   Evelyn C. White, ed., *The Black Women's Health Book: Speaking for Ourselves* (Seattle: Seal, 1990).

11   Alexandra Dundas-Todd, *Intimate Adversaries: Cultural Conflict Between Doctors and Women Patients* (Philadelphia: University of Pennsylvania Press, 1989); *The New Our Bodies, Ourselves* (New York: Simon and Shuster, 1992).

12   Diana Scully, *Men Who Control Women's Health: The Miseducation of Obstetricians-Gynecologists* (Boston: Houghton Mifflin, 1980).

13   See Susan Bell, "Political Gynecology: Gynecological Imperialism and the Politics of Self-Help," *Science for the People* 11, no. 5 (1979): 8–14.

14   See Gena Corea's classic book *The Hidden Malpractice: How American Medicine Mistreats Women* (New York: Harper and Row, 1985), and Diana Scully's *Men Who Control Women's Health, supra* note 12.

15   Dr. Antonia Novello and Dr. Joycelyn Elders, who was forced to resign in late 1994 because of her outspokenness on the importance of sexuality education and access to contraception for teens.

16   Dr. Bernadine Healey, who left her position in the summer of 1993.

17   See "Breast Cancer: A National Strategy/A Report to the Nation," by the President's Cancer Panel/Special Commission on Breast Cancer, NIH, October 1993, p. 3. This same subject arose earlier at the Workshop on Opportunities for Research on Women's Health, sponsored by the Office of Research on Women's Health, September 1991, Huntsville, Md.

18   Currently, the United States and South Africa remain the only industrialized countries without such programs, a scandal that this country continues to tolerate.

19   At that time, birth control pills contained much more estrogen (and carried greater risks) than the current low-dose estrogen pill.

20   See "The Phoenix Rises: Patient Package Inserts Reborn," *Network News* [newsletter of the National Women's Health Network], 19, no. 6 (November/December, 1994): 4.

21   Cynthia Pearson, Program Director, National Women's Health Network, personal communication, February 1995.

22   Allan Chase, "American Indian Women Not Fully Informed FAO Study Finds," *Medical Tribune*, August 10, 1977, 1, 6; Allan Chase, "Passing the Word on Sterilization 1933–1977," *Medical Tribune*, September 21, 1977, p. 1.

23   The hearings were held before the Department of Health, Education and Welfare during 1978; a federal hearing was conducted on January 17, 1978, and accompanied by numerous regional hearings.

24   Stanley K. Henshaw and Jennifer Van Vort, "Abortion Services in the United States, 1991 and 1992," *Family Planning Perspectives* 26, no. 3 (May/June 1994): 112.

25   Interestingly, in a country like Australia, where services are largely state supported, public funding has ensured the continued existence of women's health centers. Women in Melbourne even succeeded in obtaining approximately $400,000 from the Victorian government to start a women's health information center. The women's health movement in Australia is in many respects stronger than its American counterpart because of its ability to influence government expenditures and create a more stable financial base for women-directed services and advocacy.

26   See Susan Rennie, "Breast Cancer: The Latest Conference Results," *Network News* 10, no. 6 (November/December 1985): 3.

27   See Susan Ferraro, "The Anguished Politics of Breast Cancer," *New York Times Magazine*, August 15, 1993, 25; Monte Paulsen, "The Profits of Misery/Breast Cancer and the Environment: How the Chemical Industry Profits from an Epidemic It May Be Causing," *Detroit Metro Times*, May 19–25, 1993, 12; " The Politics of Breast Cancer," *Ms.*, May/June 1993, 37–60.

28   See "The Politics of Breast Cancer," *Science* 259 (January 29, 1993): 616–617.

29   It should be noted that this project was funded during the tenure of the first female director of NIH, Dr. Bernadine Healy. Dr. Healy is now editor of the *Journal of Women's Health*, which receives substantial funding from the pharmaceutical industry.

30   See Paulsen, "The Profits of Misery," *supra* note 27, a series that ran in the *Detroit Metro Times* in May 1993. Is it a coincidence that Imperial Chemical Industries (ICI), a major producer of pesticides (which contain organochlorines), paid for the educational materials used for National Breast Cancer Awareness Month during a year when *no* mention of the environment appeared on the posters and pamphlets distributed?

31   Tamoxifen has been most notable for its success in the treatment of estrogen-dependent breast cancer in postmenopausal women.

32   See Adrienne Fugh-Berman and Samuel Epstein, "Tamoxifen: Disease Prevention or Disease Substitution," *Lancet* 340 (November 7, 1992): 1143–1145.

33   In 1993, women's health advocates meeting at a European conference began a campaign to halt contraceptive vaccine research and to reallocate research funds to support more female-controlled barrier methods. Their reasons included: abuse potential; the belief that manipulation of the immune system for contraceptive purposes is unlikely ever to be harmless and involves many potential risks, such as induction of autoimmune diseases and immune disturbances; and a high risk of fetal exposure to ongoing immune reactions. For a complete copy of the campaign statement, contact the Women's Global Network for Reproductive Rights in Amsterdam or send a SASE to the Boston Women's Health Book Collective, P.O. Box 192, West Somerville, MA 02144.

34   The REALITY female condom became available in the U.S. in late 1993. Two types of cervical caps, the FemCap and Lea's Shield, continue to undergo clinical trials, while a Brazilian feminist who has developed a unique silicone diaphragm (which doesn't produce an off-odor, as rubber does) pursues possible distribution of this diaphragm in the United States and elsewhere.

35   See FDA, "Guidelines for Premarket Testing of Women-controlled Contraceptives which Prevent STDs" (Rockville, Md., April 1990).

36   For a report of one such dialogue, see "Creating Common Ground: Women's Perspectives on the Selection and Introduction of Fertility Regulation Technologies" (Geneva, Switzerland: World Health Organization and International Women's Health Coalition, 1991).

37   See Julia R. Scott, "A Dangerous Combination: Norplant and Teens," *Vital Signs* [newsletter of the National Black Women's Health Project], no. 1 (January–March 1993): 30–31.

38   For a lengthy discussion of women's experiences with Norplant in several different countries, see Women and Pharmaceuticals Project of the Women's Health Action Foundation (WHAF), *Norplant: Under Her Skin* (Amsterdam: WHAF, 1993).

39   Cynthia Pearson, Program Director of the National Women's Health Network, personal communication February 1995.

40   The film *Something Like a War* graphically documents how, even today, family planning "motivators" in India have their salaries withheld if they do not bring in the requisite number of "cases" for sterilization. See also *Political Environments* 1 (Spring 1994), published by Committee on Women, Population and the Environment, c/o Population and Development Program, Hampshire College, P.O. Box 5001, Amherst, MA 01002.

41   See Marge Berer, "The Quinacrine Controversy One Year On," *Reproductive Health Matters* 4 (November 1994): 99–106.

42   Preparatory (prepcom) meetings in New York City, April 1993 and 1994; "Reproductive Health and Justice: International Women's Health Conference for Cairo '94" in Rio de Janeiro, January 1994; statement of the Committee on Women, Population and the Environment, signed by over 300 organizations and individuals around the globe.

43   This document was published in 1994 by the Women's Institute for Childbearing Policy. It is available from the Boston Women's Health Book Collective, P.O. Box 192, West Somerville, MA 02144.

44 See *Reproductive Rights Network Newsletter,* Summer 1993, for a complete discussion of the abortion-provider shortage. For more information on the Abortion Access Project of the Reproductive Rights Network, contact R2N, P.O. Box 686, Jamaica Plain, MA 02130.

45 See Kary Moss, "Substance Abuse during Pregnancy," *Harvard Women's Law Journal* 13 (spring 1990): 278–299. See also Wendy Chavkin et al., "Drug Abuse and Pregnancy: Some Questions on Public Policy, Clinical Management, and Maternal and Fetal Rights," *BIRTH* 18, no. 2 (June 1991): 107–112; and Wendy Chavkin, "Mandatory Treatment for Drug Use During Pregnancy," *Journal of the American Medical Association* 266, no. 11 (September 18, 1991): 1556–1561.

46 The case of in vitro fertilization (IVF) represents a good example. Several states have mandated third-party reimbursement for IVF, thus recognizing it as a nonexperimental, legitimate therapy, but some women's health advocates believe this has been an unfortunate development.

47 See "Special Report: Women as Wombs," *Ms.* 6, May/June 1991, 28–47. For example, the internal fetal heart monitor represents a case where a technology was introduced as the standard of care before adequate technology assessment was carried out. Now, after scientific assessment, considerable evidence challenges not only the routine use of electronic fetal heart monitoring but also its use in high-risk situations. Nonetheless, it will be a monumental task to change the prevailing medical practice. The consequences for both quality of care and costs are obviously substantial.

48 S. Riger, "Challenges of Success: Stages of Growth in Feminist Organization," *Feminist Studies* 20, no. 2 (summer 1994), 275–300.

49 For a complete copy of this statement, contact the Massachusetts Women's Health Care Coalition, c/o BWHBC, P.O. Box 192, West Somerville, MA 02144.

50 See Judy Norsigian, "Women and National Health Care Reform: A Progressive Feminist Agenda," in *Reframing Women's Health*, ed. Alice J. Dan (Thousand Oaks, Calif.: Sage, 1994), 111–117.

8

5

FOR WOMEN'S HEALTH

*Uncoupling Health Care Reform
from Tort Reform*

Joyce E. McConnell

Introduction

When President Clinton thrust health care reform into the vortex of the 1992 campaign, others demanded that tort reform be treated as indispensable to achieving universal health care. The growing public perception that the civil justice system generally, and the tort system specifically, is responsible for many of the problems in the current health care system, increasing health care costs and decreasing pharmaceutical availability, forced reformers to couple health reform of health care to tort reform. This effort linked the tort system, the law and procedure by which a person seeks compensation for injuries caused intentionally or negligently by another, to other social and legal changes characterizing the development of tort law.[1]

To support this position, politicians accused "greedy plaintiffs" and "avaricious lawyers" of stifling product development, bankrupting hospitals, and disillusioning physicians.[2] They did not reveal, however, that many of the so-called "greedy" plaintiffs were women who sued pharmaceutical companies and doctors to recover for reproductive and fetal harm. For behind the political cry to couple health care reform to tort reform are women who have suffered substantial injuries and who have turned to the tort system to be compensated for their injuries and to prevent other women from being injured by the same products and doctors.

Women must concern themselves with a health care reform strategy that links tort reform to health care reform. Proposals to trade new limitations on tort liability for universal health care coverage are key to this strategy. Some of these trade-offs may be worth it to women, others may not. Women must inform themselves about possible linked reform efforts as well as the potential impact of these efforts on women's health. To aid this process, this chapter sets forth the most common tort reform proposals linked directly to health care in a manner accessible to the widest possible audience and examines them with one question in mind:[3] How will the reforms affect women's health care?

To answer this question it is necessary to put the current political imperative to link tort reform to health care reform into recent historical context. The first section of this chapter does this by examining the convergence of events in the tort liability system in the late 1970s and 1980s to which the "crisis" is attributed.[4] Many of these involved women's health, particularly their reproductive health. Women's reproductive health was affected both by defective medical products, such as the Dalkon Shield and diethylstilbestrol (DES), as well as by inadequate gynecological and obstetrical care. These correspond to the two areas of tort law most often targeted for reform: products liability and medical malpractice. Consequently, the remaining sections of the chapter analyze various proposals to reform liability for defective products or negligent medical care. Sometimes these proposals affect only one or the other. Often, however, they affect both. Reform proposals that cut across tort liability categories in this way suggest that linking tort reform to health care reform could have significant consequences for women who seek civil remedies for reproductive wrongs caused by defective medical products or medical malpractice.

What these consequences may be is very difficult to predict. This chapter explores four proposals typical to tort reform efforts and their possible consequences. Ultimately, however, it advises that there is insufficient information at this time to conclude that the reforms proposed will benefit women. The evidence reviewed here suggests the following: that the tort system serves an essential role as a last-resort arbiter of accountability; that despite this, it is a woefully inadequate and inefficient system; and that no current proposal includes an adequate alternative. Ultimately, I conclude that in the absence of alternative systems of accountability, the reform proposals should not be adopted.

Historical Background: The Myth of a Crisis

Cases that received media attention in the 1980s, the period most oft described as the prime of the "explosion" in liability and the peak of the "crisis,"[5] include lawsuits brought by thousands of women for reproductive harm caused by defective products. The two most famous are the suits against the manufacturers of diethylstilbestrol (DES)[6] and the manufacturer of the Dalkon Shield.[7]

DES was prescribed in the 1950s and 1960s as miscarriage-prevention medication for pregnant women.[8] When the daughters of these women reached adolescence, some of them developed adenocarcinoma, a deadly form of cervical and vaginal cancer, commonly referred to as clear cell carcinoma.[9] Their cancers and other reproductive injuries were found to have been caused by the DES prescribed for and taken by their mothers.[10] Later some of the sons of mothers who took DES developed testicular cancer and genital tract abnormalities. Many believe their cancers and abnormalities are also linked to their mothers' use of DES.[11] The DES-injured offspring brought thousands of lawsuits against the pharmaceutical manufacturers and alleged that the manufacturers had failed to test the drug adequately and were therefore liable for their injuries.

Another product widely used by women in the early 1970s to prevent pregnancy, the Dalkon Shield intrauterine device, became the subject of thousands of lawsuits. Shortly after its entry into the market, the manufacturer began receiving reports that the Dalkon Shield caused death, pelvic inflammatory disease, septic abortions, infertility, and other reproductive harms.[12] The first women to discover that they had been seriously injured by the Dalkon Shield sued their doctors for medical malpractice. They assumed that the product itself was fine, but that their doctors had inserted the Dalkon Shields negligently.[13] As soon as the women and their lawyers learned, however, of a large number of women suffering similar injuries from the Dalkon Shield, the lawsuits were brought against the manufacturer for producing a defective product and for failing to warn of its hazards as soon as the company learned of them.[14] So many women had been harmed by the time that the Dalkon Shield was removed from the market that the manufacturer filed for bankruptcy.[15] Injured women are now paid out of a trust fund established by the bankruptcy court.[16]

When such a large number of lawsuits are brought against a single defendant or defendants who engage in similar conduct, they are referred to as mass torts.[17] In the 1980s, mass torts, such as these affecting women and others like those filed against asbestos manufacturers and the manufacturers of the herbicide Agent Orange, fueled the perception of a tort liability crisis.[18]

At the same time that mass torts captured public attention, other alleged changes in the tort system fed the perception that the tort system was being abused by greedy lawyers and clients. Physicians openly attributed their disappointment with practicing medicine to the rise in lawsuits against them and increases in medical malpractice premiums. The medical practice hit the hardest was obstetrics. Obstetricians across the country claimed that they were driven from their obstetric practices due to the rise in lawsuits and increased insurance premiums. While the mass quality of individual medical malpractice lawsuits is not immediately apparent, physicians, their professional organizations, and the insurance industry regarded them as a phenomenon similar in size and significance to the other mass tort cases.[19]

With public attention focused on the tort system, reports of excessive jury verdicts and anecdotes about undeserving plaintiffs receiving compensation took on mythological power.[20] Critics of the tort system focused on the jury system.[21] They characterized juries as too sympathetic, anti–big business, distrustful of doctors, misled by unscrupulous plaintiffs' attorneys, duped by expert witnesses, and incapable of understanding the sophisticated and complex scientific, medical, and technological evidence of the contemporary lawsuit.[22] When mass torts, medical malpractice lawsuits, increased insurance premiums, excessive jury verdicts, and compensated but perhaps undeserving plaintiffs converged, the perception of a crisis in tort liability was born, and reform efforts were launched at the state and federal levels.[23]

These reform efforts, however, were targeted at a crisis created not by fact but by what law professor Michael J. Saks of the University of Iowa calls "anecdotes, assumptions and unsupported assertions."[24] While there is certainly not enough research on the tort liability system and the way in which it responds to economic and social pressures, there is some well-designed and respected research that demonstrates that there is no "crisis." This conclusion has been borne out in a number of studies of the problem.

For example, a recent study conducted by the Rand Corporation on the cost of accidents found that Americans suffered $175.9 billion in medical expenses and lost wages in a year, but received only $7.7 billion in compensation.[25] Thus, injured Americans are grossly undercompensated. Rather than there being a liability crisis, the cost of which is borne by the business and medical community, there is a crisis of uncompensated victims potentially dependent on public support.[26]

Other studies challenge widely held, yet paradoxical, assumptions. Take the assumption that there is rampant medical malpractice. A 1993 Harvard Study, commissioned by the New York State Legislature as part of a bargain over medical malpractice reform, reported that in the hospitals included in the study only about 1 percent of hospital patients each year are injured as a result of medical malpractice.[27] While this is a low rate, the 1 percent translates into 27,000 victims of malpractice a year. Half of the injuries were minor. Of those that were serious, about a quarter resulted in serious disability or death. The paradox is that while the real rate of malpractice is low, given the large numbers of patients treated, the number of those seriously injured (13,500) is high. Nationwide, 75,000 deaths each year result from medical malpractice.

The Harvard Study indicates some other interesting characteristics. Those who suffer the least serious injuries are more likely to sue and to receive several times their actual losses in compensation. In contrast, the most seriously injured are less likely to sue and ultimately receive far less than their losses.[28]

Even these seemingly large numbers of patients injured by medical malpractice do not result in a high rate of lawsuits. Only about 2 percent are pursued. Further, those who are harmed by malpractice rarely receive significant compensation. Finally, the compensation is generally considerably less than the financial loss. Only 35 percent of those lawsuits filed result in a settlement or judgment for the plaintiff. The remaining 65 percent are either lost or dropped. Of all medical malpractice claims only 15 to 20 percent result in trial.[29]

These figures force us to reconsider the claim that there exists a tort liability crisis and to see that the problems that do exist are complex and not necessarily to be remedied by tort reform. Some observers of the tort system believe that any "crisis" that exists was actually created by the insurance industry restructuring for higher profits.[30]

However created, real or unreal, the "crisis" has seized the American imagination. Calls for reform are now commonplace, not only from the business and medical community, but also from the average person who accepts its existence as a matter of faith, which cannot be rocked by validly conducted studies demonstrating the contrary.

Reform on the Horizon

Faith in the existence of the "crisis" has led to many reform efforts at both the state and federal levels.[31] Attempts at the state level have been very successful, predominately because the substantive and procedural laws governing medical malpractice and products liability generally are governed by state law.

Despite the fact that the state is the locus of these laws, the business, medical, and insurance communities have put pressure on the federal government to pass sweeping reforms that would apply uniformly to the states. Until the Republicans took control of both the United States House of Representatives and the Senate in the fall of 1994, however, there seemed little chance that federal tort reform legislation would succeed, out of federal respect for the right of the states to make their own decisions regarding tort liability and reform.

In the fall of 1994, however, the Republicans in their "Contract With America" made civil justice reform generally, and tort reform specifically, a cornerstone of their platform. Despite this, all attempts in both the House and Senate failed.[32] Their proposals were typical of past state and federal reform efforts. One would have made a party to a lawsuit who rejects an offer and either loses the lawsuit or receives a judgment for less than the offer, pay the opposing party's attorney's fees.[33] The other would have capped punitive damages in products liability lawsuits and permitted judges to sanction parties that bring allegedly frivolous lawsuits.[34]

Had these typical tort reforms passed, they would have impacted significantly on women seeking compensation for harm from defective products or medical malpractice. Take, for example, the early DES and Dalkon Shield cases, both of which were extremely risky cases to bring at the time because of the novel legal and medical issues involved. Plaintiffs and plaintiffs' attorneys would be deterred from bringing these cases if they had to face the specter of paying the opposing side's attorney's fees or the possibility of judge-imposed sanctions, if the suit was determined to be frivolous. Lawsuits such as these, which test legal waters, would be less likely to be pursued where the risk of litigation outweighs possible success. The preventative role of such suits would be lost, leaving women with fewer ways to hold accountable those who impair women's health.

These most recent reform attempts must be understood as only the most recent in a long-term national struggle to balance universal access to health care with cost control. While health care reform may recede from national attention for short periods of time, health care remains a pressing national issue. Health care reform has become the most recent and well-known vehicle to drive federal tort reform. The American Medical Association, for example, recognizing the promise of coupling tort reform to health care reform, indicated that it would be more likely to support health care reform if national tort reform were part of a complete reform package.[35]

While the urgency of health care reform may subside temporarily, the debate will continue, along with pressure to couple it with tort reform. Possibilities are numerous. Most pertain to medical malpractice. It is difficult to determine, however, the extent to which reforms will be limited to medical malpractice lawsuits or will also extend to tort liability generally, and thereby impact upon products liability lawsuits. Either way, the changes have the potential to impact upon women's health and their legal rights to sue where their health is damaged by negligent doctors or defective products.

Women's health care advocates must study health care policy carefully and examine critically the links made between health care and tort reform. Such reforms may or may not be good for women. There will be trade-offs that must be evaluated to determine whether they are beneficial or detrimental to women generally or only to some women specifically. Factors to consider in this evaluation are the race, age, disability, socioeconomic, and immigrant status of the women affected.

To frame the salient reform possibilities, it is useful to describe in exaggerated form the two opposing sides in the reform debate. On one side are plaintiffs and their lawyers and on the other are businesses, insurance companies, and physicians. Each side is also joined by sympathetic organizations. Plaintiffs and their lawyers want no reforms that limit liability and damages. Businesses, insurers, and physicians want the opposite. Remember this statement is exaggerated to facilitate analysis.

Option 1: Liability vs. Coverage

Take for a moment the business/insurer/physician position that to limit liability as part of health care reform will benefit all because it will keep health care costs lower and make health care available to all. Assuming for the moment that this is true, this may be beneficial to some women and not to others. For poor women, universal health care coverage may be more important than whether they have the right to sue their doctors for medical malpractice. These women have gone without health care and are unlikely to sue even if they have the right to do so. Studies on claiming behavior suggest that middle- and upper-class women are much more likely to sue.[36]

Women must not accept the linkage uncritically, however. Advocates of health care reform should be wary of trading off liability for coverage. Even though on the surface such a trade-off seems worthwhile, particularly in light of the benefit of gaining coverage for poor women, there may be significant but less immediately tangible losses. The specter of liability creates the incentive to develop, produce, and distribute products carefully and to provide competent medical services. The loss of such an incentive would be a critical one in the battle to insure quality medical care. So, although women who now receive no medical care would benefit from universal coverage, they, like all the other women who are covered under the current scheme, must be concerned about reforms that remove a factor that promotes quality control without replacing it with provisions that will insure competent health care and coverage for treatments that may be necessary when a woman is harmed by incompetent health care provision or defective medical products.

In an environment in which women — particularly low-income women, women of color,[37] and immigrant women — are less likely to be insured, to receive quality health care, and to obtain their share of medical research attention, it must concern us that current reform efforts linking health care and tort reform may remove one of the few incentives for being careful in manufacturing medical and pharmaceutical products and providing health care. State licensing boards, responsible for policing doctors, are notorious for lack of enforcement. The federal government through the Food and Drug Administration regulates manufacturers of pharmaceutical and medical devices but has done so ineffectively; it has neither the money nor the authority to do all that needs to be done. Remove liability, and little remains in the state or federal legal or regulatory structures to govern the conduct of manufacturers and physicians. Yet reform proposals do not address this risk.

Under the current health care system, tort litigation is a last resort for women who have been harmed by defective products or negligent medical treatment and who seek compensation to pay for necessary medical treatment, lost wages, and pain and suffering. This is particularly true for women who are not eligible for Medicaid and who lack health insurance. It is precisely this group that the current health care reform proposals are said to benefit the most. To the extent that these persons will, under a reformed system, receive medical treatment, they will benefit from the reforms. With the DES, Dalkon Shield, and medical malpractice cases as examples, however, it becomes apparent that limitations on liability as part of health care reform should be viewed skeptically.

While health care reform could result in a health care system in which women would not have to turn to litigation to pay for their health care needs after a wrongfully caused injury, there has been little attention paid to women's need for compensation for loss of wages during illness, for fertility treatments and surgeries, for the loss of reproductive capacity, and for the pain and suffering that accompanies such illness and loss.

Manufacturers and physicians, however, suggest that they are not removing the potential for liability, they are merely proposing reforms that will insure that the lawsuits that reach the courts are not frivolous. The American Medical Association recommends that all cases of alleged medical malpractice be reviewed by panels that would serve as gatekeepers of litigation.[38] If they find proof of medical malpractice, the panels would refer the case for mandatory arbitration, thereby taking the medical malpractice case out of the liability system entirely. Manufacturers and insurers, along with physicians, also recommend other reforms, including enterprise liability,[39] no-fault liability, and various bans or caps on damages, among them the exclusion of pain and suffering from awards and the elimination of punitive damages.

Reforms such as these demand scrutiny from those concerned about women's health generally and their reproductive health specifically. To facilitate this process of policy formation, the remainder of this chapter examines in more detail the various reforms characteristic of proposals to link tort and health care reform.

Option 2: Enterprise Liability

Health maintenance organizations and other types of aggregate health care enterprises have become more prevalent and increasingly popular. They serve as a model for health care reform, but they also raise questions about tort liability for negligent patient care. Traditionally, a physician is liable for his or her own negligent conduct. With the increase in health care enterprises and the probability that health care reform will spawn more, reformers have suggested that the liability of the individual doctor or health care practitioner shift from the doctor or practitioner to the provider group or plan covering the injured patient.[40] An injured patient would then sue the plan and not the person from whom she received treatment.

Shifting liability away from the individual doctor or health practitioner implicates two significant and interrelated policy concerns. The first is the need to keep health care costs down. The second is to provide patients with good health care. Enterprise liability potentially affects both.[41]

Many who advocate health care reform believe that health care costs increase as liability increases. While this may not be accurate, the belief that it is by those interested in developing and investing in provider groups and plans raises fears that patients will view the group or plan as a "deep pocket" with the resources necessary to pay substantial damages. They predict that this could give rise to a greater number of frivolous lawsuits because of the perception that the enterprises are resource rich. They also express concern that patients may be more likely to pursue cases in which the defendant is a business entity rather than an individual physician with whom the patient has had a previous and possibly long-term professional relationship.

Inserting the provider enterprise into the relationship between physician and patient also raises the second policy issue. Assuming that individual physician and health-care practitioner liability serves as an incentive to provide good health care, the shift of liability away from the individual to the enterprise may diminish this effect. While most doctors care about their patients and strive to provide their patients with the best care, for those who do not, enterprise liability may provide a shield from individual liability.

In addition, physicians and the American Medical Association are concerned that when health care organizations attempt to control health care costs, they will excessively and detrimentally interfere in a physician's exercise of medical judgment. Physicians and the American Medical Association also worry that to limit costs further, health care organizations may go so far as to exclude from provider lists excellent and caring physicians who provide high-quality care that involves expensive procedures.[42]

For women, the effects of enterprise liability are ambiguous. While it may serve as a disincentive for physicians to provide the best care possible, it may simultaneously force provider groups and plans to create a system of accountability that will result in better health care for women. It might also, however, under the cover of cost control, allow micromanagement of a physician's best medical judgment. To insure quality care and to take adequate precautions against conditions that could give rise to enterprise liability, groups and plans will need to exercise the utmost care in selecting and maintaining providers. They will also have to attempt to control costs without jeopardizing the full health care services that a patient needs. Thus, they must take affirmative steps to maintain quality medical care and to reduce the risk of liability. These might include screening, monitoring, and training policies to insure that all employees provide quality medical care while still leaving room for physicians to exercise independent decision making.

While health care enterprises will adopt such policies to limit their liability, advocates for women's health care should propose uniform policy standards that insure excellent women's health care. For example, one might propose a mandate that each health care enterprise develop and use policies that provide for escalating negative sanctions, including termination, when a physician or other employee provides care that falls below that which is commonly and professionally acceptable. Or, in contrast, one might call for treatment protocols that allow physicians flexibility in treatment options, including new and possibly expensive procedures. Uniformly applicable mandates to provide continuing education and training on topics such as the stages of women's reproductive health and breast cancer could be a significant opportunity for women's health care advocates to put into place policies that will serve the long-term interests of women and their health. If enterprise liability is adopted, such policy proposals should accompany health care reform, to insure that women receive quality health care.

Option 3: No-Fault Liability

No-fault liability systems, such as those adopted in many states for automobile accidents and in all states for workers' compensation, create alternatives to the civil tort system.[43] Generally, they establish a claims system that operates as the exclusive forum for claimants who seek damages for injuries. They have extremely limited exceptions that allow claimants to file claims in the courts, outside the exclusive no-fault system. In exchange for these systems, which are intended to provide a quicker monetary recovery than the torts system, claimants can enter the torts system only under narrow exceptions. The two most common in automobile no-fault systems are for severe injuries or large monetary losses.[44] In workers' compensations systems there is generally only one exception and that is where a claimant's injuries are caused by the grossly negligent, intentional, or criminal misconduct of the employer.[45]

If one accepts, as many do, that health care costs are escalating due to large tort awards for medical malpractice, a no-fault system to compensate injured patients is extremely attractive. A typical medical malpractice no-fault system might operate as follows: injured patients submit claims to an internal claims payment system rather than filing civil medical malpractice actions in state courts; claims are processed and reconciled exclusively through this system; when the claim meets the established criteria, the individual is compensated; when the claim does not meet the criteria, the patient pursues her claim through an alternative dispute resolution system.[46] At this final stage, a hearing officer or arbitrator decides the matter based on evidence produced by the claimant and the defendant. Based on the hearing officer's or arbitrator's conclusions, the claimant is or is not compensated. After this final stage is complete, a claimant may be able to appeal inside or outside the claims system. Appeals outside the claims system would be to the courts.

Many policymakers argue that, for most women, such a system would be positive. Women are the primary users of health care and as a result expose themselves to the possibility of medical malpractice more often than men.[47] Under a no-fault system, injured women presumably could receive compensation for their injuries more quickly than they are now able to do through the tort system. For example, in many populous states with large urban centers, like New York, it is at least three years before an injured woman with a nonfrivolous complaint can obtain a trial date. Recently, local bar associations in New York raised the possibility that given the burden on the courts created by the increase in crime, courts will no longer be able to accommodate civil litigation. This same sentiment was expressed by a federal judge in New York. Given the long delay that exists already in obtaining a trial date, a no-fault system is appealing to policymakers and to women who cannot wait for compensation.

As attractive as the no-fault system sounds, the workers' compensation system provides some evidence to support skepticism about its merits for women. First, a no-fault system requires a bureaucracy to process and decide claims. If the no-fault system for health care is designed similarly to other existing no-fault systems, it will most likely be with the goal that claimants need not be represented by counsel. The impetus for creating such a user-friendly system will be fueled by the perception that lawyers are unscrupulous and one of the causes of high liability costs. Despite such intentions, however, a no-fault system for health-care disputes will likely evolve into one in which claimants either need lawyers to navigate the complex system or believe that lawyers are essential to guarantee the highest possible award. This is true for workers' compensation even though it was designed originally to eliminate the need for claimants to be represented by lawyers. A health care no-fault system would have to be structured differently to gain the confidence of women's health care advocates.

Also of concern are the damage limitations that accompany a no-fault system of compensation. No-fault schemes generally require a trade-off between expediency on the one hand and compensation for pain and suffering and punitive damages on the other.[48] For women with serious and disabling injuries who currently can sue in the tort system with some possibility of success, such a trade-off is not desirable. However, for women with less serious injuries who cannot sue, in part because they cannot find lawyers willing to take their cases because of the prospect of small damage awards, the trade-off may be a desirable one.

Another factor, other than the severity of injury, that advocates must consider, is the socioeconomic class of the injured women. A recent study reveals that poor women are much less likely to sue when there is medical malpractice.[49] For these women, to trade away the right to be compensated for pain and suffering and to receive punitive damages may not be a loss, given that they are less likely to sue than are their middle- and upper-class counterparts. For low-income women, a no-fault compensation system may be more accessible and may actually provide an increased chance to receive compensation for injuries. On a cautionary note, however, women's health care advocates should not trade away rights of the least privileged without first considering whether there are alternative reforms that will provide women the full compensation that they deserve when their health is injured through negligent health care.

Option 4: Limiting Damages for Pain and Suffering

Proposals that accompany no-fault liability systems and call for limiting damage awards are only one example of such attempts. Most proposals for health care reform contain provisions for changing the tort liability rules for damages. Of these, the most common proposal is to either limit or eliminate damage awards that compensate victims for pain and suffering. For some advocates, to do either is simply to act in the best interest of the society as a whole. They argue that to compensate for pain and suffering is simply too costly. To continue to permit it in an era of universal coverage would lead to something akin to national health care bankruptcy.

This position — that health care will be bankrupted without limits or a complete bar on damages for pain and suffering — does not square, however, with the statistics on the low rates of malpractice and the even lower rates of settlements or awards for plaintiffs. Nor can these claims be reconciled with the actual value of awards, which more often than not fall below the actual loss that the injured individual suffers. Despite these contradictions, those who advocate for limits and bars have succeeded in creating a myth about the crisis of large damage awards and their potential to destroy actualization of the dream of universal health care.

Another view supporting control of damages for pain and suffering raises significant philosophical issues about what is considered "real" harm. This is a different argument entirely from the one in which advocates concede that pain and suffering constitute actual harm, but contend that the health care system simply cannot afford to compensate for it. This is the view of skeptics who believe that pain and suffering is a contested reality. They posit that it may or may not be "real" in any given situation and that because of the inherent inability of medicine to measure it objectively, it should not be a part of damage awards.[50]

Over the last two decades much has been done to try to understand the nature of pain and suffering both theoretically and physically. The body and the effects of harm have been the focus of theorists. Similarly, the reality of pain and its significant impact on human functioning have occupied physicians. Pain and suffering have become legitimate subjects of inquiry at the same time that a move to limit damages for them has emerged.

In the theoretical realm, postmodernists and feminists have placed the question of the body at the center of philosophical inquiry. Postmodernists, particularly Michel Foucault, have focused their attention on the body as being socially constructed.[51] Feminists have challenged the Enlightenment position that experiences like pain and suffering, which cannot be objectively observed and rationally proved, cannot be "real." Instead, feminist theorists suggest that philosophical positions that separate the psychological, intellectual, and emotional from the physical body are incomplete.[52] It could appear that these two positions are contradictory, that on the one hand there is no body, only a discursive text constituted by society and culture. On the other hand, the body is real and inclusive in its unmeasurable experiences. Despite appearances, these positions can be reconciled. Both philosophical positions honor the uniqueness of each body and the body's experience and context — or situatedness.

This intersection of postmodern and feminist theory is an important one for the philosophy of pain and suffering. Both suggest that each body has its own unique experience of disease, injury, pain and suffering. While there may be no objective measures of that which cannot be observed, there is a philosophical base from which to reason that social policy, like health care reform, must begin from a place that honors the individual's experience of the body's intangibles. To remove or limit pain and suffering awards does the opposite.

Another equally important connection occurs between the physical and the philosophical where theorists suggest that the body — a woman's body — is defined, constructed, and interpreted as the "Other" by subjects who occupy sites of power and who dismiss women's experience of pain as inventions. For example, one woman's cramping caused by the Dalkon Shield intrauterine device was characterized by her male physicians as "a nervous breakdown."[53] This mild discomfort was actually, "extremely painful," signaling serious disease and injury of the uterus.[54] The injuries resulting from the Dalkon Shield included death, septic abortions, pelvic inflammatory disease, infertility, and loss of reproductive organs. So many women were seriously injured that the large number of lawsuits resulted in mass tort liability of the manufacturer. Despite the lessons to be learned by the medical community from the Dalkon Shield experience, physicians still do not take complaints of pain seriously enough. Women report that they are described as "hysterical" because of their reports of pain and suffering. Very real pain and suffering from menstrual cramping is often dismissed as "exaggeration." Postpartum depression is diagnosed as "failure to bond" rather than being attributed to the precipitous hormonal changes that affect some women after they give birth. This tendency to dismiss women's reports of pain is dangerous. To limit damages for pain and suffering is dismissive in the extreme.

Women's experience as the Other and the frequency with which women consume medical care suggest that limiting damages for pain and suffering will be to women's detriment. Damage to women's reproductive health carries with it significant pain and suffering. To the extent that negligent health care or defective medical products or pharmaceuticals damage women's reproductive health, a limitation on pain and suffering will have a disproportionate impact on women. This is particularly true in light of their more frequent use of physicians and reproductive products and pharmaceuticals, particularly because of their gynecological and obstetrical needs. Efforts to limit damages for pain and suffering must be evaluated in this context.

Physicians suggest that the experience of pain affects physical and mental functioning. Any of us who has ever been in pain could testify to this. Most of us can report a time in our lives when severe pain interfered with our ability to concentrate and to perform an intellectual task. Pain can also affect our ability to carry out simple tasks of life — grocery shopping, working, or taking care of children. Significantly, chronic pain can depress even the most resilient among us. At a time when psychology is recognizing the role of pain in psychological functioning, proposals to limit or bar damages for pain and suffering mark a movement against a trend toward greater understanding and recognition of the role pain and suffering play in functioning. This trend legitimates the need for damages for pain and suffering; without them, there can never be adequate compensation to an injured person.

As part of this trend, the United States Department of Health and Human Services in 1985 commissioned a panel of medical, legal, and ethical experts to examine the role that pain should play in disability determinations for federal social security disability benefits.[55] An important step in public policy occurred when the panel determined that pain itself could constitute disability and that the social security disability determination had to take into account the injured claimant's subjective reports of her own pain. This resulted in a policy change on the part of the Social Security Administration and a change in the regulations governing how disability is determined.[56]

Arguments that deny pain and suffering as legitimate factors in damage awards are a departure from a larger trend that acknowledges their philosophical, psychological, and medical significance. There is more medical research now than there has been in the past on the experience of pain and suffering by patients and the role that both play in the healing process and in the delay of death. It appears from the literature that research on objectively unprovable medical events — like pain and suffering or the fact that individuals with a similar disease or injury can have dissimilar outcomes — is more plentiful than ever. This is consistent with trends in other disciplines and indicates an openness to the existence of pain and suffering as "real" harm. Tort reform that includes denying or limiting pain and suffering defies this trend. If pain and suffering is to be limited or eliminated, reformers must attend to this discrepancy and be accountable to the public about whether trading off individual interests is worth the public benefits.

Option 5: Punitive Damages

When plaintiffs win lawsuits, they are awarded damages to compensate them for their losses. Very few receive large compensatory damage awards.[57] On rare occasions a plaintiff receives damages above the amount necessary to compensate or to punish a tortfeasor. Punitive damages punish the defendant for engaging in egregious, almost criminal conduct. Such awards are extremely unusual, but they have captured the attention of tort reformers, who seek to eliminate or, at minimum, limit them. One possible explanation for this is that because liability insurers typically exclude punitive damages from coverage, punitive damages must be borne by the individual defendant. All other damages of concern to medical and pharmaceutical communities are generally covered by liability insurance and impact physicians, hospitals, and manufacturers only through a resulting increase in premiums. This is not to deny that defending oneself or one's company from a lawsuit is not a time-consuming and stressful event. It is an experience that no one seeks, but for physicians and companies it is cushioned by the insurance carriers who represent them in the lawsuit. Even under the worst of situations, where the physician or company must employ counsel separate from the insurance company because of potential conflict, the legal expenses are fully deductible as business expenses.

Punitive damages stand out as the most frightening aspect of liability because there is no indemnity and no protective cover of insurance company counsel. For physicians and pharmaceutical manufacturers this fear is flamed by reports of excessive punitive damage awards. Anecdotal accounts of such awards create a myth with immense power — a power sufficient to withstand the reality that punitive damage awards are rare and represent a fraction of total damages awards in the small number of cases that actually reach a trial and verdict for the plaintiff.

If punitive damages are rare, why then would it be against the interests of women to limit or eliminate them? The answer is connected more to the role that punitive damages play overall in the tort system than in individual cases. Punitive damages serve primarily two goals. First, they serve to punish. In this role they fulfill a purpose that historically has been left to the criminal law. Yet, for those cases in which a jury determines that the wrongdoing is done with maliciousness, or at least wanton or reckless disregard, should not the civil defendant be punished? The only tool available is the award of punitive damages. Punitive damages also deter the individual and others from engaging in the same tortious activity. They deliver a message that the wrongful activity will not be tolerated. As stated earlier, punitive damages are particularly suited to this goal because insurance carriers do not indemnify conduct that gives rise to punitive damages. The cost is borne by the wrongdoer.

Second, punitive damages serve to finance risky litigation. Cases with problematic factual and legal issues are not attractive to lawyers because the compensatory damages are frequently too small to cover the time and expenses involved in a complex or uncertain case. A good example of the role of punitive damages in products liability arises out of the Dalkon Shield litigation. There, punitive damages served as an incentive for lawyers to take early cases. They also played a significant role in making the corporation respond to the threat of thousands of lawsuits, because the threat of punitive damages loomed over the corporation's continued financial viability.

With the promise of punitive damages, lawyers are more willing to take risks. This is important, particularly in the products liability context, where the problem of investigating possible corporate wrongdoing often exceeds the resources available to the average private practitioner. With this in mind, some propose abandoning the punitive goal of punitive damages and adopting in its stead a compromise that would meet the deterrence and financing needs without punishing.[58] Such suggestions are notably absent from the current tort reform proposals accompanying health care reform. Until deterrence and financing are addressed, policymakers who wish to create conditions to promote and protect women's health should be wary of eliminating punitive damages without providing an adequate substitute.

Conclusion

For women's health care advocates, attempts at health care reform present an opportunity and a challenge to press for policies that meet the needs of all women. The opportunity is here to create a system of health care in this country in which every woman will receive quality health care. The challenge is to understand that all women do not have the same needs and that certain health care reform proposals may be good for some and bad for others. For women currently without access to health care, a trade-off between universal coverage and tort liability may seem like an excellent one. For women at the bottom of the economic ladder, who do not receive health care, concern about whether or not they will be able to sue for medical malpractice is far less pressing than their more immediate need to receive health care in the first place. Women's health care advocates and policymakers must be wary, however, of bargaining away the system of accountability provided by tort liability, which operates to protect women against negligent health care and defective products that can cause and have caused serious injuries, particularly to reproductive health.

While it may be tempting to buy the argument that tort liability is a benefit only for middle- and upper-middle class women, advocates and policymakers must be vigilant about insuring that a system exists to facilitate the manufacture of safe reproductive products and the delivery of quality medical care. Our current tort liability system does not do this well, but it should be maintained until an effective system of accountability replaces it. Advocates and policymakers must insert into any discourse about health care reform the need for additional mechanisms to mediate corporate and medical accountability. Women's health must be protected, and universal coverage and access to medical care is not enough to accomplish this goal.

A women's health agenda must include preservation of the tort liability system and more. It should include more effective state controls on the licensing, monitoring, and sanctioning of physicians. Stricter federal regulations governing testing of medical products and pharmaceuticals and their effects on women, pregnant and not pregnant, must be part of the agenda as well. An agenda for the twenty-first century will be incomplete without attending to the consequences of the new biogenetic and other testing technologies available to be used by women and on women. It has almost become trite to say that these technologies develop more quickly than our ability to understand the ethical implications of them. Women's health care advocates and policymakers must continue to push state and federal lawmakers and the medical profession and pharmaceutical industry to attend to these implications.

The twenty-first century will bring with it new products and new medical technologies and treatments that are now only imaginable. To link tort reform with health care and to make the latter's creation depend on the former's destruction is to eliminate for the future the primary form of professional and industrial accountability provided by the legal system. Women's health advocates and policymakers must be vigilant to insure that future generations of women have the right to quality health care along with the right to hold accountable professionals and manufacturers who fail to provide it.

Notes

1   G. Edward White, *Tort Law in America: An Intellectual History* (New York: Oxford, 1980).

2   Vice President Quayle inserted tort reform into national political discourse in a speech to the American Bar Association on August 13, 1991, in which he described the

fifty reforms of the civil justice system recommended by the President's Council on Competitiveness. Vice President Danforth Quayle, "Agenda for Civil Justice Reform in America," Address before the American Bar Association, August 13, 1991.

3   To make this chapter accessible, I limit referential and explanatory endnotes to those that are essential. I omit legal jargon where possible and include basic definitions in the text with expanded explanations in endnotes where necessary. I recognize that when an author makes this choice, she runs the risk of her work being taken less seriously by the academic community. I knowingly accept this risk with the hope that by reaching out to a wider audience, my ideas will have greater impact on women's health.

4   Michael J. Saks, "Do We Really Know Anything About the Behavior of the Tort Litigation System — and Why Not?" *University of Pennsylvania Press Law Review* 140 (April 1992): 1147, 1154.

5   Congress responded to the crisis with legislative action and political rhetoric. For example:

> *Mr. McConnell:* Mr. President, I am introducing legislation today that will put the brakes on the lawsuit crisis that is running amok in this country. My bill is called the Lawsuit Reform Act of 1989, because its purpose is to reform the "sue-for-million" mentality that has gripped our civil justice system.

135 *Cong. Rec.* S5989-02 (June 1, 1989).

6   *Hymowitz v. Eli Lilly & Co.*, 73 N.Y.2d 487, 539 N.E.2d 69, 541 N.Y.S.2d 941 (1989).

7   *Tetuan v. A. H. Robins Co.*, 241 Kan. 441, 738 P.2d 1210 (1987).

8   The Food and Drug Administration (FDA) first approved DES in 1941, but for medical conditions that were not pregnancy-related. In 1947, the FDA approved the drug as a miscarriage preventive. It concluded in 1951 that DES was safe for use in pregnancy. *Hymowitz v. Eli Lilly & Co.*, 73 N.Y.2d 487, 541 N.Y.S.2d 941, 944 (1989).

9   In 1971, the FDA banned the use of DES in pregnancy, finding that it had "harmful latent effects . . . upon the offspring of mothers who took the Drug." Ibid.

10 In *Enright v. Eli Lilly & Co.*, 77 N.Y.2d 377, 382, 568, 570 N.E.2d 198, 200, N.Y.S.2d 550, 552 (1991), plaintiffs allege, "in utero exposure to DES has since been linked to other genital tract aberrations in DES daughters, including malformations or immaturity of the uterus, cervical abnormalities, misshapen Fallopian tubes and abnormal cell and tissue growth, all of which has caused . . . a marked increase in the incidence of infertility, miscarriages, premature births and ectopic pregnancies."

11 Research on men exposed to DES in utero reveal a higher incidence of genital tract abnormalities. See, for example, Hembree, Nagler, Fang, Myles, and Jagiello, "Infertility in a Patient with Abnormal Spermatogenesis and In Utero DES Exposure," *International Journal of Fertility* 3 (1988): 173, 176; Shy, Stencherer, Karp, Berger, Williamson, and Leonard, "Genital Tract Examinations and Zona-free Hamster Egg Penetration Tests from Men Exposed In Utero to Diethylstilbestrol," *Fertility and Sterility* 42 (1984): 772, 777.

12 Richard B. Sobol, *Bending the Law: The Story of the Dalkon Shield Bankruptcy* (Chicago: University of Chicago Press, 1991).

13 As an early and misguided defense strategy, A. H. Robins Company chose to persuade women that the product itself was not the source of their problems, but that medical malpractice was. Ibid., 11–12.

14 Ibid., 12.

15 Ibid., 47.

16 Ibid., 287–325.

17 Legal theorists agree that mass torts involve a large number of lawsuits arising out of the similar, and sometimes related, conduct of defendants. They disagree as to the finer points, however. One states that she uses " 'mass torts' as a catch all phrase to represent widespread, multi-victim personal injuries caused by corporate for-profit conduct." Leslie Bender, "Feminist (Re)Torts: Thoughts on the Liability Crisis, Mass Torts, Power and Responsibilities," *Duke Law Journal* 848 (1990): 849.

18 Whether enough is known about the tort litigation system to determine whether there is a crisis is the subject of an exhaustive article by Michael J. Saks, which summarizes both the sources of the public perception of the crisis as well as the empirical data on the subject. See Michael J. Saks, "Do We Really Know Anything About the Behavior of the Tort Litigation System — and Why Not?" *University of Pennsylvania Law Review* 140 (April 1992): 1147–1292.

19 James R. Posner, "Trends in Medical Malpractice Insurance, 1970–1985," *Law and Contemporary Problems* (spring 1981): 37; U.S. Department of Health and Human Services, *Report of the Task Force on Medical Liability and Malpractice* (Washington, D.C.: GPO, 1987).

20 Two anecdotes that grossly distort the facts of the cases on which they are based have become staples in reform rhetoric. The first mischaracterizes as a burglar a student who climbs onto a school roof to fix a floodlight and falls. The second, in which a man recovers damages from the telephone company when a car strikes him while inside a phone booth, omits the fact that the man saw the car coming and desperately tried to get out of the phone booth but was trapped when the door jammed. Anecdotes are used in this way in Peter W. Huber, *Liability: The Legal Revolution and its Consequences* (New York: Basic Books, 1988).

21 Stephen Daniels and Joanne Martin, "Jury Verdicts and the 'Crisis' in Civil Justice," *Justice System Journal* 11, no. 3 (winter 1986): 321.

22 Ibid.

23 Professors Henderson and Twerski provide a state-by-state chart indicating that all fifty states undertook tort reform in the years 1986 to 1991. James A. Henderson, Jr. and Aaron D. Twerski, *Products Liability: Problems and Process*, 2d ed. (Boston: Little, Brown, 1992), 859–862. U.S. Senator Hatch argues that the country needs federal tort reform because states have "discarded traditional concepts of tort law that require negligence or recklessness in order to recover in favor of an expanded doctrine of strict liability." *Cong. Rec.* (daily ed., September 25, 1986), 648–701.

24 Michael J. Saks, a social psychologist and law professor at the University of Iowa, uses this phrase to describe the basis for policymakers' collective faith in the existence of the tort liability crisis. "Malpractice Roulette," *New York Times*, Saturday, July 3, 1993, sec. 1.

25 Deborah R. Hensler, *Compensation for Accidental Injuries in the United States* (Santa Monica, Calif.: Rand, 1991).

26 Researchers for the Rand Institute for Civil Justice compared awards and settlements in aviation accident cases and in others to determine whether they exceeded the plaintiffs' economic losses. They discovered that the "compensation, on average, falls far below economic loss." Elizabeth M. King and James P. Smith, *Economic Loss and Compensation in Aviation Accidents* (Santa Monica, Calif.: Rand, 1988), vii.

27   Harvard Medical Practice Study, "Patients, Doctors, and Lawyers: Medical Injury, Malpractice Litigation, and Patient Compensation in New York," *Report of the Harvard Medical Practice Study to the State of New York* (1990), 3.

28   Ibid., 6.

29   David S. Rubsame, *The Obstetrician's Professional Liability: Awareness and Prevention* (Calif.: Professional Liability Newsletter, Inc., 1993), 171.

30   Saks, "Do We Really Know Anything," *supra* note 18, 1148, 1152.

31   Ibid., 1153.

32   On Thursday, March 9, 1995, the House of Representatives passed H.R. 988, "The Attorney Accountability Act of 1995," which requires a party that has first rejected a settlement offer and then either loses entirely or wins a judgment below the offer to cover the opposing side's legal fees. This legislation is described as the "loser pays" bill. The next day, Friday, March 10, the House passed two more bills; H.R. 1058, which tightens requirements for bringing securities-fraud lawsuits; and, H.R. 956, "The Common Sense Legal Standard Reform Act of 1995, "which caps punitive damages in products liability cases at $250,000 and allows judges to sanction parties that bring frivolous products liability lawsuits.

33   See H.R. 988, "The Attorney Accountability Act of 1995," March 9, 1995.

34   See H.R. 956, "The Common Sense Legal Standard Reform Act of 1995," March 10, 1995.

35   Dana Priest, "Hillary Clinton Takes Her Case to AMA," *Washington Post*, Monday, June 14, 1993, sec. 1.

36   Saks, "Do We Really Know Anything," *supra* note 18, 1186–1187.

37   Vernelia L. Randall, "Racist Health Care: Reforming an Unjust Health Care System to Meet the Needs of African-Americans," *Case Western Reserve University School of Law, Health Matrix: Journal of Law–Medicine* 3 (1993): 127.

38   Dana Priest, "White House Considers AMA's Prescription for Malpractice Relief," *Washington Post*, Saturday, June 12, 1993, sec. 1.

39   Ibid.

40   Early in his administration, President Clinton floated a trial balloon to test the medical and insurance interests' reaction to enterprise liability. Enterprise liability was used by the administration to describe the health care organization's liability for a health care provider's malpractice. The trial balloon was shot down when "69 groups representing medical specialties publicly protested" the administration's proposal. Dana Priest, "White House Considers AMA's Prescription for Malpractice Relief," *supra* note 38.
     The administration's retreat from enterprise liability is of less consequence than one might assume, because institutions like provider plans, hospitals, and clinics will remain open to liability under the corporate negligence doctrine, which is well-established and accepted in many jurisdictions. The doctrine permits plaintiffs to sue a health care organization for permitting incompetent providers to use its facilities. *Darling v. Charleston Community Memorial Hospital*, 33 Ill. 2d 326, 211 N.E.2d 253 (1965); *Insinga v. LaBella*, 543 So. 2d 209 (Fla. 1989). (The latter case surveyed the states in 1989 and found seventeen jurisdictions that approved the doctrine.)

41   A 1986 symposium on health care cost containment offers an extensive review of strategies for cost containment and their affect on health care and liability: "The Legal Implications of Health Care Cost Containment," *Case Western Law Review* 36 (1986): 605–1233.

42   Robert Pear, "A.M.A. and Insurers Clash Over Restrictions on Doctors," *New York Times*, Tuesday, May 24, 1994, sec. 1. To address these issues, Senator Paul Wellstone of Minnesota introduced the Patient Protection Act, mandating that health plans disclose the standards used to select and exclude doctors and provide a right to appeal exclusion. The legislation also requires that only physicians in the same specialty area approve or deny authorization for payment for medical services.

43   There are hundreds of law review articles and books that explore alternative compensation systems. For an overview of the topic, see Dan B. Dobbs, Robert E. Keeton, and David G. Owen, *Prosser and Keeton on Torts* (St. Paul, Minn.: West, 1984), 584–615.

44   *Licari v. Elliot*, 57 N.Y.2d 230, 441 N.E.2d 1088, 455 N.Y.S.2d 570 (1982).

45   *Martin v. Lancaster Battery Co., Inc.*, 530 Pa. 11, 606 A.2d 444 (1992).

46   Priest, "White House Considers AMA's Prescription," *supra* note 38.

47   In 1986, women constituted 51 percent of the United States population but accounted for 60 percent of visits to physicians and approximately 60 percent of users of pharmaceuticals and vitamins. Cynthia Taeuber, ed., *Statistical Handbook on Women in America* (Phoenix, Ariz.: Oryx, 1991), 221; 244, Table C4-3.

48   Saks, "Do We Really Know Anything," *supra* note 18, 1153.

49   Ibid., 1186–1187.

50   Ellen Smith Pryor, "Compensation and the Ineradicable Problems of Pain," *George Washington Law Review* 59 (1991): 239–306.

51   Bryan S. Turner, *Regulating Bodies: Essays in Medical Sociology* (London: Routledge, 1992).

52   Martha Albertson Fineman and Nancy Sweet Thomadsen, eds., *At the Boundaries of the Law: Feminism and Legal Theory* (New York: Routledge, 1991).

53   Morton Mintz, *At Any Cost: Corporate Greed, Women, and the Dalkon Shield* (New York: Pantheon, 1985), 13.

54   Ibid.

55   The Social Security Administration administers federal benefits for disability. In 1985, it established the Commission on the Evaluation of Pain. The Commission's charge was to study pain in consultation with the National Academy of Sciences and to make findings and recommendations for future policies regarding pain.

56   The final agency regulations to evaluate pain were published in the Federal Register. 56 F.R. 57928, Thursday, November 14, 1991. They were promulgated as 20 C.F.R., Sec. 404–416.

57   Saks, "Do We Really Know Anything," *supra* note 18, 1214, 1220.

58   Dan B. Dobbs, "Ending Punishment in 'Punitive' Damages: Deterrence-Measured Remedies," *Alabama Law Review* 40 (1989): 831–917.

6

WOMEN, GIRLS, AND THE HIV EPIDEMIC

. . . .

Catherine Teare and Abigail English

Introduction

The HIV epidemic, socially and medically devastating in all of its manifestations, is currently evolving to affect most severely women and adolescent girls, particularly those from racial and ethnic minority groups who are living in poverty. Understanding this evolution requires placing the issues associated with HIV clearly in the broader context of women's lives.

We do not pretend in this chapter to address all the important issues associated with women, girls, and the HIV epidemic. In particular, there are pressing concerns related to the HIV epidemic's effect on women and girls worldwide, but this chapter primarily addresses issues within the United States. Here we focus on three issues that are critically important in their own right and that we believe reflect trends in the legal and policy responses to the HIV epidemic in women and girls. These issues are: (1) how AIDS and HIV disease are defined for purposes of case reporting and disability determination, (2) HIV testing policies, and (3) access to health care and clinical trials. Policies or laws in these areas have recently changed or are likely to change in response to activism, biomedical advances, epidemiologic shifts, or these forces in combination.

In writing this chapter, we have tried to be aware of certain biases common to discussions of HIV and women. The first of these is the tendency to define women as mothers, as evidenced in testing policy by the near-exclusive preoccupation with perinatal transmission. Summing up this problem, critics have charged that women "are regarded by the public and studied by the medical profession as vectors of transmission to their children and male sexual partners rather than as people with AIDS who are themselves frequently victims of transmission from the men in their lives."[1] Women's own risk for infection and their experiences with the continuum of HIV disease have been minimized or ignored in a number of arenas, including those of law and policy that we discuss here.

This is not to suggest that mothering and reproductive decision making are not critical issues for many women with HIV. Most women infected with HIV are of childbearing age, and many have children. Levine and Dubler, among others, have described insightfully the social, cultural, and political contexts of reproduction for women with HIV, among them the importance of reproduction to women living in poverty in this country.[2] In addition, some of the most important public policy issues in the years to come will involve the children of mothers who die of AIDS. While we do not discuss these issues in depth in this chapter, we recognize that they are foremost in the minds of many women who, upon finding out that they are infected or ill with HIV, worry first about their children's futures.[3]

We also approach this topic having worked for some time on issues related to HIV in adolescents. Legal and policy discussions often see "adolescents" and "women" as exclusive categories, and we attempt in this chapter to show that a person with HIV can be both. This approach is made more urgent by the trend toward infection at younger ages, particularly among women. In this effort, we use the term "girls" to refer to adolescent women, both to emphasize that adolescents may, because of their status as minors, face issues and barriers different from those faced by adult women, and also as a reminder that many females affected by and infected with HIV are, in fact, very young.

Epidemiology

AIDS and HIV Infection — Number of Cases
Through December 1994, 58,428 cases of AIDS in adult women and adolescent girls had been reported to the federal Centers for Disease Control and Prevention (CDC), comprising 13 percent of the total adult and adolescent cases.[4] AIDS in women and girls is growing rapidly: in 1992, the number of women with AIDS rose 9.8 percent, compared to 2.5 percent for men.[5] Estimates of the number of women and girls infected with HIV but not diagnosed with AIDS are more difficult to derive, but the numbers are certainly many times higher. Preliminary data from the National Health and Nutrition Examination Survey (NHANES III) estimates HIV seroprevalence at approximately 500,000, with a range

from 300,000 to 1.2 million, in the United States household population. According to this estimate, approximately 123,000 U.S. women were infected by 1994.[6]

Rapid Increase among Poor and Minority Women and Adolescents
The disease affects racial and ethnic minority women — African-American and Latina women specifically — disproportionately compared to their numbers in the general population.[7] Black and Hispanic women and girls accounted for 75 percent of all cases of female adult/adolescent AIDS reported to the CDC in 1993. In 1993, the AIDS case rate was approximately fifteen times higher among black women and seven times higher among Hispanic women than among white women (73, 32, and 5 cases per 100,000 population, respectively).[8]

Young women are most at risk of HIV infection, and age at infection is dropping. Researchers at the National Cancer Institute report that between 1987 and 1991 the median age at infection dropped to 25 (from 30 in the early 1980s). One of every four people newly infected with HIV between 1987 and 1991 was under 22.[9] While 12 percent of all people with AIDS are women, by the end of 1994 women made up 23 percent of the AIDS cases in people 20–24 years old and 34 percent of the cases among adolescents.[10] Studies show consistently high rates of infection among some groups of adolescents, including Job Corps applicants, military recruits, patients at sexually transmitted disease (STD) clinics, and homeless and runaway teenagers, with male and female infection rates roughly equivalent in many cases.[11]

The epidemic is also evolving into one that affects rural as well as urban women and girls. While ten metropolitan areas accounted for more than half (51.5 percent) of reported cases among women in the U.S. through the end of 1992, infection is spreading rapidly outside these mostly coastal urban areas.[12] A study in Mississippi of adolescents attending STD clinics found infection rates of 4 per 1,000 for both male and female subjects, with rates in rural areas similar to those in the most populous counties.[13]

Finally, women and girls with HIV are poor. The concentration of the epidemic in African-American and Latino communities is in fact a marker of poverty. Relatively little information has been collected that links economic status to health status.[14] However, the AIDS Cost and Service Utilization Survey (ACSUS), which follows 1,949 adults and adolescents with HIV/AIDS in ten cities, found that women in the sample are very poor — poorer than the men in the study. Fifty-five percent of the women had before-tax incomes of less than $5,000 in 1990, and only one percent had before-tax incomes greater than $40,000. (Comparable percentages for men in the survey were 31 percent under $5,000 and 12 percent over $40,000.)[15] The poverty of HIV-infected women has a profound impact on all the legal and policy issues discussed here.

Routes of Transmission

Injection drug use has been the predominant factor in women's infection with HIV, although heterosexual transmission is increasing in frequency and will likely continue to do so. Through 1994, injection drug use (IDU) was the risk factor for infection in nearly half the AIDS cases in women (48 percent). Another 19 percent of cases in women are attributed to sex with an injection drug user.[16]

In 1992, for the first time, heterosexual transmission surpassed injection drug use as the leading cause of new AIDS cases in women;[17] in 1993, heterosexual contact cases in women increased 139 percent over 1992.[18] Heterosexual transmission is more common for both sexes in younger age groups.[19] Female-to-female transmission of HIV appears to be rare, although some cases have been reported and it is a potential means of transmission.[20]

As important as injection drugs in women's HIV infection has been the explosion of crack cocaine use since the mid-1980s. Smoking crack is associated with sexually transmitted diseases and high-risk sexual behaviors, including high numbers of sex partners and acts of unprotected sex, exchanging sex for money, and using drugs before or during sex. Women crack users in one study averaged 11.5 sex partners in the previous 30 days, versus the men's average of 3.3.[21] Drugs of all kinds affect sexual behavior and may increase HIV transmission risk: a recent study shows that unsafe sexual practices are common among people with drinking problems.[22] Drugs and sex come together in particularly dangerous ways for young women: in one study, 78 percent of adolescent women surveyed reported that they felt it was "easier to have sex" when using alcohol or other drugs.[23]

It is difficult to glimpse through these statistics the social and cultural contexts of the women and girls who live with HIV infection and how, for the majority, these risk factors overlap. Anastos and Marte have written that "for many women, their address alone places them at risk. . . . [P]oor black and Latina women are at unduly high risk for infection, whatever their life-style, because poverty and lack of resources and opportunity keep them in areas of high HIV seroprevalence."[24] Many poor women confront HIV in contexts so fraught with other dangers that the risk of HIV may be, if not minimized, then deferred. According to Levine and Dubler, "[w]omen's risks — of abuse, violence, loss of housing, illness, discrimination — are daily fare. To them, AIDS is just another, and less immediate, risk."[25]

Natural History of HIV Infection
Basic research on the natural history of HIV infection in women — gynecologic manifestations, the effect of pregnancy on disease progression and on treatment, the effects of hormones on the course of the disease, and other topics — has begun in earnest only recently. For some time, however, clinicians have noticed that HIV manifests and progresses differently in women than in men.[26]

As in men, AIDS in women generally features opportunistic infections: Pneumocystis carinii pneumonia (PCP), candida esophagitis, cryptococcal meningitis, wasting syndrome, herpes simplex virus (HSV) disease, cytomegalovirus (CMV) disease, tuberculosis, toxoplasmosis, and lymphoma are all reported commonly in women. Women rarely develop Kaposi's sarcoma (KS), a common opportunistic infection in gay men,[27] but are more likely than men to experience bacterial pneumonia, endocarditis, and septicemia.[28]

Earlier in the course of HIV disease in particular, women's symptoms are very different from men's. As many as 42 percent of HIV-infected women may experience one or more manifestations of gynecologic disease, often very early in the course of the disease. Recurrent and severe vaginal candidiasis often appears even without any indicators or symptoms of immunosuppression, such as lowered T-cell counts.[29] Cervical manifestations are also common. In a study of 310 HIV-infected women attending methadone maintenance and sexually transmitted disease clinics in New York City and Newark, New Jersey, for example, cervical dysplasia was confirmed in approximately 22 percent of cases, a prevalence rate ten times greater than that found among women attending family planning clinics in the United States.[30] Cervical disease also seems to progress more rapidly to advanced stages in HIV-infected women than in uninfected women.[31] Women who are infected with both HIV and human papillomavirus (HPV) apparently run a particular risk of developing cervical cancer, probably because HIV-induced immunodeficiency allows the expression of HPV, which can lead to cervical lesions and cancer.[32] HPV disease recurs more frequently and responds less well to treatment in HIV-infected women, and women with both infections have shorter survival times than women who are infected only with HPV.[33]

Early reports suggested that women die faster after an AIDS diagnosis than men do, but in most subsequent studies the gender differential disappeared after controlling for certain variables, including zidovudine (AZT) use and/or the initial AIDS-indicator disease.[34] The largest scale study to date, however, found that women did have shorter survival times, even after adjusting for baseline differences and even though rates of disease progression did not differ between women and men.[35] The reasons for this differential require further study, but it may be due to women's poorer access to health care, greater poverty compared to men, homelessness, substance abuse, domestic violence, or nutrition.

Regardless of survival time, AIDS has become a major killer of women. In 1992, a dozen years into the epidemic, HIV became the leading cause of death for men 25–44 years old. In the same year it became the fourth leading cause of death for all women 25–44, and the second leading cause of death for black women in this age group. In 1991 (the most recent year for which mortality data are available for Hispanic ethnicity and for other races), HIV infection was the third leading cause of death among Hispanic women in this age group (12.4 percent of deaths). In 1992 the death rate from HIV infection for women 25–44 was 12 times as high for black women (38.0 per 100,000) as for white women (3.3 per 100,000).[36]

Changes in Official Definitions of AIDS and HIV: Policy and Implementation

CDC AIDS Case Definition

Women's exclusion from AIDS research, services, and funding was and remains a multifaceted issue, but can be traced in some part to the fact that many women have become sick because of HIV and died from it but never had "AIDS." The AIDS surveillance case definitions of the U.S. Centers for Disease Control and Prevention (CDC, formerly the Centers for Disease Control), first announced in 1982 and revised in 1985 and 1987, drew substantial criticism as the epidemic evolved because of their failure to take into account gender differences in the manifestation of HIV disease. An AIDS diagnosis is important: from an individual perspective, it may qualify women for services and benefits, including access to research protocols, reserved for people with AIDS; on a community level, a count of people with AIDS is used to disburse funds from the Ryan White CARE Act, a major source of federal funding for HIV services, and other programs. Changing the definition thus became a priority for women and a major campaign for activists and advocates.[37]

On December 18, 1992, the CDC issued a revised classification system for HIV infection and expanded the surveillance case definition for AIDS in adolescents and adults.[38] The definition was expanded to include HIV-related immunosuppression below certain levels (fewer than 200 CD4+ T-lymphocytes/μL, or a CD4+ T-lymphocyte percentage less than 14, even in the absence of opportunistic infections). The expanded definition also added three new clinical conditions — pulmonary tuberculosis, recurrent pneumonia, and invasive cervical cancer — to the twenty-three AIDS-defining conditions in the 1987 case definition.

The impact of the revision has been dramatic. In 1993, the first year of the new definition, 103,500 new AIDS cases were reported to the CDC, an increase of 111 percent over 1992. The 1993 increase was greater among women and girls (151 percent) than among men and boys (105 percent), and greater among blacks and Hispanics than among whites. The largest percentage increases in case reporting over 1992 occurred among adolescents (214 percent) and people 20–24 years old (133 percent). Most of the increase was due to cases of HIV-related immunosuppression. Women, blacks, heterosexual IDUs, and persons with hemophilia were more likely than others to be reported with the three illnesses added to the definition in 1993, and pulmonary tuberculosis was the most common of these. Only 151 cases — less than 1 percent of the cases based on the new illnesses — were reported based on HIV-related cervical cancer.[39]

Despite the new CDC definition, underdiagnosis in women continues, and some commentators have asked whether a female-specific AIDS definition is necessary.[40] As an example of the continuing inadequacy of the definition for women, there is the large number of HIV-infected women whose primary manifestations are gynecologic infections. Some of these women can meet the AIDS definition because of a depressed T-cell count, but, as noted above, severe infections can occur even with normal immune function. Further, even when their T-cell counts are very low, women are less likely to have access to the laboratory testing needed to document it. Finally, the perception that AIDS is a male disease continues: physicians do not expect women to have HIV disease and are not alert to its symptoms. Delay in diagnosis leads to delay in treatment and, sometimes, to a faster death.[41]

SSA Definition of HIV-Related Disability

Pressure on the CDC to change its AIDS definition was directed simultaneously at the Social Security Administration (SSA), leading to an important revision of SSA's HIV policies. SSA administers two long-term disability programs that provide cash assistance for individuals who are unable to work due to their medical conditions. The first is Social Security Disability Insurance (SSDI), an insurance program tied to contributions paid by workers. The second is Supplemental Security Income (SSI), a need-based program that provides a monthly benefit payment to low-income disabled individuals, regardless of work history. The programs are important to women not only for the cash benefits they entail, but also because of the linkage they provide to health insurance coverage — Medicare (after two years of SSDI) or Medicaid (upon determination of SSI eligibility, in most states).[42]

In the early years of the epidemic, the SSA regulations followed the CDC AIDS definition, reflecting the illness as it appeared in gay and bisexual men, primarily, and excluding claimants whose HIV disease presented differently. Despite SSA's move to "unlink" the disability determination process from the CDC definition in 1987 by broadening the definition of HIV-related disability to include people without AIDS diagnoses, many people disabled as a result of HIV disease were still denied benefits. In 1990, nineteen New York State residents, many of them women, filed a class-action complaint asserting that they had been denied benefits under SSA regulations even though they were disabled by HIV-related conditions.[43] As a result of that lawsuit and other pressure from advocates, SSA published new regulations for determining eligibility in December 1991 and revised them into final form in July 1993.[44]

Unlike the CDC AIDS definition, the final SSA regulations do not include a depressed CD4+ T-cell count as a disabling condition. However, they do include some diseases and conditions absent from the CDC definition, among them pelvic inflammatory disease, vulvovaginal candidiasis, and condyloma caused by HPV (genital warts).[45] The regulations explicitly recognize that these conditions affect girls as well as adult women and include them in both the childhood and adult listings.[46] Even more important, individuals can qualify based on *any* manifestations of HIV disease that occur repeatedly and are accompanied by functional impairment. This provision recognizes that HIV often presents as an ongoing series of medical problems, none necessarily disabling on its own, but severely limiting in combination and succession.

On paper, the new listings are a significant improvement. Unfortunately, advocates are finding that many biases that were part of the old regulations continue to make it difficult for women to receive benefits. In particular, people who have manifestations that are not exclusively HIV-related — such as bronchitis, yeast infections, or diarrhea — find that disability evaluators trivialize the disabling nature of their illnesses and do not approve them for benefits.[47] This pattern of denials, if it continues, will affect women particularly severely, since they are often disabled by exactly these conditions and less frequently experience the more exotic opportunistic infections that clearly qualify a person for SSI or SSDI.

The CDC's revised AIDS surveillance definition and SSA's HIV-related disability regulations are examples of long-term advocacy on multiple levels resulting in policy changes that make a significant difference for women. They represent the first real victories for women activists in the epidemic and, as such, are models for further advocacy on women's issues. However, there is much work still to be done before the real world of service delivery and disability evaluation catches up to the definitions on paper.

HIV Testing Policies

The availability, beginning, in 1985, of a test to determine the presence of antibodies to HIV engendered numerous proposals and controversies in the medical, legal, and public policy arenas. Many of these proposals and controversies focused on women.[48] The most pressing questions embodied the inevitable tensions concerning the rationales for testing, the locus of control and decision making about testing, and the relationship between testing and treatment. In 1994, advances in antiviral treatment to prevent perinatal HIV transmission brought these issues to the fore once again, and they will likely continue to dominate HIV testing policy in the decades to come.

Number of Women Tested

Large numbers of women — about a third of the population — have been tested for HIV to date. Including tests done as part of the blood donation process since 1985, by 1990 35 percent of women aged 15–44 in the U.S. had been tested for HIV infection.[49] Black women were two and a half times more likely than white women to report having been tested at clinics, and were also more likely to have received an HIV test as part of a medical examination.[50] White women and women with higher incomes were more likely to be tested through blood donations and, therefore, presumably less likely to receive counseling or other services than women tested at clinics.

Rationales for Testing

The reasons proffered for testing women and adolescent girls run the gamut from punitive to benevolent. Some testing proposals view women primarily as vectors of transmission and posit as the goal the protection of others, while others view women as individuals in their own right and focus on the protection of their health. At one end of the spectrum are proposals for mandatory testing of women prostitutes for the purpose of protecting their clients. At the other end are proposals to make HIV testing available to women on a voluntary basis so that they can seek appropriate health care early enough to improve their quality of life and slow the progression of their disease. Somewhere in between lie the suggestions that women should be tested in order to facilitate their reproductive decision making or to further the health of their infants, or even their fetuses.

Protecting the health of women themselves provides the most direct and straightforward justification for testing. Offered on a voluntary basis, HIV testing can provide a woman the opportunity to increase her knowledge of her own health status so that she can make decisions about lifestyle and health care to maximize her own health.[51] Thus far, testing of women on an *involuntary* basis to protect their own health has not been seriously urged. Despite the importance of protecting women's own health — both to them as individuals and to their families, friends, and others who know and care for them — this rationale is cited less frequently than others as a basis for testing.

More common in discussions of testing individual women or screening groups of women for HIV are the rationales that focus on women as vectors of transmission. By far the most common are the justifications related to reproductive decision making and protecting the health of a woman's fetus or infant child.[52] Until recently, the risk of transmission of HIV from an infected woman to her fetus has not been widely seen as justifying routine screening or mandatory testing of women.[53] Voluntary testing of pregnant women has been widely encouraged, however. Shortly after the HIV antibody test became available, for instance, the CDC recommended that it be made available to women in five "high risk" groups,[54] and the National Academy of Sciences and other experts have recommended that "[a]ll pregnant women and new mothers should be informed about HIV infection and the availability of HIV testing for themselves and their newborns."[55] Most recently, the CDC has amended its recommendations to endorse routine HIV counseling and voluntary testing for all pregnant women.[56]

Some experts in ethics have suggested that if a therapy existed that would help or at least not harm the pregnant woman and that was beneficial to the fetus, its existence would provide a stronger reason for women to be tested and treated while continuing the pregnancy than has existed in the past.[57] In 1994, the results of a study were released suggesting that AZT taken during pregnancy and delivery may fulfill those criteria, although numerous questions remain to be answered. In a double-blind, placebo-controlled study of 477 HIV-infected pregnant women, of the 53 babies born with HIV infection, 40 were born to mothers who had received the placebo, while only 13 were born to mothers who had received the AZT;[58] the transmission rates in the two groups were 25.5 percent and 8.3 percent, respectively.[59] This study, AIDS Clinical Trials Group Protocol 076 (hereafter the "076 trial"), raises major ethical and legal questions about how and when women should be tested for HIV, although its overall impact ultimately will depend in large measure on the results of further research concerning the validity of the initial findings, as well as the short- and long-term effects on pregnant women and their fetuses of administering AZT during pregnancy. Already, however, the possibility of reducing the likelihood that an infant would be infected has led to a spate of legislative and policy proposals on testing of pregnant women and the disclosure of newborn HIV surveillance data.

Within months of the release of the study results, for example, legislation was introduced in the U.S. House of Representatives to undo the confidentiality of the newborn HIV surveillance data collected anonymously by the CDC.[60] (Subsequently, the CDC terminated its newborn seroprevalence study, rendering the pending legislation moot.)[61] In the states, legislation was introduced to require HIV-test counseling (e.g., New York) and an offer of voluntary testing for pregnant women (e.g., New York and Michigan).[62] Other states can be expected to follow suit with similar legislation, as well as with proposals for mandatory testing of pregnant women.

There are at least two alternative approaches that are frequently considered as ways to use HIV testing to reduce perinatal transmission of the virus: testing of newborns, or of women at the time of delivery or immediately postpartum; and testing of pregnant women. While each of these approaches has apparent, if superficial, appeal, at least since the results of the 076 trial have been made known, neither is without problems.

All infants of infected mothers will test positive for HIV antibody initially, even though only a small number are themselves infected.[63] Thus, testing of newborns is in effect testing their mothers, and policies that would mandate such testing would mean that childbearing women are tested without their consent. Even if this serious legal and ethical problem did not exist, however, to the extent that proposals focus on disclosing newborn's test results or require testing to be offered at delivery or postpartum, they will not reduce perinatal transmission. The 076 protocol requires AZT administration during the second trimester of pregnancy and during birth, and to the infant before she or he is six weeks old.[64] Testing the mother or the infant at birth is too late to prevent maternal-fetal transmission.

HIV testing *early* in pregnancy could be more directly related to prevention of perinatal transmission, but only if a number of factors are present. First, it would have to be the case that pregnant women learning of their infected status would alter their behavior, choosing either to terminate their pregnancies or to take AZT (or any other drug that may in the future be identified as reducing the risk of perinatal transmission). Second, even assuming that women were to choose one of these alternatives, their ability to effectuate their choice would depend on the existence of accessible, affordable abortion services and accessible, affordable AZT treatment. The accessibility and affordability of neither can be assumed. Nevertheless, after extensive consultation with experts and women with HIV infection, in July 1995 the CDC issued new recommendations for universal HIV counseling and voluntary testing of pregnant women, articulating its reasons for doing so as follows:

> For uninfected women, such HIV counseling and testing programs can reduce their risk for acquiring HIV; for women who have HIV infection, these programs can enable them to receive appropriate and timely medical intervention for their own health and for reducing the risk for perinatal . . . and other modes of HIV transmission. These programs also can facilitate appropriate follow-up care and services for HIV-infected women, their infants, and other family members.[65]

To the extent that mandatory testing — either of the woman directly or by proxy through her newborn — is an element of proposals pending now or introduced in the future, many commentators have raised the concern that such coercive approaches will drive women away from health care.[66] Moreover, the efficacy of mandatory testing of women during pregnancy might ultimately depend upon a willingness to mandate not only testing but also treatment. In light of the many open questions that remain about the short- and long-term effects — for women and fetuses — of AZT administered during pregnancy, such a course would fall well outside the framework of ethically acceptable approaches. According to one commentator,

> [h]owever great the potential benefit, there is no ethical warrant for the imposition of a treatment that would entail five doses of AZT a day for months, as well as an intravenous dose of AZT during delivery. It is virtually never ethically acceptable to coerce a woman to undergo treatment to benefit her child, even when undergoing such treatment would be the morally right thing for her to do. In this instance, when there may be some risks for the mother, and when there are unknown risks to the child who would have been born infected, the case against mandatory treatment is stark. Additionally, sheer pragmatics preclude the adoption of a compulsory regime.[67]

As yet, there have been no serious proposals to mandate antiviral treatment for pregnant women. The CDC recommendations for counseling and testing for pregnant women specifically anticipate these pressures, however, stating that "HIV-infected pregnant women should not be coerced into making decisions about ZDV therapy. . . . A woman's decision not to accept treatment should not result in punitive action or denial of care."[68]

The promising results of the 076 trial have led both to policy proposals and media accounts that perpetuate the notion of a conflict between women's rights and their infants' health and which risk driving women and children away from care, and to policy recommendations that specifically address issues of women's autonomy and access to treatment. For example, the American Academy of Pediatrics has issued a policy statement recommending that "[t]esting programs for HIV antibody must be confidential, voluntary, and accompanied by cultural [sic] and ethnically-appropriate information regarding HIV infection. Such programs should be universally available."[69] In addition, the Academy has recommended that education about HIV infection and testing must be "part of a comprehensive program of health care for women" and that "comprehensive, HIV-related medical services should be accessible to all infected mothers, their infants, and other family members."[70] In this line of thinking, women's interests can be seen as coinciding, rather than competing, with those of their children.[71] The 076 trial could thus serve as an impetus to see that women are brought into care *before* they become pregnant, that they receive care early in their pregnancies if they become pregnant, that they are offered testing on a voluntary basis, and that they and their children are linked to treatment — HIV-related care and primary care — if it is medically indicated. Whether this model will prevail remains to be seen.

Almost as frequent as the reproductive rationales for testing are the justifications related to protecting the health of other third parties with whom women have contact: sexual partners (including the clients of female prostitutes) and needle-sharing contacts. While most of the recommendations for testing women in order to reduce the likelihood of transmission to others have involved *voluntary* testing, prostitutes have been a target for *mandatory* testing. The issue of whether prostitutes should be subjected to mandatory HIV testing, either upon arrest or upon conviction, has attracted considerable attention in the media[72] as well as in the state legislatures.[73] Between 1988 and 1990, an increasing number of states enacted laws mandating HIV testing of sex offenders, including prostitutes,[74] and this trend has continued.[75] In some states, prostitutes have been subject not only to involuntary testing for HIV but also to punitive measures, including criminal sanctions, when they fail to conform to public health injunctions to practice safe sex and to warn partners, according to anecdotal reports.[76]

Informed Consent and the Decision to Test

Although "voluntary" and "mandatory" testing are often posited as the two options for how the testing decision is made for an individual or a group, in fact there is a continuum of voluntariness, which includes completely mandatory, conditionally mandatory, routine without notification, routine with notification, and voluntary testing.[77] While there is a considerable body of opinion among medical experts, ethicists, and advocates that the decision of whether or not to be tested for HIV should ultimately rest with a woman herself, departures from this principle have occurred. These departures have included statutory requirements for completely mandatory HIV testing (such as for prostitutes, prisoners, and persons convicted of drug-related offenses);[78] conditionally mandatory HIV testing programs (such as for Job Corps applicants and military recruits);[79] and the routine HIV testing that occurs in some hospitals without patients being notified of their test results.[80]

These examples aside, however, for women and girls many of the troublesome issues associated with the decision to be tested for HIV arise in a context in which it is *assumed* that the test will be administered only with the informed consent of the woman herself. As of 1990, at least thirty-four states had enacted statutes requiring that HIV testing generally be based on the informed consent of the subject of the test.[81] In addition, the federal Ryan White CARE Act (discussed more extensively in the next section) contains a provision requiring states that receive funds under the Act to have in place informed-consent requirements for HIV testing.[82] Nevertheless, testing often occurs — or is omitted — without a truly voluntary decision by the woman as to whether or not she wishes to know her serostatus.

First, despite the fact that a significant percentage of women have already been tested for HIV either at clinics or when donating blood, many women simply do not have access to HIV testing. They may receive no primary health care at all or may obtain it at a site where they are not informed about the option of HIV testing.[83] For example, half the women counseled at the Women and AIDS Resource Network of New York learned that they were infected only when their children were diagnosed with HIV disease.[84] Second, many women who are told about the availability of the test do not receive appropriate pre-test counseling to enable them to make an informed choice. In fact, many women are given directive counseling, both pre- and post-test, particularly in an effort to influence their reproductive decisions.[85]

Many adolescent girls do not have the opportunity to make a voluntary decision about HIV testing. Access to testing for adolescents is even more limited than for adult women. Age appropriate pre- and post-test counseling is rarely available, even though it has been cited by a multidisciplinary group of experts as an essential element of HIV testing for adolescents.[86] Moreover, there is a widespread lack of understanding of whether adolescent girls who are legally minors are or are not authorized to give their own consent for an HIV test. In actuality, in more than half the states a statutory basis exists for minors to give consent for their own HIV test on one of three grounds: an explicit statute authorizing minors to consent to an HIV test; a statute authorizing minors to consent to diagnosis and treatment of sexually transmitted or venereal disease combined with a classification in state law of HIV or AIDS as STD or VD; or a statute authorizing minors to consent to diagnosis or treat-

ment of infections, contagious, or communicable diseases and a classification in state law of HIV or AIDS as such a disease.[87] In addition,
states have other laws on the books that authorize minors to consent to
medical treatment based on their status (as pregnant minors or runaway
youth, for example) or the services they seek (pregnancy-related care or
diagnosis and treatment related to a sexual assault), which might also
enable a girl to consent to her own HIV test.[88]

Thus, for the vast majority of women and adolescents, a legal framework is in place that ought to assure that they will not be tested without
their voluntary informed consent. Nevertheless, this is frequently not
the case, in part because of the exceptions to the informed-consent law,
in part because of the pressures exerted on women of reproductive age,
and in part because of the lack of an adequate linkage between testing
and treatment.

Testing and Treatment
In recent years the availability of therapies for HIV and related illnesses
has been viewed as an important reason for an individual woman or girl
to learn her serostatus,[89] but this has not been accompanied by any
assurance that the therapies will be actually available to women who
undergo the test. As discussed above, in the case of women, particularly
pregnant women, arguments for more widespread testing based on advances in treatment are being revived with even greater urgency since
the release of results of the 076 trial. However, the validity of treatment
availability as a justification for HIV testing depends on a number of
factors, one of the most significant of which is the degree to which there
is an actual link between HIV testing and follow-up treatment. For a
woman who does not wish to know her serostatus, it remains possible for
her to practice preventive measures to avoid becoming infected if her
status is negative and to avoid infecting others if she is infected. If she
would choose to seek treatment were she infected, she must learn her
HIV status, however; but the knowledge will not necessarily guarantee
that she will be able to obtain the treatment.

While it is easy for policymakers and others to call for greater use and
availability of testing, it is far more difficult to assure that those who are
tested will be able to receive appropriate treatment should they test
positive. Moreover, significant questions remain about many of the
therapies that are currently available, and these questions can have a
significant bearing on a woman's decisions concerning her medical care.
For example, there are ongoing questions about the quality of life for

those who choose to take AZT,[90] about the efficacy of AZT in prolonging the life of infected individuals, and about the best time in the course of illness to take the drug. Even though the 076 trial means, in the words of one clinician, that "we know more of AZT in pregnancy than any drug save penicillin,"[91] the effects of AZT on *women* were not a primary focus of the trial, and a protocol to follow the women was only belatedly added to the study plan.[92] The women in the 076 trial were at an earlier stage of HIV infection than that for which AZT has been considered therapeutically useful, and the effect of this early AZT use on disease progression — for instance, whether use during pregnancy might increase the development of AZT-resistant viruses, compromising its effectiveness later — remains unknown.[93]

Questions such as these suggest that even among women who do have access to therapies for HIV, different choices might be made by individual women about how to act on the news of seropositivity. Thus, while it is critically important for policymakers to strive to make both HIV testing and follow-up treatment available to women and girls, it is equally important that their ability to make informed voluntary choices for themselves about both testing and treatment be carefully safeguarded.

Treatment

While no cure for HIV disease or AIDS is on the horizon, therapeutic advances can be expected to increase survival times for infected individuals, primarily through improvements in the treatment of opportunistic infections and also through the continued development of antiretroviral agents that slow disease progression.[94] Survival time clearly is affected by early entry into treatment and by quality of care. A study in Georgia found that women with AIDS in metropolitan Atlanta lived longer than women with AIDS in other, mostly rural, areas in the state (400 days vs. 296 days), even when their diagnoses were identical. According to researchers, the difference in survival time was most likely attributable to the fact that women in the rural areas had poorer access to medical care than women in Atlanta.[95]

Access to Primary and Reproductive Health Care

The fact that most women and girls with HIV are poor, African-American or Latina, and involved with drugs directly or indirectly means that they have uneasy relationships with the health care system. According to one commentary,

[t]hese women are accustomed to discriminatory treatment and therefore do not readily seek or trust service providers in a system they perceive as hostile and punitive. . . . These factors lead women to come to the attention of care providers later in disease processes of all kinds, including HIV-related ones.[96]

Because of the stigma associated with HIV/AIDS, because concern over HIV in women has been so heavily weighted toward transmission and away from women's own health status, and because of punitive policies, women's mistrust of the health care system may be compounded when the medical condition in question is HIV.

The problem is not primarily women's attitudes toward care, however, but rather the attitudes of health care systems and providers to the women who are at greatest risk of contracting HIV. Indeed, a recent study of primary-care physicians found that they were considerably less likely to provide reproductive health services — gynecologic, contraceptive, prenatal, or abortion — to women with HIV than to other women.[97] Ensuring women's and girls' access to care thus becomes one of the greatest challenges for advocates and providers.

Access to primary care for women and girls is especially limited if they are low-income or members of racial and ethnic minority groups. Because they are more likely to be uninsured and because of the shortage of providers in poor neighborhoods, low-income women and women of color are less likely to have a regular source of health care or to receive preventive services, and more likely to use an emergency room when they do seek care.[98] Even programs that are designed to increase access for women and girls have frequently failed to do so. For example, of all the federally funded Maternal and Child Health (MCH) programs in the fifty states and the District of Columbia, only five had a women's health component (gynecologic and primary care).[99]

Reproductive health care is especially important because many women — regardless of socioeconomic or HIV status — seek health care services primarily in the context of gynecologic and reproductive care. Reproductive health settings thus become critical sites for HIV-related prevention, testing, and treatment. For adolescents, reproductive health settings are particularly important sites for health care because under state law in most states minors have independent access to contraception, pregnancy-related care, and diagnosis and treatment of STDs but not necessarily to other routine preventive care,[100] and consequently they may be more likely to seek services in reproductive health settings.

However, access to reproductive health care for all age groups remains extremely limited. According to one study, the unmet need for OB-GYNs in poor areas of New York is 62 percent greater than the unmet need for all primary-care providers.[101] Moreover, under current practice, HIV counseling and testing are not routinely offered in all reproductive health care settings.

Women who are pregnant and HIV infected face particular obstacles in accessing care, whether they decide to continue or terminate their pregnancies. More than 1 million of the 3.9 million women who gave birth in the U.S. in 1988 did not receive any prenatal care during the first three months of pregnancy, considered a critical time for the health of the mother and the baby; 6.1 percent received care only in the last trimester or not at all.[102] Access for women with HIV infection is even worse. A 1989 study at 36 AIDS clinical trial centers found that only 17 percent of identified HIV-infected women began prenatal care during the first trimester. Of the remainder, 43 percent made their first contact during the second trimester, 22 percent during the third trimester, and 17 percent had no prenatal care at all.[103] Policy debates over testing pregnant women so that they can be treated with AZT in order to diminish the chances of transmitting infection to their infants must take these statistics into account. Although an infected woman may now theoretically be in a position to make informed decisions regarding pregnancy and risks and benefits of drug therapy for herself and her infant, unless she has access to early prenatal care, is identified as HIV-infected, and can get and afford AZT, these advances in treatment are empty victories.

Some women who discover that they are HIV-infected and pregnant want to terminate their pregnancies; many will have difficulty carrying out their plans. The high cost of abortion makes it unavailable to some women in states where public funds will not pay for the procedure. Even with a 1993 federal requirement that state Medicaid programs pay for abortions in cases of rape or incest, at least nine states initially refused to do so.[104] More than half the states have passed laws mandating parental consent or notification before a minor can obtain abortion services, and as of 1992, these laws were being enforced in at least eighteen states.[105] In addition, since the 1992 decision in *Planned Parenthood of Southeastern Pennsylvania v. Casey*,[106] a number of states have passed laws requiring waiting periods, state-designed counseling, and other "nuisance" provisions designed to make it more difficult for women to obtain abortions.

The number of abortion providers in the country is dropping. A survey by the Alan Guttmacher Institute found that 83 percent of U.S. counties (51 percent of metropolitan counties and 93 percent of non-metropolitan counties) have no abortion provider.[107] Even where abortions are legally and geographically available, HIV-infected women may not be able to find a provider willing to treat them. In a 1990 study of New York City abortion facilities, approximately 42 percent responded that they either would not treat HIV-positive women or that they would charge a higher price for the procedure.[108] Two years later, following action by the New York City Commission on Human Rights, this percentage had dropped to 4 percent, but similar situations may exist in other communities.

Limitations on access to abortion services are ironic and cruel in the context of efforts to control HIV-infected women's childbearing. As Levine and Dubler write,

> HIV-infected women — the same class of women who have traditionally been encouraged or coerced to limit reproduction, on grounds either of benefit to themselves and their families or of benefit to society — are now being encouraged to limit reproduction to prevent transmission of disease to their children and on grounds of costs to society. However, at the same time their options for making this choice independently are being restricted. Women placed in this no-win situation, not surprisingly, cannot win.[109]

In the same way, women who are discouraged from terminating their pregnancies are likely to be foreclosed from the prenatal care and OB-GYN services that could improve their chances of healthy birth outcomes and protect their own health.

Access to HIV-related Care and Clinical Trials

Lack of access to primary care, including reproductive health care, translates, not surprisingly, into lack of access to specialized treatments for HIV disease and AIDS. A recent analysis of health services usage by women with HIV found that asymptomatic women are 20 percent less likely than asymptomatic men to receive AZT, a result that agrees with previous studies of AZT use in women.[110] (Asymptomatic study participants were significantly more likely to receive AZT if they had private or public insurance than if they were uninsured.) Women with symptomatic HIV infection or AIDS were more likely to use outpatient services — emergency room, hospital and community clinics, and private doctor visits — than men, but women with AIDS were less likely than men with AIDS to be hospitalized.[111] The author of this study suggests that the women's lower use of health services — a finding that remains after adjusting for income, race, insurance, and geographic differences — may be due to their greater family responsibilities, to superior health status compared to men in the study, or to discrimination against them as women with HIV.[112]

Another study of HIV-infected women with infants found that while 73 percent of the *infants* had adequate immunizations by nine months of age, less than half of the *mothers* (46 percent) had sought health care from specialized HIV clinics during their pregnancies or by twelve months postpartum. Moreover, women whose infants were infected were twice as likely to receive health care for themselves as women whose infants were not.[113]

Even when women do have access to reproductive health care and other primary care, it may be poorly integrated with HIV-related care. In 1994, the Alan Guttmacher Institute surveyed health care facilities that provide mainly HIV services (grantees under Title IIIb of the federal Ryan White CARE Act — see discussion below) and family planning clinics that provide at least some HIV services. The study found that neither type of provider saw HIV care and gynecologic care as integrated services. While most Ryan White grantees provided HIV testing and counseling and some gynecologic care, they spent only small amounts on reproductive health services and provided them almost exclusively to HIV-positive women. The family planning agencies, by contrast, revealed that they believed that their role in HIV-related care was limited to counseling and testing and encouraging condom use, and, although they provided a broad range of gynecologic and reproductive health services, they did not see those services as falling under the rubric of HIV/AIDS care.[114] This conceptual split, between HIV-infected women who need HIV-related care and childbearing women who need gynecologic and reproductive care, is extremely troublesome, given that gynecologic and reproductive health services can, according to the study's author, "help prevent HIV transmission to women and by women, identify women's gynecologic manifestations of HIV infection and AIDS and diminish the impact of gynecologic problems for infected women."[115]

In addition to the forces that limit women's access to primary care, access to AZT and other AIDS treatments may be affected by women's exclusion from HIV/AIDS research. Women's exclusion from research has serious implications, both for them individually — given that trials have been a major source of access to new therapies and to comprehensive care for many people with HIV/AIDS, especially gay men — and for HIV research generally, by stalling the expansion of knowledge of pharmacokinetics, safety, and efficacy of interventions. For example, because they lack information on the effects of investigational agents in HIV-infected women of childbearing age, clinicians have been hesitant to prescribe antiretrovirals and other HIV-related treatment even after their approval.[116] According to one commentator, women with HIV are denied access to HIV-related research on four counts: first, their reproductive capacity; second, their minority status and lack of access to health care generally and to research in particular; third, their drug use and presumed noncompliance with research protocols; and fourth, their ineligibility for trials focusing on AIDS itself, since many do not meet the AIDS definition.[117]

The first of these reasons, women's reproductive capacity, has been the basis for a complex regulatory scheme that has barred most women from all kinds of research, not only that which is HIV-related. Research involving human subjects is regulated by the Department of Health and Human Services (DHHS). DHHS Protection of Human Subjects policies[118] establish requirements for the protection of human subjects of research funded by the DHHS, and almost all institutions that conduct research, whether or not they are funded by DHHS, have adopted these rules.[119] Subpart B of the DHHS regulations — "Additional Protections Pertaining to Research Development, and Related Activities Involving Fetuses, Pregnant Women, and Human in Vitro Fertilization" — states that no pregnant woman may be a research subject unless the purpose is to meet the mother's health needs and the fetus will be placed at risk only to the minimum extent necessary to meet these needs, or the risk to the fetus is minimal.[120] In addition, such research generally requires the informed consent of the mother and the father, except where the purpose of the research is to meet the mother's health needs, the father cannot be found or is not available, or the pregnancy is a result of rape.[121] While the regulations do not completely exclude women from research, they emphasize the potential risk to fetuses and take a protectionist attitude toward pregnant women. In combination with pharmaceutical companies' concerns over liability for teratogenic drugs, the rules have effectively kept many women — pregnant and not — out of clinical trials.[122]

The same federal regulations, in Subpart D which contains the "Additional Protections for Children," also address the participation of adolescents in research studies (including clinical trials).[123] These regulations establish criteria under which research involving varying levels of risk is acceptable, and would be particularly relevant in evaluating research on adolescents that involves HIV testing of subjects or clinical trials of drugs with significant side effects. The Additional Protections ordinarily require both parental permission and the assent of the adolescent in order for adolescents who meet the definition of children under the regulations to participate in research. However, the regulations also provide for the requirement of parental permission to be waived if the research is "designed for conditions or for a subject population for which parental or guardian permission is not a reasonable requirement."[124] Thus the requirement might be waived, for research related to HIV, if under state law minors may consent to HIV testing and/or treatment or if the adolescent research subjects are capable of giving informed consent, and the research does not entail more than minimal risk.[125] In order for adolescents to benefit from participation in HIV clinical trials and research studies, research protocols must be designed to ensure that adolescents' participation is voluntary and that a mechanism is in place to ensure that those who choose to be involved are linked with services they need.[126]

A second set of federal rules applies to drug studies that will result in submissions for marketing approval to the Food and Drug Administration (FDA), a component of DHHS. In 1993 the FDA issued an update of its guideline for clinical research on women, liberalizing an earlier policy's recommendation against including women "of childbearing potential" in early-phase studies of most drugs except when the drug was intended as a life-saving or life-prolonging measure.[127] Admitting that the prior blanket exclusion of women of childbearing potential "appeared rigid and paternalistic," the new regulations — which cover private pharmaceutical company research — urge that women of all ages be studied in all stages of drug development and state that "exclusion of women from early trials is not medically necessary because the risk of fetal exposure can be minimized" — through pregnancy testing, contraception, and provision of full information about potential fetal risks to prospective study subjects.[128] However, the regulations do not *require* pharmaceutical companies to enroll women in early-stage studies, and the FDA admits that the change in policy only removes the "Federal impediment" to women's participation.[129]

The FDA further states that it is drug companies' fears of liability that have led to the paucity of studies among pregnant women, and in turn to a situation in which "many drugs are ultimately administered during pregnancy without reliable data on their maternal and fetal effects."[130] While the revised FDA guideline does not address the question of participation in research for women who are already pregnant or who become pregnant, several expert panels recently have called for pregnant women's inclusion in investigational treatments. The Agency for Health Care Policy and Research (AHCPR) clinical practice guidelines for early intervention in HIV disease encourage the development of new clinical trials policies to address pregnant women's access to investigational drugs, which

> should avoid *a priori* exclusion of pregnant women and should specify an approach that includes assessment of stage and gravity of the disease; specific drug characteristics, including risks associated with the drug; phase of the proposed study; and availability of other treatment options.[131]

The Institute of Medicine, part of the National Academy of Sciences, also recently issued new recommendations on women's participation. In a February 1994 report, the Institute said that pregnant women should be able to participate in medical research, provided they are fully informed of the risks.[132]

Even with the regulatory barriers diminished, funding for research on HIV in women is scarce. In recent years, calls for equity in research have become more insistent, and as a result, Congress has codified an earlier policy of the National Institutes of Health (NIH) calling for inclusion of women in research studies in numbers proportionate to their number in the affected population(s).[133] In addition, the federal government has increased its efforts to include in clinical trials underrepresented populations such as women, minorities, adolescents, and injection drug users. Since 1989, the National Institute for Child Health and Human Development (NICHD) has funded twenty-eight sites to conduct clinical trials in HIV-infected, predominantly minority children, adolescents, and pregnant women in collaboration with the AIDS Clinical Trials Group (ACTG), the federal network that coordinates clinical trials of experimental AIDS therapies involving drug companies, university hospitals, and government agencies.[134] The ACTG itself recently developed programs targeting certain populations, particularly women and adolescents.[135]

As of mid-1995, ACTG studies had enrolled a total of 40,475 people — adults, adolescents, and children. Nineteen percent of the total enrollees were female. Among adults, women represent 13 percent of all enrollees. Among adolescents, the female-to-male ratio is more favorable, with girls accounting for 44 percent of all enrollees aged 13–18. Overall, however, adolescents make up only 1 percent of the total enrollees. People of color are not well represented, either: among adults, 68 percent of enrollees to date are white; among adolescents, 40 percent are. Thirteen percent of adult entries, and only 2 percent of adolescent entries, are current or former injection drug users.[136]

Women and girls should have better access to clinical trials through a newer research initiative, the Terry Beirn Community Programs for Clinical Research on AIDS (CPCRA), established by the National Institute for Allergy and Infectious Disease (NIAID) in 1989 in order to involve community-based providers and their patients in clinical trials. The program's goal is to make experimental drugs available to patients who may not have access to clinical trials located at university-based medical centers.[137] Enrollment of women has been much higher than in the ACTG: nearly one-fifth of the 7,460 enrollees in these trials through September 1993 were women (although only 14.5 percent of all enrollees were under age 29 and only 0.1 percent were adolescents); 80 percent of all female enrollees were Latina or African-American.[138]

Even where research programs that admit or even seek out women exist, however, significant economic, cultural, and practical barriers remain. In part these are the same as those that limit access to primary care: family and child-care responsibilities, transportation difficulties, language and cultural differences, and mistrust of the health care system. In addition, increased requirements for investigators and institutions when women participate in research (pregnancy testing, the disenrollment of women who become pregnant, the cost of providing child care) have limited the enrollment of women in studies;[139] concerns about adolescents' ability to participate without parental involvement have effectively shut them out of research altogether.

Financing and Costs of Treatment
In 1993, an AHCPR study estimated that the lifetime cost of treating a person with HIV from the time of infection until death is approximately $119,000. This amount does not reflect the cost of treating women or girls specifically: estimates of the duration of the stages of illness were obtained from a study of homosexual and bisexual men, and the model assumes that a person begins treatment at the earliest possible time after infection.[140] Women, for whom the natural history and progression of

HIV disease are unknown and who enter care later than many men, may have lower overall costs. (Alternatively, they may have higher costs: another recent study found that injection drug users had longer and more expensive hospital stays than noninjecting homosexual patients; no statistically significant differences by gender were observed.)[141] Regardless, HIV is a financially burdensome illness, and most people are not equipped to pay for the treatment it requires.

By 1992, an estimated 38.5 million Americans were without health insurance.[142] The problem is greater for the HIV-infected population. Nearly 30 percent of persons with AIDS lack any form of health coverage, public or private. At primary health care facilities funded under the Ryan White CARE Act, more than 40 percent of the patients are reported to be uninsured.[143] Even if some version of state or national health care reform ultimately brings about positive change, in the interim the existing sources of funding need to be made to work better for women and girls. Currently, the primary sources of public funding, apart from some specialized state programs, are Medicaid[144] and the Ryan White CARE Act.[145]

Medicaid is available primarily to two groups of low-income persons: (a) individuals who are aged, blind, or disabled; and (b) pregnant women, children, or members of families with dependent children. The eligibility of these groups has been dependent on their status as recipients of cash assistance under the Supplemental Security Income (SSI) or AID to Families with Dependent Children (AFDC) program. Despite the expansion of the federal disability standards for HIV/AIDS, described earlier in this chapter, which will enable more people to qualify for Medicaid through SSI, the majority of women and girls with HIV are more likely to qualify through the second category, based on their linkage to AFDC.[146] Although some expansions of Medicaid eligibility, increasing the number of eligible pregnant women and young children, were enacted by Congress during the 1980s, eligibility for adolescents lags behind. Unless they are eligible for AFDC, many adolescents living below the federal poverty line will not be covered until the year 2002.[147] Moreover, significant changes to both the AFDC and the SSI programs are under consideration in Congress and at the state level in many states as part of ongoing "welfare reform" efforts. Many women and girls who would be eligible for Medicaid under the eligibility criteria in place in early 1995 may no longer be able to qualify once the welfare reform changes have taken place.

Medicaid — in the structural form that has characterized the program in the first thirty years of its existence — has one significant advantage as a funding source. To the extent that women and girls can establish eligibility, they are entitled to whatever services Medicaid covers in their state — in contrast to other programs that provide services but do not create any entitlement. Moreover, for Medicaid-eligible children and adolescents, the amendments to the Early and Periodic Screening, Diagnosis, and Treatment (EPSDT) program enacted by Congress in 1989 entitle them to any medically necessary, federally reimbursable Medicaid service, whether or not their state generally provides it for Medicaid-eligible adults.[148] Disadvantages of Medicaid include the difficulty in qualifying, even for many poor people, and limitations in coverage such that Medicaid often does not cover some of the services most needed by women and girls, particularly nonmedical, health-related services (such as case management). While the legislative changes enacted by Congress during the 1980s represent important expansions of Medicaid eligibility, the continued focus on pregnancy as the eligibility trigger for low-income women serves to reinforce the view of women's health as important only insofar as they are mothers.

In addition, in many states Medicaid reimburses primary-care providers at less than half what they would receive under either Medicare or private insurance. Low reimbursement rates may discourage physicians from accepting Medicaid or, potentially, from accepting HIV-infected patients whose care may be more intensive and take much longer.[149] In response to the shortage of Medicaid providers for HIV-infected people, some states have increased reimbursement rates to providers for a variety of HIV-related primary-care activities; others have elected to cover case management services under their Medicaid programs.[150] Several states have received waivers of basic federal Medicaid requirements to provide a broader range of home- and community-based services to individuals with AIDS than would ordinarily be available under the state's Medicaid plan.[151] States have broad discretion in designing these AIDS waivers, and their effectiveness in meeting the needs of women and girls depends on the specific provisions of each state's program, including level of diagnosis (HIV infection or AIDS) and type of services offered.

The second major source of public funding has been the Ryan White Comprehensive AIDS Resources Emergency (CARE) Act of 1990,[152] which authorizes funding for a system of comprehensive HIV care for individuals and families to be provided by cities, states, and other public and private entities.[153] For the first year of this program, FY 1991, Congress authorized a total of $875 million but appropriated only a quarter of that — $220 million. For FY 1994, the Act was funded at $633 million, still significantly short of the original authorization.[154]

Women and girls are specifically considered under two of the Act's four funding streams, or "Titles." Under the Emergency Relief Grant Program (Title I of the Act), which funds comprehensive treatment and case management services in geographic areas hardest hit by the epidemic, one half of the funds is awarded as supplemental grants to areas that provide assurances that their use of funds will include appropriate allocations for infants, children, women, and families.[155] Under the Comprehensive Care Grant program (Title II) — which supports a broad range of health services, support services, and home- and community-based services — at least 15 percent of the funds must be used for services to infants, children, women, and families.[156] For both programs, it is essential that women, girls, and their advocates be involved — through the HIV Health Services Planning Councils, which establish priorities for the allocation of Title I funds, or through other channels — in ensuring that programs serving women and girls actually receive the monies.

The Early Intervention Services program (Title III) also has the potential to support services — including counseling, testing, referrals, clinical and diagnostic services, periodic medical evaluations, and therapeutic services — that are needed urgently by women and girls with or at risk for HIV infection.[157] They will benefit, however, only if programs such as STD clinics and substance abuse treatment programs that are eligible for these funds ensure that their services are accessible to and appropriate for these populations.

Originally a separate program administered by the Maternal and Child Health Bureau in the Health Resources and Services Administration, the Pediatric/Family AIDS Demonstration Projects were incorporated as Title IV of the Ryan White CARE Act in FY 1994.[158] Now known as the Pediatric/Adolescent Services and Research program, projects funded through Title IV are mandated to provide comprehensive, community-based, family-centered care for children and families affected by HIV. In the first few years of the projects, only a few were specifically targeted to adolescents, although the ability to serve adolescents has since become an important criterion in selecting projects for funding. As part of Title IV, the projects are required to provide or phase in voluntary access for HIV patients to clinical research on therapies "for pediatric patients with HIV disease as well as pregnant women with HIV disease."[159] The fact that research under this Title will be conducted within comprehensive care systems bodes well for expanding women's and girls' access to biomedical, behavioral, and psychosocial research.

Ultimately, the ability of women and girls to obtain specialized, HIV-related health care, as well as primary and reproductive services, will be closely linked to the outcome of health care reform efforts. Although the effort by the Clinton administration and the Congress to enact comprehensive national health care reform legislation in 1994 was not successful, health care "reform" developments continue at a rapid pace. The possibility continues to exist that some form of national health care reform legislation, perhaps very modest in scope, will be enacted by Congress in the future. Whether or not that happens, however, numerous developments are already occurring at the state level, particularly in the redesign of state Medicaid programs, to expand eligibility, restrict benefits, and require Medicaid recipients to enroll in managed care arrangements. Congress is simultaneously considering major changes in Medicaid, such as "capping" the total amount of federal expenditures for the program and granting states even greater flexibility. The degree to which any of these developments will include effective mechanisms for ensuring that women and girls can receive the services they need remains a wide-open question.

While it is inevitable that the health care financing landscape will change, the degree to which that change is in a positive direction will depend on a number of factors: whether coverage is universal, whether there is a mandated comprehensive benefit package that includes services needed by infected women and girls, and whether home- and community based services are financed, to mention only a few of the critically important issues. Under any circumstances, however, strategies for financing and access must reflect a more systemic and long-term approach and rely less on AIDS-specific approaches and funding sources. At the same time, advocates must continue to press for the inclusion of women and girls in clinical trials of new AIDS drugs and in the HIV-specific programs that do exist.

Conclusion

In order to meet the needs of women and girls affected by the HIV epidemic effectively, policymakers will be required to make rapid and serious progress on a challenging agenda. This agenda cuts a broad swath across several fields: health care and research, child welfare, and law, among many others. Several of the most urgent tasks to be included in that agenda for women and girls are the following:

1. We must expand access to primary care for women and girls, especially those with low incomes.
2. We must expand access to and ensure funding for clinical trials and research studies for women and girls.
3. We must expand research on the natural history of HIV disease in women and girls.
4. We must expand access to specialized treatment for HIV disease and substance abuse.
5. We must limit mandatory testing of women and girls.
6. We must expand access to appropriate HIV counseling and voluntary testing for women and girls.
7. We must ensure that adolescent girls have independent, confidential access to health care services.
8. We must continue to advocate for making AIDS definitions used for epidemiological and disability determination purposes reflect women's experience of HIV disease.
9. We must increase financial support for HIV-infected women, their children, and their caretakers.
10. We must involve infected and at-risk women and girls in developing policies that meet their needs.

The rapid spread of the HIV epidemic among women and girls makes this agenda ever more urgent. A failure to address it effectively and soon will be a failure of our entire society, once again, to address the needs of some of its most vulnerable members.

Notes

1   Kathryn Anastos and Carola Marte, "Women: The Missing Persons in the AIDS Epidemic," *Health/PAC Bulletin*, Winter 1989, 10.
2   Carol Levine and Nancy Neveloff Dubler, "Uncertain Risks and Bitter Realities: The Reproductive Choices of HIV-Infected Women," *Milbank Quarterly* 68 (1990): 321–351.
3   See, for example, Catherine Teare, "Advocates Struggle to Develop Placement Options for AIDS Orphans," *Youth Law News* 15, no. 3 (1994): 1–7; Carol Levine, ed., *A Death in the Family: Orphans of the HIV Epidemic* (New York: United Hospital Fund, 1993).
4   Centers for Disease Control and Prevention (CDC), *HIV/AIDS Surveillance Report* 6, no. 2 (1995): 12.
5   Centers for Disease Control and Prevention (CDC), "Update: Acquired Immu-

nodeficiency Syndrome — United States, 1992," *Morbidity and Mortality Weekly Report* 42 (1993): 549.

6   Sandra Surber Smith, Public Affairs Office, National Center for Health Statistics, personal communication, April 1, 1994. The study on which this estimate is based (NHANES III) did not include people in hospitals or institutions or homeless people, and had a low response from young men and injection drug users. Ibid.

7   We use the terms "African-American" and "Latina," except when referring to sources that use other terminology.

8   Centers for Disease Control and Prevention (CDC), "AIDS Among Racial/Ethnic Minorities — United States, 1993," *Morbidity and Mortality Weekly Report* 43 (1994): 644.

9   Philip S. Rosenberg, Robert J. Biggar, and James J. Goedert, "Declining Age at HIV Infection in the United States," *New England Journal of Medicine* 330 (1994): 789.

10 CDC, *HIV/AIDS Surveillance, supra* note 4, 14. There were 661 cases in girls aged 13–19 and 3,775 in women aged 20–24 through December 1994. Ibid.

11 Don C. Des Jarlais et al., "AIDS and Adolescents," in *AIDS: The Second Decade*, ed. Heather G. Miller, Charles F. Turner, and Lincoln E. Moses (Washington, D.C.: National Academy Press, 1990), 147–167.

12 New York City, West Palm Beach, Ft. Lauderdale, Newark, Miami, San Juan, Baltimore, Washington, Chicago, and Los Angeles, with case rates ranging from a high of 41.5 down to 4.5 per 100,000. CDC, "Update: AIDS," *supra* note 5, 549. A number of states have reported the spread of HIV beyond the central cities. Shari Wasser, Marta Gwinn, and Patricia Fleming, "Urban-Nonurban Distribution of HIV Infection in Childbearing Women in the United States," *Journal of Acquired Immune Deficiency Syndromes* 6 (1993): 1040–1041.

13 Ronald A. Young et al., "Seroprevalence of Human Immunodeficiency Virus Among Adolescent Attendees of Mississippi Sexually Transmitted Disease Clinics: A Rural Epidemic," *Southern Medical Journal* 85 (1992): 462.

14 U.S. Congress, Office of Technology Assessment, *Adolescent Health — Volume 1: Summary and Policy Options* (Washington, D.C.: U.S. Government Printing Office, 1991), 1-21.

15 Fred J. Hellinger, "The Use of Health Services By Women with HIV Infection," *HSR: Health Services Research* 28 (1993): 552.

16 CDC, *HIV/AIDS Surveillance, supra* note 4, 12. Current reporting probably overestimates IDU and underestimates sexual transmission. A significant number of persons with AIDS classified as injection drug users also reported heterosexual contact with a person at risk, but these cases are all classified as IDU, which is considered a more probable mode of transmission. Centers for Disease Control and Prevention (CDC), "Heterosexually Acquired AIDS: United States, 1993," *Morbidity and Mortality Weekly Report* 43 (1994): 159.

17 CDC, "Update: AIDS," *supra* note 5, 549.

18 CDC, "Heterosexually Acquired AIDS," *supra* note 16, 157. The 1993 case reports reflect the use of the new CDC definition of AIDS; see discussion below in the section titled "CDC AIDS Case Definition."

19 Ibid., 156–157. In the South, heterosexually transmitted AIDS cases among women aged 20–29 increased 165.5 percent between 1988 and 1992. CDC, "Update: AIDS," *supra* note 5, 550.

20   Susan Y. Chu et al., "Epidemiology of Reported Cases of AIDS in Lesbians, United States 1980–89," *American Journal of Public Health* 80 (1990): 1381; Susan Y. Chu et al., "Female-to-Female Sexual Contact and HIV Transmission" (letter), *Journal of the American Medical Association* 272 (1994): 433.

21   Robert E. Booth, John K. Watters, and Dale D. Chitwood, "HIV Risk-Related Sex Behaviors among Injection Drug Users, Crack Smokers, and Injection Drug Users Who Smoke Crack," *American Journal of Public Health* 83 (1993): 1144–1148.

22   Andrew L. Avins et al., "HIV Infection and Risk Behaviors among Heterosexuals in Alcohol Treatment Programs," *Journal of the American Medical Association* 271 (1994): 515–518.

23   Susan G. Millstein et al., "Female Adolescents at High, Moderate, and Low Risk of Exposure to HIV: Differences in Knowledge, Beliefs, and Behavior," *Journal of Adolescent Health* 14 (1993): 133.

24   Anastos and Marte, "Women: The Missing Persons," *supra* note 1, 10.

25   Levine and Dubler, "Uncertain Risks," *supra* note 2, 331.

26   Catherine Hankins and Margaret Handley, "HIV Disease and AIDS in Women: Current Knowledge and a Research Agenda," *Journal of Acquired Immune Deficiency Syndromes* 5 (1992): 957–971.

27   Ibid., 959.

28   Daniel Daley, "Reproductive Health and AIDS-Related Services for Women: How Well Are They Integrated?" *Family Planning Perspectives* 26 (1994): 264.

29   Hankins and Handley, "HIV Disease and AIDS in Women," *supra* note 26, 959–962.

30   Centers for Disease Control and Prevention (CDC), "1993 Revised Classification System for HIV Infection and Expanded Surveillance Case Definition for AIDS Among Adolescents and Adults," *Morbidity and Mortality Weekly Report*, 41, no. RR-17 (1992): 7.

31   Agency for Health Care Policy and Research (AHCPR), *Evaluation and Management of Early HIV Infection*, Clinical Practice Guideline no. 7, January 1994, 60.

32   Ibid., 63.

33   Hankins and Handley, "HIV Disease and AIDS in Women," *supra* note 26, 961–962.

34   Ibid., 966.

35   Sandra L. Melnick et al., "Survival and Disease Progression According to Gender of Patients with HIV Infection," *Journal of the American Medical Association* 272 (1994): 1915–1921.

36   Centers for Disease Control and Prevention (CDC), "Update: Mortality Attributable to HIV Infection Among Persons Aged 25–44 Years — United States, 1991 and 1992," *Morbidity and Mortality Weekly Report* 42 (1993): 869–872.

37   Carol Levine and Gary L. Stein, "What's in a Name? The Policy Implications of the CDC Definition of AIDS," *Law, Medicine & Health Care* 19 (1991): 278.

38   CDC, "1993 Revised Classification System," *supra* note 30, 1–19.

39   Centers for Disease Control and Prevention (CDC), "Update: Impact of the Expanded AIDS Surveillance Case Definition for Adolescents and Adults on Case Reporting — United States, 1993," *Morbidity and Mortality Weekly Report* 43 (1994): 160–170.

40   Hankins and Handley, "HIV Disease and AIDS in Women," *supra* note 26, 958.

41 Nan D. Hunter, "Complications of Gender: Women and HIV Disease," in *AIDS Agenda: Emerging Issues in Civil Rights*, ed. Nan D. Hunter and William B. Rubenstein (New York: New Press, 1992), 10. See also the discussion of treatment issues later in this chapter.

42 Irwin E. Keller, "Social Security's HIV Disability Regulations: Slow Bureaucratic Machine Eludes Fast Virus," *San Francisco Barrister,* April 1994, 11.

43 *S.P. v. Sullivan*, No. 90 Civ. 6294 (MGC) (S.D.N.Y., complaint filed 1990).

44 58 Fed. Reg. 36008 *et seq.* (July 2, 1993).

45 SSA did not, however, adopt other recommendations related to symptoms of HIV disease in girls and women, such as revising the listing-level criteria for invasive cervical cancer to stage IB (it remains at stage II) or adding cervical dysplasia and chronic headaches to the listings.

46 The regulations also allow adolescents to be evaluated under the adult listings if the childhood listings do not apply. Catherine Teare, "New SSI Regulations Expand Eligibility for Minors with HIV," *Youth Law News* 15, no. 1 (1994): 11–12.

47 Keller, "Social Security's HIV Disability Regulations," *supra* note 42, 14–15. In one case, a woman who had involuntarily lost more than seventy pounds in nine months was told that she had now reached a "normal" weight and thus did not qualify for benefits based on HIV-related wasting. She eventually received benefits based on gynecologic manifestations. Ibid.

48 See, for example, Ruth Faden, Gail Geller, and Madison Powers, eds., *AIDS, Women and the Next Generation: Towards a Morally Acceptable Public Policy for HIV Testing of Pregnant Women and Newborns* (New York: Oxford University Press, 1991).

49 Jacqueline B. Wilson, "Human Immunodeficiency Virus Antibody Testing in Women 15–44 Years of Age: United States, 1990," *Advance Data from Vital and Health Statistics* no. 238 (Hyattsville, Md.: National Center for Health Statistics, 1993), 1–13.

50 Ibid.

51 See, for example, Leroy Walters, "Ethical Issues in HIV Testing During Pregnancy," in *AIDS, Women and the Next Generation*, ed. Faden, Geller, and Powers, *supra* note 48, 276.

52 See, for example, Working Group on HIV Testing of Pregnant Women and Newborns, "HIV Infection, Pregnant Women, and Newborns: A Policy Proposal for Information and Testing," *Journal of the American Medical Association* 264 (1990): 2416–2420; published in an expanded version in Ruth R. Faden et al., "HIV Infection, Pregnant Women, and Newborns: A Policy Proposal for Information and Testing," in *AIDS, Women and the Next Generation*, ed. Faden, Geller, and Powers, *supra* note 48, 331–358.

53 Marcia Angell, "A Dual Approach to the AIDS Epidemic," *New England Journal of Medicine* 324 (1991): 1498–1500.

54 Centers for Disease Control (CDC), "Recommendations for Assisting in the Prevention of Perinatal Transmission of Human T-Lymphotropic Virus Type III/Lymphadenopathy-associated Virus and Acquired Immune Deficiency Syndrome," *Morbidity and Mortality Weekly Report* 34 (1985): 721–726, 731–732.

55 Faden et al., "HIV Infection, Pregnant Women, and Newborns," *supra* note 52, 332.

56 Centers for Disease Control and Prevention (CDC), "U.S. Public Health Service Recommendations for Human Immunodeficiency Virus Counseling and Voluntary

Testing for Pregnant Women," *Morbidity and Mortality Weekly Report* 44, no. RR-7, (1995): 1–15.

57 Walters, "Ethical Issues in HIV Testing During Pregnancy," *supra* note 51, 278. Some commentators have noted that, while the justification for testing women of childbearing age for HIV has been the hope that they would avoid pregnancy as a result, the justification for testing *pregnant* women — which in the minds of some would be the hope that they would end the pregnancy through abortion — has, for political reasons, not been clearly stated. Wendy Chavkin, Vicki Breitbart, and Paul H. Wise, "Finding Common Ground: The Necessity of an Integrated Agenda for Women's and Children's Health," *Journal of Law, Medicine & Ethics* 22 (1994): 262–269.

58 "In Major Finding, Drug Limits H.I.V. Infection in Newborns," *New York Times*, February 21, 1994, A1.

59 Centers for Disease Control and Prevention (CDC), "Zidovudine for the Prevention of HIV Transmission from Mother to Infant," *Morbidity and Mortality Weekly Report* 43 (1994): 285–287.

60 "Newborn Infant HIV Notification Act," H.R. 4507, 103d Cong. 2d Sess. (introduced May 26, 1994) (Rep. Ackerman, D-N.Y.). Similar legislation had previously been introduced in New York State: 1993 Assembly Bill No. 6747, New York 215th General Assembly — First Regular Session (introduced March 30, 1993) (Mayersohn). This legislation was later amended to provide for mandatory HIV-test counseling for pregnant women and for voluntary testing.

61 "CDC Suspends Testing of Newborns," *AIDS Policy and Law* 10, no. 10 (June 2, 1995): 1.

62 Elizabeth Cooper, J.D., "An Exploration of the Medical, Ethical, and Legal Arguments against Mandatory HIV-Antibody Screening of Newborns and Parturient Women," presentation at the American Public Health Association 122nd Annual Meeting and Exhibition, Washington, D.C., October 31, 1994.

63 Lynne M. Mofenson and Anne Willoughby, "Transmission of Human Immunodeficiency Virus in Children and Women," in *Management of HIV Infection in Infants and Children*, ed. R. Yogev and E. Connor (St. Louis, Mo.: Mosby-Yearbook, 1992), 63–87.

64 Centers for Disease Control and Prevention (CDC), "Recommendations of the U.S. Public Health Service Task Force on the Use of Zidovudine to Reduce Perinatal Transmission of Human Immunodeficiency Virus," *Morbidity and Mortality Weekly Report* 43, no. RR-11 (1994): 3.

65 CDC, "U.S. Public Health Service Recommendations for HIV Counseling and Voluntary Testing for Pregnant Women," *supra* note 56, 1.

66 Lisa Merkel-Holguín, "The Facts on Mandatory Testing," *Children's Voice* 4, no. 1 (1994): 18; Chavkin et al., "Finding Common Ground," *supra* note 57, 264.

67 Ronald Bayer, "Women's Rights, Babies' Interest: Ethics, Politics and Science in the Debate of Newborn HIV Screening," unpublished manuscript, Columbia University, School of Public Health, HIV Center for Clinical and Behavioral Studies, May 1994, 20.

68 CDC, "U.S. Public Health Service Recommendations for HIV Counseling and Voluntary Testing for Pregnant Women," *supra* note 56, 10.

69 Provisional Committee on Pediatric AIDS, "Perinatal Human Immunodeficiency Virus (HIV) Testing," *AAP News*, December 1994, 30

70 Ibid.

71 See Chavkin et al., "Finding Common Ground," *supra* note 57, 263–264.

72 See, for example, "Should Prostitutes be Tested for AIDS?" *San Francisco Daily Journal*, February 20, 1991, 4.

73 See, for example, "Manual Appendix A: State Laws Concerning Reporting of Names of Persons Testing Positive for HIV Antibodies; Informed Consent Requirements for HIV Antibody Testing; Confidentiality of Information Concerning HIV Status; Anonymous Testing; Quarantine; Mandatory Testing of Prisoners and Persons Charged with or Convicted of Crimes; Criminal Laws Concerning Transmission of HIV and Defendants with HIV; and Related Statutes," in *AIDS Practice Manual: A Legal and Educational Guide*, ed. Paul Albert et al., 3d ed. (San Francisco: National Lawyers' Guild AIDS Network, 1992), A.1–A.26.

74 "State AIDS Legislative Trends, 1983–1990," *Intergovernmental AIDS Reports* 3, no. 5 (1990): 1, 3.

75 See, for example, Lisa Bowleg, *A Summary of HIV/AIDS Laws from the 1992 State Legislative Sessions* (Washington, D.C.: Intergovernmental Health Policy Project, 1993), 38; *A Summary of HIV/AIDS Laws from the 1993 State Legislative Sessions* (Washington, D.C.: Intergovernmental Health Policy Project, 1994), 41.

76 See, for example, Elizabeth B. Cooper, "When Being Ill Is Illegal: Women and the Criminalization of HIV," *Health/PAC Bulletin*, Winter 1992, 10–14.

77 Ruth R. Faden, Nancy E. Kass, and Madison Powers, "Warrants for Screening Programs: Public Health, Legal, and Ethical Frameworks," in *AIDS, Women, and the Next Generation*, ed. Faden, Geller, and Powers, *supra* note 48, 4.

78 "State AIDS Legislative Trends," *supra* note 74, 3.

79 Karen Hein, "Mandatory HIV Testing of Youth: A Lose-Lose Proposition," *Journal of the American Medical Association* 266 (1991): 2430–2431.

80 Anita L. Allen, "Legal Issues in Nonvoluntary Prenatal HIV Screening," in *AIDS, Women, and the Next Generation*, ed. Faden, Geller, and Powers, *supra* note 48, 184.

81 David A. Hansell, "HIV Antibody Testing: Public Health Issues," in *AIDS Practice Manual*, ed. Albert et al., *supra* note 73, 3–5.

82 42 U.S.C. § 300 ff. 61(b)(1) (West 1991).

83 Hunter, "Complications of Gender," *supra* note 41, 12–13.

84 Ibid., 13.

85 Ibid., 18–19.

86 Abigail English, "AIDS Testing and Epidemiology for Youth: Recommendations of the Work Group on Testing and Epidemiology," *Journal of Adolescent Health Care* 10 (1989): 52S.

87 Abigail English, "Adolescents and HIV: Legal and Ethical Questions," in *The HIV Challenge*, ed. Marcia Quackenbush and Kay Clark, 2d ed. (Santa Cruz, Calif.: Network Publications, 1995), 259–285; Abigail English, "Expanding Access to HIV Services for Adolescents: Legal and Ethical Issues," in *Adolescents and AIDS: A Generation in Jeopardy*, ed. Ralph J. DiClemente (Newbury Park, Calif.: Sage, 1992), 265–266.

88 English, "Expanding Access," *supra* note 87, 266–267.

89 "Experts on AIDS, Citing New Data, Push for Testing," *New York Times*, April 24, 1989, A1.

90 William R. Lenderking et al., "Evaluation of the Quality of Life Associated with

Zidovudine Treatment in Asymptomatic Human Immunodeficiency Virus Infection," *New England Journal of Medicine* 330 (1994): 738–743.

91   Janet L. Mitchell, M.D., M.P.H., "An Exploration of the Medical, Ethical, and Legal Arguments against Mandatory HIV-Antibody Screening of Newborns and Parturient Women," presentation at the American Public Health Association 122nd Annual Meeting and Exhibition, Washington, D.C., October 31, 1994.

92   Chavkin et al., "Finding Common Ground," *supra* note 57, 264.

93   CDC, "Recommendations on the Use of Zidovudine," *supra* note 64, 4–5.

94   National Commission on AIDS, *An Expanding Tragedy: The Final Report of the National Commission on AIDS* (Washington, D.C.: National Commission on AIDS, 1993).

95   Bruce M. Whyte and Jane C. Carr, "Comparison of AIDS in Women in Rural and Urban Georgia," *Southern Medical Journal* 85 (1992): 574–577.

96   Denice Benson and Catherine Maier, "Challenges Facing Women with HIV," *Focus: A Guide to AIDS Research and Counseling*, December 1990, 1.

97   Centers for Disease Control and Prevention (CDC), "HIV Prevention Practices of Primary-Care Physicians — United States, 1992," *Morbidity and Mortality Weekly Report* 42 (1994): 989.

98   Jane Perkins, "Race Discrimination in America's Health Care System," *Clearinghouse Review* 27 (1993): 373–375.

99   Chavkin et al., "Finding Common Ground," *supra* note 57, 263.

100 Patricia Donovan, *Our Daughters' Decisions: The Conflict in State Law on Abortion and Other Issues* (New York: Alan Guttmacher Institute, 1992), 10–14.

101 Levine and Dubler, "Uncertain Risks," *supra* note 2, 340, citing C. Brellochs and A. B. Carter, *Building Primary Health Care Services in New York City's Low-income Communities* (New York: Community Services Society of New York, 1990).

102 Sara Rosenbaum, Christine Layton, and Joseph Liu, *The Health of America's Children* (Washington, D.C.: Children's Defense Fund, 1991), 9–12.

103 Pamela Stratton, Lynne M. Mofenson, and Anne D. Willoughby, "Human Immunodeficiency Virus Infection in Pregnant Women Under Care at AIDS Clinical Trials Centers in the United States," *Obstetrics and Gynecology* 79 (1992): 366–367.

104 "Suit Planned to Seek Abortion Payments," *New York Times*, April 3, 1994, 15.

105 Donovan, *Our Daughters' Decisions*, *supra* note 100, 14.

106 *Planned Parenthood of Southeastern Pennsylvania v. Casey*, 505 U.S. 833 (1992).

107 Stanley K. Henshaw and Jennifer Van Vort, "Abortion Services in the United States, 1987 and 1988," *Family Planning Perspectives* 22 (1990): 106.

108 Cooper, "When Being Ill Is Illegal," *supra* note 76, 14, note 8.

109 Levine and Dubler, "Uncertain Risks," *supra* note 2, 342.

110 Hellinger, "Use of Health Services," *supra* note 15, 543–561. Gender was not a significant variable for symptomatic people or for people with AIDS.

111 Ibid., 553–557.

112 Ibid., 559.

113 Arlene M. Butz et al., "HIV-Infected Women and Infants: Social and Health Factors Impeding Utilization of Health Care," *Journal of Nurse-Midwifery* 38 (1993): 106.

114 Daley, "Reproductive Health and AIDS-Related Services for Women," *supra* note 28, 264.

115 Ibid., 268.

116 AHCPR, *Evaluation and Management, supra* note 31, 72.

117 Carol Levine, "Women and HIV/AIDS Research: The Barriers to Equity," *Evaluation Review* 14 (1990): 449.

118 45 C.F.R., Part 46 — Protection of Human Subjects (1989).

119 Levine, "Women and HIV/AIDS Research," *supra* note 117, 450.

120 45 C.F.R. § 46.206(a)(2) (1989).

121 45 C.F.R. § 46.207(b) (1989).

122 Levine, "Women and HIV/AIDS Research," *supra* note 117, 454.

123 Additional Protections for Children Involved as Subjects of Research, 45 C.F.R. Part 46, Subpart D (1989).

124 45 C.F.R. § 46.408(c) (1989).

125 National Commission for Protection of Human Subjects of Biomedical and Behavioral Research, *Research Involving Children: Report and Recommendations* (Washington, D.C.: U.S. Government Printing Office, 1977), 17–19.

126 English, "Expanding Access," *supra* note 87, 262–283.

127 AHCPR, *Evaluation and Management, supra* note 31, 71.

128 58 Fed. Reg. 39406–39416 (July 22, 1993).

129 58 Fed. Reg. 39408 (July 22, 1993).

130 Food and Drug Administration, "Women in Clinical Trials," *FDA Medical Bulletin,* December 1993, n.p. Under the previous (1977) FDA guidelines, pregnant women could be granted access to experimental drugs under life-threatening circumstances, and this mechanism remains available under the new guidelines. AHCPR, *Evaluation and Management, supra* note 31, 72.

131 AHCPR, *Evaluation and Management, supra* note 31, 73.

132 "Pregnancy Called No Bar to Tests," *New York Times,* February 27, 1994, A13.

133 National Institutes of Health Revitalization Act of 1993, Pub. L. No. 103-43, 107 Stat. 122 (1993).

134 National Institute of Allergy and Infectious Diseases (NIAID), "Where Do AIDS Drugs Come From?" July 1992, n.p.

135 AHCPR, *Evaluation and Management, supra* note 31, 72.

136 National Institutes of Health, "Demographic Summary of ACTG Study Entries From Beginning to 7/7/95," July 11, 1995, 1.

137 NIAID, "Where Do AIDS Drugs Come From?" *supra* note 134.

138 Community Programs for Clinical Research on AIDS (CPCRA), "CPCRA Patient Demographics," October 8, 1993, n.p. Received from ACTIS.

139 AHCPR, *Evaluation and Management, supra* note 31, 72.

140 Fred J. Hellinger, "The Lifetime Cost of Treating a Person with HIV," *Journal of the American Medical Association* 270 (1993): 474–478.

141 George R. Seage III et al., "The Effects of Intravenous Drug Use and Gender on the Cost of Hospitalization for Patients with AIDS," *Journal of Acquired Immune Deficiency Syndromes* 6 (1993): 831.

142 S. Snider and S. Boyce, *Sources of Health Insurance and Characteristics of the Uninsured: Analysis of the March 1993 Current Population Survey,* EBRI Special Report No. SR-20; Issue Brief No. 145 (Washington, D.C.: Employee Benefit Research Institute, January 1994).

143 AHCPR, *Evaluation and Management, supra* note 31, 101.

144 42 U.S.C. §§ 1396 *et seq.* (West 1992 & Supp. 1994).

145   Pub. L. No. 101-381, 104 Stat. 576 (Aug. 18, 1990), 42 U.S.C. §§ 300 ff. *et seq.* (West 1991 & Supp. 1994).

146   AHCPR, *Evaluation and Management, supra* note 31, 102.

147   42 U.S.C. § 1396a(1)(1)(D).

148   42 U.S.C. § 1396d(r)(5) (West 1992).

149   AHCPR, *Evaluation and Management, supra* note 31, 103.

150   Ibid.

151   Abigail English, "The HIV-AIDS Epidemic and the Child Welfare System: Protecting the Rights of Infants, Young Children, and Adolescents," *Iowa Law Review* 77 (1992): 1557. By late 1992, fifteen states had approved waiver programs for persons with HIV infection, and other applications were pending. Ibid.

152   Pub. L. No. 101-381, 104 Stat. 576 (Aug. 18, 1990), 42 U.S.C. §§ 300 ff. *et seq.* (West 1991 & Supp. 1994).

153   Abigail English, "New Federal Law May Help Children and Adolescents with HIV," *Youth Law News* 12, no. 2 (1991): 1.

154   San Francisco AIDS Foundation, *HIV Policy Watch* (August 1995): 6.

155   42 U.S.C. § 300ff-13(b)(1)(E) (West Supp. 1994).

156   42 U.S.C. § 300ff-22(b) (West 1991).

157   42 U.S.C. §§ 300ff-41 to 300ff-67 (West 1991).

158   59 Fed. Reg. 4086–4087 (January 28, 1994).

159   National Pediatric HIV Resource Center, "Background Memorandum — Title IV of the Ryan White AIDS CARE Act: Implementation Issues Related to HIV Research," November 6, 1993, 1–4.

7

HEALTH CARE ACCESS FOR IMMIGRANT WOMEN

Janet M. Calvo

Introduction

Elizabeth is a young woman recently married to a citizen of the United States. She herself had come to the United States as a child. Although her mother had tried to legalize her immigration status, the process took a long time because of lost documents, and Elizabeth unwittingly made herself ineligible through the relationship with her mother by marrying. Although Elizabeth is eligible for a legal status through her marriage to a citizen, her husband has not yet filed the correct petition for her. He lost his job shortly after Elizabeth discovered she was pregnant. They have no health insurance. Elizabeth knows she needs medical care to assure the health of her baby, but has no funds to pay for it.

∎

Maria has two children, one a United States citizen and one an "undocumented alien," like herself. She and her husband came over the border to the United States with their first child to escape civil strife and poverty. Her husband died when she was pregnant with her second child in the United States. She works long hours in a hot dusty factory. She has developed a persistent cough and would like to have a doctor look at it. She would like to get health care for her children as well. She has been told that they need to be immunized to keep them healthy and that she should take them to a doctor or clinic. There have been cases of children with whooping cough and measles in her community. But Maria is afraid. She fears that the health care provider will report her to the Immigration and Naturalization Service (INS).

∎

Shaid is married to a legal permanent resident. She met him through friends of her family who lived in the United States and encouraged her to come to the U.S. to meet him. Her husband started hitting her six months after they were married. At first, he slapped her occasionally, but the violence is getting heavier and more frequent. He threatens he will have her deported if she tells anyone.

He recently twisted her arm and punched her in the face and stomped on her when she fell. She tried not to cry out but the pain was too bad. A neighbor heard and called the police.

■

Sean is a recent legal permanent resident. She became a legal permanent resident through the diversity program. She works as a word processor at several temporary jobs, none of which provide health insurance. One night, on her way home from work, she fell in front of a subway train. Her life was saved, but she became a paraplegic as a result of injury to her spinal cord. The hospital wants to transfer her to a rehabilitation facility where she could learn to care for herself. Sean's resources soon were depleted by her health care needs. She lies in a bed in an acute-care hospital that cannot meet her needs but costs more per day than the rehabilitation facility.

■

Evelyn came to the United States when she was 20 to visit an older sister who is a permanent resident, then stayed when their mother died during that visit. Evelyn works for a family and makes just enough to cover rent, food, and necessities. She takes care of the elderly grandmother in the household and keeps an eye on the two grandchildren when they come home from school. Evelyn has had some nursing training but has been unable to get a job that would serve as the basis for a legal immigrant status. Evelyn has not seen a doctor since she came to the United States five years ago.

These situations illustrate the plight of many women living in the United States whose health care access is restricted or threatened because of their immigration status. In addition to the direct harm suffered by these women, there are severe adverse consequences to the public health. Health care and welfare reform proposals made by federal and state legislators and the president do not hold the promise of making the situation better. On the contrary, health care access for these women, and the adverse public health consequences, will become significantly worse if these proposals are implemented. Some federal legislators even propose limiting health care access for immigrants even after they become naturalized citizens.

"Alien" women are currently caught in a double layer of invisibility that has severe consequences for them and for the public as a whole. The notion that the norm of the human body is male still persists and is reflected in a lack of attention to the effects of health care and welfare reform on women's health. The invisibility of women in general is compounded by the invisibility of women as immigrants; the norm of an immigrant is a young man.[1] As a result, public debate does not address the consequences for these women and for the public health of restricting their access to health care.

Women currently comprise almost half the immigrants entering the United States. When young male children are added, women and children predominate.[2] Similarly, almost half of the refugees and asylees granted permanent resident status are women.[3] Moreover, in recent years, studies have found that women have comprised an increasing proportion of the "undocumented," in one year, for example, ranging from 60 to 80 percent of the "undocumented" population.[4] The 1990 census figures show that 49.44 percent of all the noncitizen, foreign-born individuals living in the United States are female.[5] Together, women and children aged 14 or younger comprise 55 percent of this group.[6] Barriers to health care for immigrants in general therefore have a substantial impact on the access of women to health care. Further, there are particular barriers that predominately adversely affect women.

Some barriers to health care for immigrants are caused by language, cultural differences, limited medical knowledge, and different perceptions of medical treatment. However, many current and proposed barriers are based on immigration status. These barriers harm the individual women involved, but they also have a substantial adverse impact on family, community, public health, and the cost of health care. Understanding the barriers to health care and their consequences requires a fairly sophisticated understanding of immigration law and status.

Immigration Status

Aliens enter the United States in one of several ways. The first is with some type of temporary visa, also called a nonimmigrant visa (for example, as a tourist or student).[7] Others enter the United States as legal permanent residents.[8] And others enter as refugees. Refugees are aliens who have been screened outside the United States and are found to have a well-founded fear of persecution in their countries of origin.[9]

Other aliens may enter the United States with no prescreening or documents. These people are often called "undocumented" or "illegal" aliens. Sometimes these terms are also applied to persons who come to the United States on a temporary visa and stay beyond the designated time. However, the terms, "undocumented" or "illegal" aliens, are often applied erroneously. While aliens originally enter the United States in relatively few ways, there are a larger number of potential statuses for aliens in the United States and their immigration status may change more than once.

The most secure immigration status is that of legal permanent residents,[10] who now have the greatest access to health care. However, some federal legislative proposals would substantially bar them from major sources of health care. There are several bases on which aliens can become permanent residents. These include certain family relationships to United States citizens or permanent residents,[11] certain employment or investment in the United States,[12] and nationality of countries from which there has been limited recent immigration to the United States.[13] Also eligible to become permanent residents are juvenile wards of the state,[14] aliens who have been found eligible for the "legalization program,"[15] aliens who have been refugees or asylees,[16] and certain aliens who have lived in the United States for a long time.[17]

Many aliens face a lengthy process to obtain permanent residency while they are in the United States, and they will need health care during that time. They are not necessarily "illegal" or "undocumented" during the processing time. Other aliens have statuses that allow them to live and work in the United States, but they will not necessarily become permanent residents. Some aliens may be eligible for more than one immigration status or more than one category of status. These aliens are often erroneously viewed as "illegal," and are therefore excluded from many sources of health care.

Aliens who have lived in the United States for a long time may be here legally, for example, those who are registry-eligible (having lived in the United States since 1972). Other aliens are allowed to live and work in the United States because they are fleeing persecution or other conditions in their home countries.[18] Additionally, there are "humanitarian" statuses that allow aliens to reside in the United States,[19] such as deferred action, voluntary departure, stay of deportation, and parole.[20] For example, an alien can be granted deferred-action status if she can show that her forced removal from the United States would be inhumane because she is in need of medical care that she can obtain only in this country.[21]

Finally, certain relatives of United States citizens and permanent residents are afforded special eligibility for immigration status to prevent the separation of families. They are allowed to reside in the United States while they complete the processing for permanent resident status.[22] An example is the spouses and children of legalized aliens who are waiting for a visa number to become available.[23]

Barriers to Health Care Access

Women with various types of immigrant status face diverse barriers to accessing health care. These include barriers in the health insurance system, barriers posed by limitations on alien access to publicly sponsored programs, and barriers created by the adverse impact that seeking health care can have on immigrant status.

The Health Insurance System

Immigrant women face barriers caused by a health insurance system that is heavily dependent on employment status. Except in Hawaii, employers are not required to offer or provide health insurance to their employees. Women immigrants frequently work in jobs in which health insurance is not the norm — as domestics or in factories, for example. Often, immigrants work in industries where wage, hour, child labor, and health and safety laws are not sufficiently enforced, making the need for health care all the more crucial.

The "employer sanctions" law has exacerbated this situation. This law, passed by Congress in 1986, made it a civil offense — and in some circumstances, a criminal offense — for an employer to hire anyone who lacks either documentation of citizenship, certain alien statuses, or specific authorization to work.[24] Work authorization, even for those legally qualified, is often difficult to obtain through the INS bureaucracy. This has resulted in situations in which aliens, unable to obtain work authorization, are often abused by employers, who can take advantage of them by requiring long hours and dangerous working conditions. Aliens are reluctant to complain for fear of putting themselves in jeopardy.

This problem is exacerbated in situations in which an employee had worked for an employer before November 1986. The "employer sanctions" rules do not apply so long as the employee continues to work for the same employer.[25] Unfortunately, some employers have used this law to force immigrant workers into worse and more health-endangering working conditions. Employees who had jobs before November 1986, because they could not legally work for anyone else, became totally dependent on their employers and thus unable to complain about unscrupulous demands. For women immigrants, these demands have sometimes taken the form of sexual harassment.

Limitations on Aliens' Access to Publicly Sponsored Programs

Very few citizens or aliens can afford to pay for health care without health insurance. Therefore, those without health insurance, or whose coverage maximums have been reached, are frequently dependent on some form of publicly sponsored health care. There are a variety of limitations on immigrant women's access to the health care provided by public programs. These limitations vary from program to program, without any real public health rationale.

Medicaid[26] is currently a major source of health care for the otherwise uninsured in this country. Medicaid has low financial eligibility levels and was designed to provide health care for people who cannot otherwise afford it. This type of coverage is extremely important for individual and community health. However, Medicaid eligibility is restricted based on immigrant status.

The federal government's attitude toward Medicaid coverage for aliens' prenatal health care is particularly problematic for women. In recent years, Congress has expanded Medicaid coverage of pregnancy-related health care, recognizing the severe health dangers for infants and the high cost for subsequent health care if prenatal care is not provided. Further, Congress has found prenatal care to be cost-effective. The Department of Health and Human Services (HHS), however, has interpreted the law to allow Medicaid to provide prenatal care only to pregnant aliens who are permanent residents or "permanently residing in the United States under color of law." This has subjected children who are born to transient aliens to the serious threats of low birthweight and lifelong disabilities. It has also increased health care costs. A lawsuit in New York that challenged the HHS interpretation resulted in a ruling prohibiting the restriction, finding that Congress did not intend to deny or delay prenatal health care based on citizenship or alien status.[27] However, HHS follows this case only in New York.

Legal permanent residents (with some limited exceptions)[28] and aliens who are "permanently residing in the United States under color of law" are eligible for full Medicaid coverage.[29] The proper interpretation of "permanently residing in the United States under color of law" has been the subject of much dispute.[30] The general definition is that of an alien living in the country with the knowledge and permission of INS "whose departure the INS does not contemplate enforcing." An alien is considered one "whose departure the INS does not contemplate enforcing" if it is the policy or practice of INS to not enforce the departure of aliens in a particular category or on all the facts and circumstances of the alien's case.

HHS has listed specific alien status categories that meet the definition of permanently residing in the United States under color of law,[31] but courts have included additional specific situations that also qualify.[32] The concept of "permanently residing under color of law" reflects the reality of immigration law. It recognizes that many aliens have a legal basis for staying in the country, and therefore should have access to health care through Medicaid for their sake and the public health.

Citizenship or alien status is not a criterion for eligibility for emergency services under Medicaid.[33] However, the application of some state residency rules has led to the denial of emergency-care coverage to aliens who have a temporary immigration status.[34] An emergency medical condition is defined as a medical condition (including emergency labor and delivery) that manifests itself by acute symptoms of sufficient severity (including severe pain) that the absence of immediate medical attention could reasonably be expected to result in placing the patient's health in serious jeopardy, serious impairment to bodily functions, or serious dysfunction of any body organ or part.[35]

Medicare, a government-sponsored insurance program for the elderly and the disabled, is tied to eligibility for Social Security benefits. Aliens who do not qualify for Medicare through Social Security cannot choose to pay to participate, unless they have been permanent residents for five years.[36] This limitation particularly affects alien women, because they are likely to have worked in jobs with no Social Security coverage, such as domestic work.

There have been several recent federal legislative proposals to further limit the eligibility of aliens for federally funded health care programs, including Medicaid. Examples from 1995 include H.R. 1214 (previously designated H.R. 4, "The Personal Responsibility Act"), which passed the House of Representatives, and S. 269, which was considered by the Immigration Subcommittee of the Senate Judiciary Committee. Some legislators seek to limit the definition of "Permanently residing in the United States under color of law" to a few categories of aliens. This approach ignores the complexity and realities of immigration law, which result in the long-term residence in the United States of many categories of aliens.

Proposals of other legislators would limit access to health care under any federal- and state-funded health programs to United States citizens and would even impose some limitations on naturalized citizens. Under these proposals, legal permanent residents, as well as aliens "Permanently residing in the United States under color of law," would have no access to publicly sponsored health care.

States and localities often implement and contribute to federal health care access programs and in doing so must impose the federal law's restrictions on immigrant access. However, individual state law often requires that additionally there be state or local health programs for the indigent. These programs differ from state to state, and include treatment at public hospitals, state medical assistance, public health programs, and particular disease treatment programs.[37] The programs tend to restrict participation on the basis of state residency, rather than alien status, but interpretation of residency had caused some access problems. Moreover, there have been recent suggestions in some states for direct and indirect limitations on aliens' access to health care that would particularly harm foreign-born women.

A state residency requirement can be problematic.[38] One argument made is that an "undocumented" alien cannot be a local resident because her presence in the United States is unlawful.[39] This position contravenes the basic notion that a residence is the place where a person lives and intends to make her home,[40] and has been largely unsuccessful in the courts.[41] However, the wording of a state statute is important. A court in California for example, found that while aliens could be residents of a California county, counties did not have to provide undocumented aliens with nonemergency care because the state statute required such care to be given to "lawful" residents.[42]

In 1994, Californians approved Proposition 187, which contains a restrictive limitation on health care access for immigrants. This law, not yet implemented because of legal challenges, allows only citizens, permanent residents, or aliens lawfully admitted for a temporary time period to receive publicly sponsored, nonemergency health care. It would exclude not only "undocumented" aliens but also all aliens who are in the process of becoming permanent residents and all aliens in an interim status that allows them to remain in the United States. Proposition 187 also requires any publicly funded health care facility to report any aliens who are ineligible for health services because of their immigration status to the Immigration and Naturalization Service. Other states are considering similar proposals.

Providing immigrant women with care for childbirth in public hospitals has caused major controversy in some states. Given the variety of expensive, difficult, and controversial medical treatments that public hospitals provide, it is odd that the simple and humane maternity care needed to guarantee an infant's and mother's health has been a special target of criticism by some public officials and news media. Critics present the scenario of a pregnant alien crossing the border for the purpose of receiving hospital care in the United States and pretending that she is a state resident without health insurance or resources to pay. This scenario, if true, instead of being considered one minor variation of fraud, somehow leads to the suggestion that the Constitution be changed so that children born in the United States not become citizens at birth.

There is no logical connection between the perceived problem and the proposed remedy. Instead, the remedy undermines an important component of democracy. The Constitution's guarantee of citizenship at birth in this country rejects the ethnic divisiveness and feudalism of the old European approach of citizenship by heritage. It is a basic component of our democracy; those born in this country and subject to its laws are its citizens, recognized for their worth as individuals, not for their family connections. Further, our laws provide a remedy for the problem of fraud. Hospitals in the United States are required to stabilize a person who is in a true emergency,[43] but this does not absolve the person of the obligation to pay for those services, nor does it prevent inquiry about payment once the emergency is treated. Moreover, fraud is a criminal offense.

Seeking Health Care Can Have Adverse Impacts on Immigrant Status
While recent publicity has focused on immigrants' utilization of health care, the real problem appears to be the opposite — the underutilization of health care by immigrants, especially of preventive and primary care. Aliens are dissuaded from getting appropriate health care by their fear that seeking medical care will lead to being reported to INS, deportation, denial of status, and inability to have family members join them. This fear is particularly strong if an alien needs publicly sponsored health care. The fear of being denied immigration status at some time in the future also leads aliens to not seek health care they cannot pay for in cash.

These fears have some basis in the law. One example that particularly affects women are immigration laws that have the effect of perpetuating domestic abuse. Abusive citizens and residents have used the immigration law to prevent alien spouses and children from seeking health care, social services, protective orders or arrest, and prosecution of their abusers.[44] While an alien spouse of a citizen or permanent resident is legally eligible to become a legal permanent resident, until recently the application process, which requires a petition, was controlled totally by the citizen or resident spouse. Without an approved petition, the alien spouse cannot legalize her immigration status, is subject to deportation, cannot work to support herself, and may be ineligible for some of the programs relied on by victims of domestic abuse. Immigrant women who are victims of domestic violence are deterred from identifying the cause of their injuries and seeking help even when the injuries from the abuse are serious.

Domestic violence is a substantial threat to the public health[45] since it is the cause of a large number of injuries for women. Spouse abuse in the United States is serious, chronic, and national in scope,[46] and the victims of domestic violence are overwhelmingly women.[47] For four years Surgeons General warned that family violence posed the single largest threat of injury to adult women.[48] One million women each year seek medical attention for injuries at the hands of male partners.[49]

The Violence Against Women Act, passed in 1994, modified, but did not eliminate, the power of citizen and resident spouses over their alien spouses immigration status. This law provides that some, but not all, abused spouses can now file petitions on their own to begin the process for gaining permanent resident status. Also, some abused spouses who have lived in the United States for at least three years may apply for suspension of deportation.[50] The biggest hurdle for an abused spouse is that she must show that she will suffer extreme hardship if deported.

The fear of losing an opportunity for permanent resident status also deters many aliens from using publicly sponsored health programs and from seeking any care for some health problems. Aliens who are eligible for resident status can lose that status if they are found to be "excludable."

The immigration law excludes aliens who are likely to become a "public charge" from becoming legal permanent residents. This economic basis for exclusion tends to harm women, particularly single parents, more than men. Women in this country on the whole earn less than men, often for the same or equivalent work. Further, the responsibility for the care of children falls more on women than men when parents split up. Generally when parents separate the economic resources of mothers diminish while those of fathers increase.

Although they are not absolute determining factors, receipt of subsidized health care and evidence of health problems do play a role in determining whether an alien will be denied permanent resident status on the public-charge basis. The potential for adverse impacts on immigration status arising from the receipt of such assistance is the greatest for aliens who are seeking to become permanent residents through close citizen or resident relatives.[51] If an alien has received medical care through a program designed to support individuals unable to provide for themselves, it is possible that she will be found likely to become a public charge. Some federal legislative proposals would go even further and consider using services like a battered women's shelter or health clinic as a factor in the public charge determination.

Ill health can also be a factor in making an alien excludable on the basis of economic status. It will be harder for an alien who is ill or has some chronic condition than for an alien who is healthy to convince government officials that she will not become a public charge. The physicians who perform medical exams of aliens applying for resident status look specifically for conditions that are significant enough to interfere with the ability to work or that may require extensive medical treatment or institutionalization in the future. If one of these conditions exists, officials may require that additional resources and health insurance be available to cover the health care costs and the living costs of the alien.

In addition to the negative immigration-status consequences from having medical conditions that impede an ability to work or are expensive to treat, having other health conditions can harm an individual's immigration status. This harm is most often suffered by those who have a legal basis to become legal permanent residents and by some permanent residents who leave the country and seek to return. This is because the application to become a resident is legally considered an "entry" into the country, even if the applicant is physically in the United States. Also, the return to the United States by a permanent resident who has left the country can be considered an entry. Therefore, several exclusion provisions based on health status may apply.

Because of the fear about immigration status, noncitizens are sometimes reluctant to admit the existence of some conditions, to the detriment of their own and others' health. Unfortunately, these conditions are also ones for which women have had difficulty in getting appropriate care and treatment. They include sexually transmitted diseases (particularly HIV infection), drug and alcohol dependence, and mental disorders. Avoiding the diagnosis of these conditions does not guarantee the grant of resident status to an applicant, because the conditions are frequently discovered in the medical examination that is required before resident status will be granted.

Aliens who have a "communicable disease of public health significance"[52] are excludable. The Secretary of Health and Human Services generally designates which diseases meet this criterion. However, Congress has amended the law to require that the HIV or AIDS virus be considered a communicable disease of "public health significance" and therefore a basis for exclusion. Under current regulations the following are the other designated communicable diseases of public health significance: chancroid, gonorrhea, granuloma inguinale, infectious leprosy, lymphogranuloma venereum, infectious-stage syphilis, and active tuberculosis.[53] An alien who tests positive for HIV infection, even without symptoms, is excludable. Further, the physician performing the immigration medical exam is directed to comply with any local laws requiring reporting of HIV-positive cases.[54]

A waiver of exclusion based on contagious disease affliction is available to certain close relatives of United States citizens or legal permanent residents. The alien must be the spouse, parent, unmarried son or daughter, or minor unmarried adopted child of a United States citizen or legal permanent resident or of an alien who has been issued an immigrant visa.[55] However, the existence of a disease, particularly HIV infection, may prompt an inquiry into whether the alien should be excluded on economic-status grounds. The inquiry would assess whether the alien will have the resources or health insurance coverage necessary for treatment and, additionally, whether the alien will have the resources for living expenses if the condition prevents work. This approach makes obtaining permanent resident status very difficult for HIV-positive aliens, even if they have obtained a waiver of the condition as exclusionary.[56]

Drug abuse and addiction can be the basis for both deportation and exclusion.[57] Further, aliens who have possessed or distributed controlled substances may have engaged in activities that could constitute a crime, thereby adding to the potential of being excluded or deported. Aliens may be reluctant to admit and get help for drug use, a fear that is warranted because drug abuse in the past can serve as the basis for an alien's deportation or denial of immigration status even if the alien is not currently a drug abuser.

Aliens with mental or physical disorders associated with certain behavior are also excludable. To form the basis for exclusion, the physical or mental disorder must be accompanied by behavior associated with the disorder that may pose or has posed a threat to the property, safety, or welfare of the alien or others. Alternatively, there must have been a history of behavior associated with the disorder that posed a threat to safety or welfare, and the behavior must be deemed likely to recur or lead to other harmful behavior.[58] The alien can demonstrate that the behavior is not likely to recur by showing that the disorder is in remission.

Alcohol abuse or dependence, by itself, is no longer a ground for exclusion, but it may be considered as an excludable mental or physical disorder. Like other physical and mental disorders, the alcoholism would have to be associated with harmful behavior. In some circumstances, exclusion based on physical or mental conditions can be waived.[59] Because existence of these disorders could have adverse consequences for immigration status, noncitizens are often reluctant to admit them and get help.

Health Care Reform Efforts and Other Proposals

While there are now many barriers to immigrant women seeking and obtaining health care, some of the recent efforts by state and federal officials to reform the health care system would make the situation worse. There seems to be a growing scapegoat mentality that blames and seeks to limit the foreign-born in education, employment, and other areas as well as health care. In the health care arena this attitude fails to acknowledge that germs and accidents do not pick their victims based upon notions of alien or citizenship status and that a community's health depends on each resident's health.

While promoting the advantages of reform, some state and federal proposals then seek to exclude various segments of the noncitizen population living in the United States. Examples include President Clinton's proposed "Health Security Act" and some state-based proposals. The usual justification for exclusion of the foreign-born is either one that expresses blatant hostility, labeling them as "other," or one that reflects misguided notions of immigration policy and "control."

Thus, proposals based on mandating employers to provide health care, like the "Health Security Act," do not always require the coverage of all aliens who have INS employment authorizations. Nor do they require coverage of the citizen family members of all alien workers. Nor do they adequately address the prevalent problem of employers who hire employees "off the books," often under health-threatening conditions. Some proposals also fail to acknowledge that there are numerous classifications of aliens who live in this country with the knowledge and acquiescence of the federal government and fail to allow the coverage of these people even to the extent currently recognized by the courts. Further, they do not guarantee three essential components of public health: universal contagious disease control, access to prenatal health care, and preventive child health care for all residents.

The proposed exclusions of noncitizens are alarming for several reasons, especially considering the proposals' promises of increased quality and cost savings by providing preventive care, early detection and treatment, and alternatives to hospital care.[60] First, there is the failure to recognize that the public health and cost-saving objectives of reform cannot be achieved if any group is excluded. Second, the adverse consequences to the public health are ignored. Third, there is a failure to recognize the reality of the country's immigration policies and practices and to include all those who are residing in the United States pursuant to those policies and practices.

Recent general sentiment against the foreign-born has also led to proposals in the guise of immigration or welfare "reform" that would impede public health, particularly for women and children. Such anti-foreign-born sentiment has occurred during various periods of American history, often during times of rapid social or economic change. Recently, this has appeared again in federal legislative proposals that have not taken into account their consequences for the public health. Some immigration "reform" proposals, such as the one considered by the Senate Immigration Subcommittee in 1995, would make noncitizens' use of public benefits for certain time periods a basis for deportation and/or denial of citizenship. The definition of public benefits or "welfare" in this proposal went far beyond the common conception of cash benefits to recipients and included the provision of health care. Health care programs that include any needs-based criteria or that limit participation by recipients of public funds could serve as the basis for deportation or denial of citizenship. This would include Medicaid but also health care provided by a public hospital or clinic on a sliding fee scale basis and programs such as battered women's shelters that receive public money.

Some "welfare" reform proposals, such as those considered by the House and Senate in 1995, would also eliminate eligibility for publicly funded, health-related programs for noncitizens and would bar certain naturalized citizens as well as aliens. Naturalized citizens would be ineligible for public health programs if they had an economic sponsor when they became a legal resident, even if the sponsor had since disappeared or refused to cooperate. This concept is particularly threatening to foreign-born women who are victims of domestic violence. For many of these women their abusive spouses were their economic sponsors. This means, for example, that they could be barred from public health care for injuries from domestic violence if the very abuser who caused the injuries did not cooperate.

The impact of limitations on health care access for the foreign born will fall heavily on women. Underlying these recent efforts is a basic blindness: there is no recognition that women and young children (who generally are in the care of their mothers) will comprise the majority of those denied access to health care.

Consequences of Barriers to Health Care Access

Immigrants are often thought of as the "others," separated from the rest of "us." But in reality, immigrants are integrated into all aspects of United States society, even at the level of the nuclear family. It is not uncommon for one spouse to be a citizen and the other an immigrant, or for a minor "undocumented" child to have a citizen sibling, as is the case with Maria's children. The barriers to one family member's health care will affect other family members. For example, the health of a citizen infant is severely threatened if an alien mother like Elizabeth does not get adequate prenatal health care.

Barriers to immigrants' health care also undermine community health.[61] An essential part of community health is contagious disease control. Since the infectious agents of diseases preventable by the use of vaccines or toxoids have not been eradicated, there is a strong public health objective for keeping immunization levels high. Any decline in these rates increases the risks of new outbreaks of these diseases with their attendant suffering, disability, and death.

Immunization for women in childbearing years is also important, not only for their health but also for the health of any children they bear. Access to health care for childhood immunization frequently depends on mothers like Maria having access to health care without fear, since mothers are predominately the primary caretakers of children.

The early detection and treatment of nonimmunizable contagious diseases are also important components of communicable disease control. For diseases such as tuberculosis, hepatitis, and venereal disease, access to primary care is essential to contain the risk of contagion. Maria, for example, should have a test for tuberculosis. Access to preventive care screenings is particularly important to avoid the spread of disease, because some diseases may be asymptomatic. These diseases need to be detected and treated in their early stages when the risk of contagion can be eliminated or reduced. For women, early detection is especially important, because there are often no early symptoms of certain sexually transmitted diseases, and pregnant women can transmit the diseases to the fetus.

Access to primary and/or preventive care for other diseases and conditions is also an important public health objective. Evelyn's situation illustrates this. Although seemingly healthy, she has not had access to health care in five years. The health of the citizen grandmother and children she cares for are intertwined with her health. Further, lack of primary medical care leads to increased costs due to delayed detection and treatment. For example, early detection and treatment of dysplasia (abnormal cell changes), accomplished through routine cervical (pap) smears, can prevent cervical cancer; receipt of prenatal care can prevent birth conditions that require expensive treatment.

Domestic abuse is also an example of broader public health concerns that are not adequately addressed when health care access is impeded. Estimates indicate that this society spends $5 billion to $10 billion a year on health care, criminal justice, and other social costs of domestic violence.[62] Shaid is harmed when she is too afraid to get help for her injuries, but the society as a whole suffers as well.

There is also an important community interest in its immigrant members' access to alternatives to inpatient hospitalizations. When a person becomes so seriously ill that inpatient hospitalization is needed, we provide health care, since as a society we do not let people die on the street. Hospitals cannot release patients until they are placed in an alternative facility or are well enough to leave the hospital. The cost of maintaining patients in acute hospitals is higher than the cost of more appropriate levels of care. These costs are paid by tax dollars or through increased hospital or health insurance rates. Further, inappropriate continuation of acute care may make inefficient use of scarce medical resources or subject the patients to unnecessary health risks, which result in additional illnesses with their attendant costs. Sean's case illustrates some potential consequences of restricting permanent residents' access to non-emergency health care. Society will pay for more costly inpatient health care, when what she needs is less expensive rehabilitation.

The United States has always been and continues to be a country of immigrants. At least half of immigrants are women, and recent studies on those labeled "undocumented" indicate that women may comprise the majority of noncitizens entering the country. Noncitizens and naturalized citizens are integrated into all parts of the United States community, even at the level of the nuclear family. The health of women and the population as a whole depends upon health care access for all its members, including the foreign-born, regardless of their citizen or alien status.

Notes

1   Houstoun, Kramer, and Barrett, "Female Predominance of Immigration to the United States Since 1930: A First Look," *International Migration Review* 18 (1984): 908, 909.

2   Immigration and Naturalization Service (INS), *1992 Statistical Yearbook of the Immigration and Naturalization Service* (Washington, D.C.: U.S. GPO, 1993), 52, Table 12.

3   Ibid., 89, Table 34.

4   J. Passel, F. Bean, and B. Edmonston, "Undocumented Migration Since IRCA: An Overall Assessment," in *Undocumented Migration to the United States, IRCA and the Experience of the 1980s*, ed. F. Bean, B. Edmonston, and J. Passel (Washington, D.C.: Urban Institute Press, 1990), 260.

5   Bureau of the Census, *1990 Census of Population, The Foreign-Born Population in the United States* (Washington, D.C.: U.S. GPO, July 1993), 1, Table 1. Of the 11,770,318 noncitizen, foreign-born individuals counted in the census, 5,819,443 were female.

6   Ibid. There were 1,266,617 noncitizen male and female children 14 years old or younger, and 5,204,481 females 15 years old and older. Women and all children 14 and younger equaled 6,471,098.

7   8 U.S.C. §§ 1101(a)(15), 1184.

8   8 U.S.C. §§ 1151, 1153, 1154.

9   8 U.S.C. § 1157.

10   Permanent residents can become naturalized citizens. 8 U.S.C. § 1427(a)(1).

11   The close relatives eligible to become permanent residents include the spouses and unmarried children of United States citizens, the parents of adult (21 or older) United States citizens, and in certain circumstances the surviving spouse of a United States citizen. 8 U.S.C. § 1151(b)(2)(A)(i). Under the immigration law, a child is a person under 21; in certain circumstances, this includes stepchildren, adopted children, orphans, and children born out of wedlock. 8 U.S.C. § 1101(b)(1). Other relatives allowed to become permanent residents are sons and daughters (adult or married children) of United States citizens, brothers and sisters of adult (21 or older) United States citizens, and the spouses and unmarried sons and daughters of permanent residents. 8 U.S.C. § 1153(a). Some federal legislative proposals would limit family-based immigrants to spouses, children, and parents of adult citizens or would eliminate sibling-based immigration.

12   There are several categories of aliens allowed to become permanent residents based on their profession or employment. These include aliens of extraordinary ability; outstanding professors and researchers; executives and managers of multinational corporations; aliens who are professionals with advanced degrees and aliens of exceptional ability in the arts, science, or business; workers who have a job offer from an employer who has filed a petition on behalf of the alien with the INS and a labor certification; some religious workers; certain nurses; and some investors in businesses in the United States. 8 U.S.C. § 1153(b).

13 Persons who are nationals of countries from which there has been limited recent immigration into the United States are also eligible to become permanent residents. This is called "diversity" immigration. 8 U.S.C. § 1153(c). Some federal legislators have proposed eliminating this provision.

14 Certain juveniles who are wards of the state can become permanent residents. If a determination has been made that it is not in the child's best interest to return to the child's native country, the juvenile is eligible for special immigrant status. 8 U.S.C. § 1101(a)(27)(J).

15 In 1986, the United States Congress passed what is known as an "amnesty" or "legalization" program. Two main groups were covered by this law: aliens who had lived in the United States since 1982 and certain agricultural workers. These aliens were eventually allowed to become permanent residents. 8 U.S.C. §§ 1160(a)(B), 1255a.

16 Aliens who have been granted asylee or refugee status are also eligible to become permanent residents. Both refugees and asylees have been determined to have a well-founded fear of persecution in their countries of origin because of their religion, nationality, political opinion, or membership in a particular social group. However, refugees have that determination made outside the United States and enter the country as refugees, while asylees make the application in the United States or at the border. 8 U.S.C. §§ 1157–1159.

17 Certain aliens with long residency in the United States can become permanent residents. Aliens who have lived in the United States since January 1, 1972, can apply for registry and become permanent residents. 8 U.S.C. § 1259(a). Also, aliens who have resided in the United States for at least seven years, who are of good moral character, and who show that their deportation would result in extreme hardship to themselves, to a United States citizen, or to a permanent resident spouse, parent, or child can be granted suspension of deportation and become permanent residents. 8 U.S.C § 1254(a).

18 8 U.S.C. § 1253(h). Another example is an alien living in the U.S. under temporary protected status. The alien is granted that status because the Attorney General has found that there are conditions in a particular country that would prevent its nationals in the United States from returning to that country—for example, armed conflict, earthquake, flood, drought, epidemic, or environmental disaster. 8 U.S.C. § 1254a.

19 This category sometimes overlaps the first and second categories because aliens who have a long United States residence or face adverse conditions in their home countries but who do not fit into a specific alien status based on long residence or a fear of persecution may nevertheless be eligible for other humanitarian-based status.

20 Aliens can be granted a status called "voluntary" departure on an extended basis because of their individual circumstances or conditions in their home countries. 8 U.S.C. § 1254(e)(1); 8 C.F.R. § 242.5. Even persons who have already been ordered deported may be granted a long-term stay of the deportation for humanitarian reasons. 8 U.S.C. § 1182(d)(5). "Parolees," "conditional entrants," and "Cuban/Haitian entrants" are aliens whom the Attorney General initially allowed to come into the United States for humanitarian reasons.

21 INS Operations Instruction 242.1(a)(22).

22 8 U.S.C. § 1255.

23 Immigration Act of 1990 § 301.

24 8 U.S.C. § 1324a.

25 Sec. 101, Act of Nov. 6, 1986, Pub. L. No. 99-603, 101 Stat. 3359, 3360.

26 42 U.S.C. §§ 1396 *et seq.*

27 *Lewis v. Grinker,* 965 F.2d 1206 (2d Cir. 1992).

28 Permanent residents who previously were temporary residents or Special Agricultural Workers (SAWs), and thereby eligible for Aid to Families with Dependent Children, are fully Medicaid eligible only if five years have passed since they were granted temporary resident SAW status; they are under 18; they are aged (65 or older); they are blind; they are disabled; or they were Cuban/Haitian entrants before becoming temporary residents or SAWs.

29 42 U.S.C. § 1396b(v)(1).

30 For a discussion of cases of permanent residence in the United States under color of law, see Robert Rubin, "Walking a Gray Line: The 'Color of Law' Test Governing Noncitizen Eligibility for Public Benefits," *San Diego Law Review* 24 (March–April 1987): 411–447; Janet Calvo, "Alien Status Restrictions on Eligibility for Federally Funded Assistance Programs," *New York University Review of Law and Social Change* 16 (1987–1988): 395, 411; Charles Wheeler, "Alien Eligibility for Public Benefits: Part I," *Immigration Briefings,* November 1988.

31 Those with status recognized by HHS as "permanently residing in the United States under color of law" includes parolees, aliens with an indefinite stay of deportation, aliens with indefinite voluntary departure, aliens on whose behalf an immediate-relative petition has been approved and their families covered by the petition, aliens who have filed applications for adjustment of status, aliens granted stays of deportation whose departure INS does not contemplate enforcing, aliens granted asylum or withholding of deportation, refugees, aliens granted voluntary departure whose departure INS does not contemplate enforcing, aliens granted deferred action status, aliens under orders of supervision, aliens who have entered and continuously resided in the United States since before January 1, 1972, aliens granted suspension of deportation, conditional entrants, and Cuban/Haitian entrants. 42 C.F.R. § 435.408; Department of Health and Human Services, *State Medicaid Manual,* Part 3, Eligibility, Transmittal No. 14 (August 1987).

32 See, e.g., *St. Francis Hospital v. D'Elia,* 71 A.D.2d 110, 422 N.Y.S.2d 104 (1979) *affirmed* 440 N.Y.S.2d 185 (1981); *Papadopoulos v. Shang,* 67 A.D.2d 84, 414 N.Y.S.2d 152 (1979).

33 42 U.S.C. § 1396b(v)(2)(A).

34 See *Salem Hospital v. Commissioner of Public Welfare,* 574 N.E.2d 385 (Mass. 1991). Contrast New York State Department of Social Services, Administrative Directive, 88 ADM 4, p. 9.

35 42 U.S.C. § 1396b(v).

36 42 U.S.C. § 1395i-2(a).

37 H.R. Rep. No. 727, 99th Cong., 2d Sess. (July 31, 1986), reproduced in U.S. Code Cong. & Admin. News 3607, pp. 3688–3689.

38 See S. Loue, "Access to Health Care and the Undocumented Alien," *Journal of Legal Medicine* 12: 271–327.

39 See L. Chavez, "Undocumented Immigrants and Access to Health Services," *Migration Today* 11, no. 1 (1983): 15–19.

40   See National Health Law Program, *Manual on State and Local Government Responsibilities to Provide Medical Care for Indigents* (Chicago: National Clearinghouse for Legal Services, 1985); Michael Dowell, "State and Local Government Legal Responsibilities to Provide Medical Care for the Poor," *Journal of Law and Health* 3 (1988–89): 1–45.

41   See *Perez v. New Mexico Dept. of Health and Social Services,* 91 N.M. 334, 573 P.2d 689 (1977) and *St. Joseph's Hospital & Med. Center v. Maricopa County,* 142 Ariz. 94, 688 P.2d 986 (1984). See also *International Health Care, Inc. v. Board of Commissioners of Blaine County,* 109 Idaho 412, 707 P.2d 1051 (Sup. Ct. 1985).

42   See *Bay General Community Hosp. v. County of San Diego,* 156 Cal. App. 3d 944, 203 Cal. Rptr. 184 (1984).

43   42 U.S.C. § 1395dd.

44   See, e.g., Hearing on Legal Immigration Reform Before the Subcommittee on Immigration, Refugees and International Law of the House Committee on the Judiciary, 101st Cong. 1st Sess., 665–668 (1989) (testimony of the Honorable Louise Slaughter, member of Congress); C. Hogeland and R. Rosen, *Dreams Lost, Dreams Found: Undocumented Women in the Land of Opportunity* (Survey Project of the Coalition for Immigrant and Refugee Rights and Services Immigrant Women's Task Force, 1990); Janet Calvo, "Spouse-Based Immigration Laws: The Legacies of Coverture," *San Diego Law Review* 28 (1991): 593–644.

45   See Council on Scientific Affairs, American Medical Association, "Violence Against Women: Relevance for Medical Practitioners," *Journal of the American Medical Association* 267 (1992): 3184–3187.

46   S. Rep. No. 545, 101st Cong., 2d Sess. (1990), 37.

47   H.R. Rep. No. 395, 103d Cong., 1st Sess. (1993), 26.

48   S. Rep. No. 138, 103d Cong., 1st Sess. (1993), 41–42.

49   S. Rep. No. 138, 103d Cong., 1st Sess. (1993), 41; S. Rep. No. 545, 101st Cong., 2d Sess. (1990), 37.

50   Pub. L. No. 103-322 6 § 241, 242.

51   Technically, this exclusion ground would also apply to an alien seeking resident status on employment-related grounds, but qualifying on such grounds generally means that the alien will have an income sufficient to preclude exclusion on the grounds of "likely to become a public charge."

52   8 U.S.C. § 1182(a)(1)(A)(i).

53   42 C.F.R. § 34.2(b).

54   Centers for Disease Control and Prevention (CDC) Technical Instructions, III-4 to III-6.

55   8 U.S.C. § 1182(g)(1).

56   See State Department cable no. 92 State-093280, reported in 69 Interpreter Releases, 516 (April 27, 1992). This cable notifies consuls that the Public Health Service has estimated that medical treatment for an HIV person through life of the illness is $85,000 and that that fact had to be considered in a determination of whether the alien would be excludable. However, the cable stated that publicly funded treatment is not always disqualifying. The alien would have to demonstrate that the treatment is available and that the government agency consented to the treatment.

57   8 U.S.C. § 1182(a)(1)(A)(iii).

58   8 U.S.C. § 1182(a)(1)(A)(ii).

59 CDC Technical Instructions, I-3.
60 See, e.g., "Health Security: The President's Report to the American People," in *The President's Health Security Plan* (New York: Times Books, 1993), 15, 17, 18, 21, 23.
61 Much of the analysis of community health is based on conversations with Victor W. Sidel, M.D.
62 S. Rep. No. 138, 103d Cong., 1st Sess. (1993), 41.

8

CULTIVATING COMMON GROUND

Women with Disabilities

. . . .

Carol J. Gill

Women and people with disabilities share some little acknowledged common ground. Both communities are large — people with disabilities number at least 43 million in this country[1] — and diverse, including all races, nations, religions, and classes. Both groups are subject to job discrimination; abuse; exposure to stressful living and working conditions; poor representation in government, media, and community institutions; personal devaluation; lack of access to leadership; physical exploitation; and paternalism in male-managed systems — much of this rationalized on the basis of biological difference. Furthermore, both groups have watched their health concerns languish on the remotest back burners of research, policy-making, and service delivery.

We who reside in the overlap of these two groups — namely women with disabilities — experience discrimination both ways. Certainly we are oppressed as women. As people with disabilities, however, we are further divested of social value, deprived even of women's traditional double-edged status of sex object on the pedestal. When a woman becomes disabled, she forfeits society's faith in her competence to produce and reproduce. Deemed unfit to make babies, households, families, and a beautiful appearance, she is left socially genderless. As illustrated in the important book *Women with Disabilities*, upon entering the world of disability, women also enter a world of "sexism without the pedestal."[2]

My own experience as a woman with a disability now spans almost four decades. My disability rights activism began in earnest about fifteen years ago, coinciding with the start of my work as a clinical psychologist in physical rehabilitation, academic, and research programs. This mix of personal, political, and professional involvement has acquainted me with people with disabilities from a broad range of backgrounds.

In the past decade, I have seen women with disabilities developing power to articulate and share our stories. Drawing strength and strategy from both the women's rights and disability rights movements, we are organizing to reject our double discrimination. Many of us work passionately to assert our rightful place in the community of all women as well as the right of all women to take their equal place in society. Much of this work focuses on health, particularly reproductive health issues. Along the way, our women, with the perseverance and creativity characteristic of the response of both the community of women and people with disabilities to oppression, have reclaimed and redefined concepts that formerly served to advance ableism and sexism.

For example, people with disabilities have begun to assail definitions of disability that are based on deficiency or the notion of individual tragedy. We have begun to recognize, even celebrate, the experiences, customs, and values we share as a community. We assert that it is society's devaluing response to the difference of disability that really handicaps people. Increasingly, people with disabilities speak of triumphing not over our disabilities but over second-rate educations, job bias, prejudice, and buildings that have stairs where ramps should be! Like women, disabled persons have had to point out that the images assigned to us are social fabrications, not natural facts of biology. Simply being physically or mentally different from average does not render someone helpless, incompetent, or suffering — any more than being a woman makes you passive, unable to compete, or brimming with maternal instinct.

Health Care in the Overlap

In the area of health, women with disabilities are doubly deprived. As women, we have suffered from the traditional disregard for women's health concerns; and as disabled people, we are often perceived as less than full human beings with less than full quality of life. Consequently, we are routinely denied health information, services, and choices that most nondisabled Americans think of as entitlements.

An additional obstacle to adequate health service delivery for disabled women is the isolation of disability within medicine. Relegated to the domain of rehabilitation medicine, disability is little studied by physicians in other areas of specialization — a compartmentalization that many disability activists view as a denial of disability as a part of life.

They complain that conditions that elude "cure" are repellent to many physicians. Furthermore, by treating disability as a unitary phenomenon, medicine neglects interacting variables such as gender.

Most medical and social scientific research on disability focuses on men. Historically, this emphasis grew out of rehabilitation medicine's concern with injured veterans returning from war. Philosophically, however, it is fueled by the notion that if disability confers passivity, dependency, and incompetence, disablement must be particularly devastating to men, whose "normal" roles are worker, sportsman, and dominant presence. For women, in contrast, disability, while unfortunate, may be viewed as conferring "more of the same" of what they already experience in their lives.

In reality, the health issues of disabled women are in many ways "more of the same" concerns that all women have. Often the obstacles we confront in obtaining health services are the problems of all women taken to the extreme. At other times, our needs differ from those of the rest of the women's community. Even when our needs are indistinguishable from those of our nondisabled sisters, the health experiences of disabled women are pertinent for all women and all health service providers.

Access
One of the first problems many women with disabilities encounter in health settings is blocked access. The barriers may be physical, such as narrow doorways that impede wheelchair use, slippery floor surfaces that aggravate walking difficulties, and examining tables that do not lower or adjust for ease in transfer and positioning. Communication barriers include lack of sign language interpreters, TTY equipment (telecommunications devices for deaf persons), signs or forms available in Braille, and instructions sufficiently clear for individuals with learning disabilities. Some barriers are programmatic, such as the staffing of clinics without assistants to help people with dressing and transfers or requiring patients to arrive for appointments too early for them to arrange for paratransit (door-to-door public transportation) where available or the services of a personal assistant. Although access barriers are preventable or remediable — there are independent living centers and other disability consumer organizations prepared to offer excellent consultation on barrier removal — they have served to exclude women with disabilities from community services, reinforcing the notion that we are so intrinsically different from all other women that we need "special" services in segregated facilities.

Privacy and Autonomy

Women with disabilities, like women in general, share horror stories of abridged health choices and of feeling treated as if the public shared ownership of our bodies. For most women, such external control focuses on protecting the socially valuable product of their uteruses and managing their power to please men. For disabled women, whose procreative and aesthetic functions are both devalued, the dynamics of control are somewhat different. Seen as too undeveloped or too damaged to fulfill our proper duties, women with disabilities are stereotyped as either perpetual children or barren crones—lacking gender in either transformation.

Our health care legacy has been a long history of medical treatment without consent, including involuntary and concealed contraception, sterilization, and abortion. Recently, a number of disabled women have been writing with considerable rage about a rarely identified form of medical abuse: being forced to disrobe and pose for display and photos in medical educational settings, often before mixed audiences of professionals and nonprofessionals.[3] Disabled women commonly report being denied critical information regarding their bodies and treatment options while being subjected to unexplained procedures and medications. Unfortunately, this is not ancient history. I have yet to attend one meeting of women with disabilities or of rehabilitation professionals where participants could not furnish current evidence of such violations.

Violence and Abuse

Personal assault is an issue of crucial concern to women with disabilities for two reasons. First, children and adults with disabilities are at significantly heightened risk for abuse compared to nondisabled people. The perceived vulnerability of disabled persons, our social isolation, and our frequent reliance on others for "hands-on" help may encourage abusers to act out their feelings of bigotry and contempt without fear of reprisal. Second, physical violence is the means by which many women acquire their disabilities in the first place. Although formal data collection has been as sparse as one might predict given disabled people's low standing in society, available reports suggest that physical and sexual abuse is the rule rather than the exception for women with disabilities.[4] An often neglected implication of this dynamic is that women who become disabled through violence enter a horrifying loop of increased risk of further assault based on their disability.[5]

Mental Health

If the average woman has difficulty developing self-confidence and positive identity in a sexist world, women with disabilities face an all-out struggle. Since self-esteem rests heavily on messages of worth from others as well as self-perception of competence and body image, women with disabilities are at a great disadvantage. We are confronted with discounting attitudes. We often receive little but discouragement even from our closest and most well-meaning friends and family regarding our appearance and our competence to work or form relationships.

Disabled women are among the most solitary of all people because, in relation not only to nondisabled women but also to disabled men, fewer marry or find permanent partners and because so many are divorced and abandoned. As one of the lowest paid and least employed groups in the country, we face the ravages of poverty and homelessness. And simply coping with the obstacles that people with disabilities face every day makes stress a way of life: lack of access to transportation, the built environment, community programs, and communication; social devaluation and defamation; inadequate education; and discrimination in jobs, housing, and services. Each day, many women with disabilities labor for hours, fighting for and worrying over their basic needs for rides, personal assistance, medical services, and adaptive equipment.

When women with disabilities experience burnout and depression, moreover, we often discover that getting the mental health services and community support we need to recover is just one more endless struggle. Many women's shelters and mental health centers are inaccessible to us due to physical and communication barriers. Residential treatment programs for substance abuse and psychiatric disorders commonly refuse women who use equipment or need physical assistance with activities of daily living. Sexual counseling, psychotherapy, and suicide intervention are rarely available from therapists who are informed about the lives of disabled people. Significantly, women with disabilities have been prominent among those receiving suicide assistance, which has garnered considerable public support. Society's apparent willingness to accept disabled women's despair while withholding support for our pursuit of a meaningful life is an ominous trend for women with disabilities who find themselves caught in the trap of depression.

Reproductive Health Issues

As it is for most women, the central reproductive health concern for women with disabilities is freedom to make our own choices. Once again, however, our experience involves some different dynamics. While our nondisabled sisters often struggle for the right to avoid or delay pregnancy, we still fight for the freedom to express our sexuality and to give birth at all. Society's discomfort with our reproductive potential is expressed as denial of our sexuality and fertility and distrust of our ability to manage our own bodies.

Consequently, decisions about our bodies are often made for us by physicians, officials, and family members. The methods of contraception most often prescribed for us are those over which we have least control: sterilization, hormone injection and implantation, and IUDs (intra-uterine devices). Not only are many of these methods associated with risk of complication for all women, but they also carry an additional unmeasured risk factor for us because the interaction of disability and reproductive health variables has never been adequately researched. We know, for example, that women with paraplegia are at greater than average risk for blood clot formation and loss of bone density. How is this level of risk affected by different forms of contraception, such as the pill, as opposed to nonhormonal methods? What changes will menopause bring to such women's lives?

Barbara Waxman, a policy analyst on disabled women's reproductive health, theorizes that society invalidates the reproductive potential of disabled women because of primitive fears that damaged women produce damaged offspring, both literally and symbolically.[6] The fear of genetic transmission of disability and the distrust of disabled women's capacity to nurture "healthy" babies lead to restrictions on our parenting options that are, according to Waxman, eugenic in intent. Keeping us genderless by discounting us as women and as sexual beings helps to prevent us from reproducing, which keeps us harmless to society. And, once we are categorized as nonbreeders, we are discarded as socially useless and join postmenopausal women in health care limbo.

Growing alarm over the eugenics threat to choice has moved some of us to challenge current practices involving prenatal screening and abortion. While few disabled women publicly endorse restricting any woman's individual right to make her own decisions about completing a pregnancy, many have expressed concerns about societal pressures on women not to bear any but physically perfect children. Several leaders in the disabled women's community have criticized the growing acceptability of "eugenic abortion" for preventing births simply on the basis of disability. They have also criticized health professionals who, acting on their own disability prejudice, fail to offer prospective parents complete and balanced information and support for raising disabled children.

The capacity of women with disabilities to express and enjoy ourselves as women is severely hampered by society's rejection of our life customs. Women who cannot or choose not to have traditional intercourse find a myriad of ways to enjoy sex with or without partners. Some of us rely on assistants to help us with preparations and positioning for lovemaking. We may negotiate with our partners to assist us with undressing, getting into bed, using adaptive equipment, and inserting contraceptive devices. In mothering our children, we operate with the same originality, flexibility, and talent for planning and problem solving. Our resourcefulness, resilience, and ingenuity could be viewed as quintessential womanhood. Yet, at almost every turn, we are told that our alternatives are illegitimate, that our ways are not the right ways. It is no wonder that so many young girls and women with disabilities feel they must hide or deny their differences and adhere to rigid, traditional sex roles to prove they can be "real" women.

Medical Negligence
In both my professional work as a clinical psychologist and my political work as a disability activist, I have been struck by the number of disabled women I have encountered whose lives were threatened by their physician's failure to investigate signs of serious conditions, including cancer, pelvic disorders, sexual dysfunction, and sexually transmitted diseases. Undoubtedly, both the tendency and the desire to view disabled women as asexual contributes to such oversight. Some women with disabilities have expressed the conviction that they are dehumanized in medical settings — viewed exclusively in terms of their disabilities, not as total persons or women.

When disability fills the lens, professionals avoid focusing on other symptoms. In working with health service providers, I have heard comments suggesting that signs of illness were overlooked in disabled persons because it was hard for the professionals to imagine "lightning striking more than once" in the same individual. In other words, the disability seemed so drastic and all-encompassing that the possibility of more illness seemed unfathomable or, perhaps, unjust. In other cases, physicians have admitted that they deliberately sidestepped disabled women's complaints, particularly those involving the reproductive system, because they felt overwhelmed by the disability and unable to handle additional problems that they judged relatively less significant. Such professionals seem uncomfortable with the idea that reproductive health problems would be "significant" to their disabled patients or that we might engage in sexual behavior like anyone else.

Disabled women commonly complain that their health service providers are unreceptive to questions about sexuality or body image. They report that their questions about subjects such as orgasm, fertility, sexual positions, childbirth, breast size, cosmetic flaws, and weight gain are often brushed off or not taken seriously. This is devastating to women who must work against social stigma to feel entitled to satisfaction with their bodies and a sense of attractiveness.

Policy Issues

Women with disabilities often find that their most basic goals are thwarted by public policies that overmedicalize and restrict their lives. A disabled woman who wants to work not only confronts discrimination in hiring and promotion on the basis of gender and disability, but if she lands a job, she may lose all her government funding for medical treatment, equipment, and personal assistance, leaving her unable to pay the inflated costs of these prerequisites to independent living. Although disability activists have been working with some success to fight such disincentives to work, many government policies still keep disabled people in the role of the dependent, needy invalid, cutting us off completely if we wish to work.

Even more irrational are policies on funds for personal assistants. For many women with disabilities, the availability of a part-time or full-time personal assistant is the deciding factor in whether or not we will be able to live in our own homes, raise families, or go to work. Whether or not funds are available for such assistance now depends on the "in-home care" policy in that person's place of residence, since each state sets its own. In many states, funds are minimal and the bureaucratic hurdles one must surmount to secure them are formidable. One of the most tragic facts of life with disability in America is that hundreds of thousands of women, men, and children with disabilities who could live in their own homes with reasonable assistance are incarcerated as "patients" in nursing homes for which the government pays many times what the personal assistance policy would cost. Disability activists across the country are joining forces to demand a national personal assistance policy that would divert funds now supporting the profitable nursing home industry into consumer-managed assistance programs that promote independence and dignity.

Another policy issue related to personal assistance funding — and one crucial to disabled women who wish to mother — is the acknowledgment of child-rearing as an "activity of daily living" for people with disabilities. Most policies governing personal assistance funding expressly exclude child care from the list of activities for which assistance is permitted. Many states are willing to pay someone to assist a disabled person with bathing, dressing, driving, food preparation, house cleaning, and even gardening, but strictly forbid any help with child care. This includes assistance as minimal as warming a bottle or helping the mother position her infant for breast-feeding. Disabled women across the country have denounced such policies as punitive and disrespectful of our right to parent as well as invasive of the private working relationship between personal assistants and the disabled persons who employ them. Because their personal assistants have been enjoined from assisting with child care tasks, some disabled mothers who lack family support and who cannot pay for private child care have permanently lost custody of their children on the grounds that they cannot provide adequate care.

National health insurance is also high on the disability rights agenda. Due to work discrimination and insurance companies that are increasingly and with impunity dropping coverage for long-term "expensive" conditions, many people with disabilities have grossly inadequate health coverage. Proposed plans to ration coverage for health care based on judgments about the effects on individuals' quality of life place some people with disabilities at great disadvantage. Disability activists are working nationally for a unified system of payment that would cover acute care not based on judgments of quality of life with disability; options for treatment and prevention; and disability-related health services, equipment, and therapy.

The passage of the 1990 Americans with Disabilities Act represented a potential improvement for people with disabilities. It mandates improved access to structures, programs, communications, and transportation, including those related to health services and information. Many women with physical, mental, and sensory disabilities are hopeful that the new law will integrate them into community services that were formerly inaccessible. Whether or not this particular dream of equality and inclusion will be realized depends, of course, on the government's commitment to implementation as well as enforcement of the act.

Future Directions

The growing empowerment of women with disabilities is visible in projects across the country that address health service issues. Several programs have been designed by disabled women to provide mentoring to adolescent girls with disabilities. Other organizations collect data on disability and parenting. The Project on Women and Disability in Boston offers, among other activities, opportunities for women with disabilities to meet in groups and share experiences, information, and consciousness about the sociopolitical issues that underlie their experiences. Programs addressing the reproductive health needs of disabled women have begun to appear in rehabilitation settings. One at the Rehabilitation Institute of Chicago is an interesting collaborative effort between community activists and rehabilitation professionals to develop medical, psychosocial, research, and resource information regarding disabled women's reproductive health.

More than ever, women with disabilities realize the importance of organizing to demand inclusion in planned and existing health programs at the same time that we continue to work collectively for policy changes that acknowledge our right to quality health services, information, and choices. Our growing consciousness and willingness to join forces promise to increase our political strength. We must also push for greater self-determination in making health decisions that affect our lives. For too long we have been forced to play the role of passive recipients, while our families and professionals made decisions about our needs. Now we are experiencing that heady realization, familiar to other minority communities, that we are the authentic experts about our own needs. We are demanding, therefore, more input and decision-making authority in the programs that serve us. We are also beginning to expect acknowledgment and compensation for our skills and efforts, and as a result we are pursuing paying jobs and positions of leadership on policy boards in, among others, the organizations that provide our services.

We must persist in communicating our experiences to other groups with whom we share common issues and, we hope, potential for collective political action. We must also continue to define and secure our place in both women's and disability organizations. Unfortunately, we are still confronting ableism in some feminist groups and sexism in some disability rights groups, both of whom frequently dismiss our issues. The successes of the DisAbled Women's Network (DAWN) in Canada in allying with women's organizations[7] and the confrontation of sexism in the disability rights movement of other countries give us hope. Most important, perhaps, is that we continue to turn to each other to validate our needs and experiences — to bolster each other's worth both as women and as people with disabilities, no longer willing to apologize on either count.

Notes

This chapter originally appeared in *Health/Pac Bulletin* 22, no. 4 (Winter 1992); it is reprinted here by permission of the publisher.

1   This figure, cited in the text of the Americans with Disabilities Act, includes people with physical, sensory, and mental impairments and chronic illnesses that substantially limit life activities.

2   M. Fine and A. Asch, eds., *Women with Disabilities: Essays in Psychology, Culture, and Politics* (Philadelphia: Temple University Press, 1988).

3   D. G. McKeen, "Such a Good Little Patient," *Disability Rag* (July/August 1992): 43; L. Blumberg, "Public Stripping," *Disability Rag* (January/February 1990): 18–20.

4   E. Bellone and B. F. Waxman, *Sexual Assault and Women with Disabilities: An Overview* (monograph) (Los Angeles: Planned Parenthood, 1983).

5   J. Panko Reis, personal communication, September 9, 1992.

6   B. F. Waxman, "Up Against Eugenics: Disabled Women's Challenge to Receive Reproductive Health Services," *Sexuality and Disability* (forthcoming).

7   B. S. Klein, "We Are Who You Are: Feminism and Disability," *Ms.* (November/December 1992): 70–74.

9

REFORMING THE PROVISION OF MENTAL HEALTH TREATMENT

. . . .

Susan Stefan

Introduction

Every year an estimated three quarters of a million women are institutionalized because of mental problems,[1] and hundreds of thousands of women receive mental health treatment.[2] The consequences for women of mental health problems, or of being labeled as having mental health problems, can be extremely severe. "Treatment" such as psychotropic medication can be imposed on an institutionalized person against her will, an act of physical intrusion that is often forced on a woman after a struggle. Negative consequences do not end with discharge or release from the hospital. A diagnosis of mental illness or a history of institutionalization may result in social stigma, destroy opportunities for employment, friendship, and romantic relationships,[3] and affect a woman's custody of her children.[4]

The problems women face in the mental health system have largely been ignored by feminists. Women's groups whose efforts are devoted specifically to health reform issues rarely include mental health as a principal part of their agenda. Even when these concerns are included, the scope of reform is usually limited to proposals for more funding for research and screening.[5] Yet many of the issues raised by mental health treatment are extremely salient to feminism: unwanted and physically intrusive treatment; coercion into roles of passivity and dependence, and punishment for stepping outside the bounds of these roles; construing "unfeminine" behavior as symptomatic and deviant; and separating women from their children. Although feminists have vocally opposed some forms of forced treatment—for example, the relatively rare unwanted cesareans performed on pregnant women—they have paid little attention to the daily imposition of unwanted electric shock, seclusion and restraint, and forcible medication in institutional settings.

It is obvious that mental health treatment raises unique questions for those who wish to reform the health care system in the United States. It is an "illness" whose very existence is questioned by some licensed practitioners in the field[6] and by many patients who were forced to accept treatment they did not want and insist to this day that they did not need.[7] Unlike other medical specialties, the conventions of the American Psychiatric Association are regularly picketed by angry ex-patients. Diagnoses such as homosexuality or proposed diagnoses such as self-defeating personality disorder are dropped as a result of lobbying and advocacy by their opponents. Meanwhile, psychiatric diagnoses such as caffeine withdrawal are being proposed.[8] Mental health is the only area of health care where treatment can be imposed on a strenuously objecting patient against her will.[9]

The frequent disagreement in the public mental health system between doctor and patient over whether the patient is actually ill or needs treatment; the power of the doctor to unilaterally impose unwanted treatment; and the political implications of some diagnostic categories make it crucial to consider whether and how mental health treatment should be included in health care reform, and its definition and scope for purposes of coverage.

This chapter begins with a look at definitions of mental illness and how these affect women. It then examines the effect of violence and threats of violence on women's emotional well-being, and the response of the mental health profession. Finally, it outlines how the delivery of mental health services might be reformed to be sensitive to the needs and concerns of women and describes where current health care reform proposals meet those needs and where they could be modified to address them.

Definitions of Mental Illness and Their Impact on Women

There exist several competing models or theories of mental illness. The "medical model" posits that mental illness is a result of neurochemical imbalances in the brain, which can be treated through biological treatments such as psychotropic medication or electroconvulsive therapy (ECT). The argument that mental illness is simply another disease is the driving argument behind the demand that benefits for mental health treatment receive parity with other health care benefits.

The older psychoanalytical model found the causes of mental illness in early childhood relations with parents and the child's attempts to cope with his or her emerging sexuality. The psychosocial rehabilitation model focuses on teaching social functioning and attributes deficits in social functioning to a variety of environmental causes, including the stresses of poverty, poor prenatal care, and experience of violence in childhood, adolescence, and adulthood. Finally, some mental health professionals and ex-patient activists argue that there is no such thing as mental illness in the medical sense: that attributions of mental illness are simply social labels for deviant and unacceptable behavior.[10]

Obviously, this summary simplifies a very complex topic: there is stronger evidence for the biological origins of some diagnoses, such as bipolar disorder, than for others, such as the personality disorders. While schizophrenia apparently is found in countries around the world,[11] anorexia, bulimia, and other eating disorders are unknown outside western cultures.[12]

In addition to the problems posed to structuring health care reform by a proliferation of models of mental illness, there is the additional problem of the unthinking stigma and discrimination against persons who have been diagnosed as mentally ill, a social reaction that leading mental health scholar Michael Perlin has called "sanism."[13] He has identified a number of stereotypes and mythologies that the public associates with mental illness, including the belief that mentally ill people will exhibit random violence or that they are childlike. These myths serve to trivialize and discredit the human being being labeled as much and in the same way as racism or sexism obscures the individuality of African-Americans and women. These constructs can be contradictory: insurance benefits for mental illness are inferior to those for "physical" illness because people believe that mental illness is easily fabricated and mental health professionals easily deceived, but at the same time society trusts the conclusions of mental health professionals on the basis of a fifteen-minute examination that an individual should be involuntarily detained and deprived of liberty, often for months or years. In addition, mental illness, like AIDS, is associated in the minds of many people with bad character; it is the only "illness" that is regularly inquired into by character investigations for professional licensing. This, too, is sanism, according to Professor Perlin.

One of the most pronounced characteristics of "sanism" is a general resistance to recognizing that people who are labeled mentally ill have a gender and sexuality. The notion that women's mental health needs might differ from those of men is rarely addressed. Even more rarely are policy questions arising out of gender and sexuality, such as contraceptive and reproductive rights of women in the mental health system, examined and resolved. This blindness to gender issues has resulted in gaps in the delivery of mental health care to women and in the proposals for health care reform in the area of mental health treatment.

The model of mental illness accepted by decision makers, and the extent to which they have absorbed and incorporated stereotypes and myths about mental illness, will make an enormous difference to the coverage accorded to mental illness under any national health care plan. Because the medical model appears to hold the most promise for funding of treatment, many have embraced it. However, a disease model for emotional distress may carry hidden problems for women and minorities and others whose distress and discontent may be due to their social circumstances, but which the disease model places squarely on deficits in their biological makeup.

When an individual's problems are accepted by herself and by society as medical — and especially psychiatric — they are rarely the impetus for action in the political sphere, either by the individual herself or by others. The sufferers are sick and not the society. This is particularly true when the illness carries the stigma and taint of mental illness. The medical model of mental illness, which by definition links the pathology to the patient, is thus not a neutral or objective perspective, but a highly political and conservative structuring of the world.

As one writer has noted about the medical model:

> what is repressed out of the medical model of mental illness is that dimension which considers the person an active social agent defined by what class, community and history have meant for him . . . disease is something going on within a person rather than in the entire relationship between the self and the world; and it is to be remedied by individual or particular action.[14]

To reject the biological disease model of mental illness does not necessarily mean that there is no place for mental health care in health care reform proposals or that mental illness itself is a social construct. There is ample precedent for a "public health" approach, such as was launched to fight tuberculosis. This approach is being pursued in the area of domestic violence. A public health approach does not deny the existence of the condition, but looks to the environment that breeds and exacerbates the problem rather than seeking to treat each patient, one at a time.

The fact that people sometimes behave in disturbed or irrational ways and that individual treatment may help some people does not necessarily mean that the only appropriate treatment is individual and medical nor that the problem as a whole can be solved by individualized treatment. The cancer caused by the Love Canal contamination, the asbestosis cases resulting after manufacturers concealed their knowledge of the dangers of asbestos, and alcoholism among Native Americans living on reservations could also be characterized as solely medical/biological problems to be treated on an individual-by-individual basis. Each case of cancer or asbestosis or alcoholism is real enough, but the big picture does not make sense until you look beyond the individual and the medical.

The psychiatrist Teresa Bernardez has proposed the following analogy, which I would like to expand upon: if you put a normal healthy foot in a shoe that is one size too small, after a while your foot will eventually have actual, genuine, medical problems.[15] This society is for many women one size too small for our energies and aspirations; violence constricts us on all sides. The answer is both to treat the foot and change the shoe. Even though the foot has real and serious medical problems, treating the foot will never help over the long haul until the shoe is changed. And if you treat the foot without changing the shoe, no treatment will help the foot after awhile.

The medical model of mental illness focuses solely on the foot. If health care reform proposals are to encompass the shoe, preventive care must be funded (in the same way that mammograms and pap smears are funded to alleviate both the suffering and expense of treatment for advanced breast and cervical cancer); psychosocial treatments and therapy must be covered, not simply medication; and coverage must be tipped in favor of community rather than institutional care. Finally, the sort of massive public education programs that succeeded in decreasing cigarette smoking and increasing use of seat belts must be targeted at explaining that violence against women is a public issue — a criminal justice priority and a public health priority — that it is neither a private nor a privileged activity. Increasingly, researchers and advocates are realizing that understanding women's mental illness almost always leads back to variations on the theme of violence in our society.

The Effects of Violence on Women's Mental Health

Women live under a constant and real threat of violence by men, especially those with whom they are intimate. In the United States, every eighteen seconds a woman is beaten; every three and one-half minutes, a woman is a victim of rape or attempted rape. More than half (57 percent, to be exact) of all violent crimes against women are committed by acquaintances (compared with 37 percent for men). Seventy-seven percent of the victims of violent crimes committed by relatives are women.[16] For a long time, domestic violence was not accepted as a reality in the mental health system, even after it was recognized as a national epidemic by others.

To this day, psychiatric hospitals admit women, provide treatment, and discharge them without ever asking whether they have been victims of sexual abuse or violence. Several studies in recent years have uncovered startling information:

–A recent survey of female psychiatric inpatients in the *American Journal of Psychiatry* revealed that 72 percent reported a history of physical or sexual abuse; 54 percent were sexually abused, of these, almost half (44 percent) reported sexual abuse before the age of 16. Most of this childhood sexual abuse was perpetrated by fathers and brothers.[17]

–A study in the *American Journal of Psychiatry* found that of the female patients in a state hospital unit who were chronically institutionalized and actively psychotic, 46 percent reported histories of childhood incest. The study discussed the implications of a possible relationship between incest and severe, intractable psychotic disorder.[18]

–Compared to nonbattered women, battered women are five times more likely to attempt suicide and three times more likely to be diagnosed with a mental disorder. Thirty-eight percent of battered women are diagnosed as depressed or having another disorder and 10 percent become psychotic.[19]

This means one of two things. Either 72 percent of women in our society are physically or sexually abused and half are victims of incest, which would mean that these women in institutions represent a fair statistical sample of women in society; or, alternatively, men's violence and sexual abuse is a very powerful determinant in driving women crazy, and driving them straight into institutions.

The failure to inquire into a woman patient's history of sexual abuse is common.[20] By ignoring histories of sexual abuse, the psychiatric profes-

sion controls the development of knowledge about the connection between sexual abuse and craziness, and shapes the way in which women
are perceived when they first enter treatment. That in turn has both
clinical and political consequences. The failure to ask about a history of
sexual assault implies that it is not relevant to the woman's current mental health problems or to her treatment. The failure to ask also means
that knowledge is not accumulated, and that lack, that absence of statistics, in turn means that officially the problem does not exist.[21]

If, as rarely happens, women answer questions that have not been
asked and tell about physical or sexual abuse, they are still ignored. Kurz
and Stark, for example, learned in 1987 that while 75 percent of battered
women volunteered the information that they had been abused, doctors
acknowledged the problem in only 5 percent of the cases.[22] When there
is a response, it is often inappropriate; battered, raped, or abused women
are given medication or shock treatment, or blamed for not leaving the
men who abuse them. One study of the quality of treatment of abused
women at general hospitals, not psychiatric hospitals, found:

> Interestingly, however, although abuse is not officially acknowl-
> edged, abused women are treated differently from other women.
> What we call an "implicit diagnosis" starts with denial of care or the
> prescription of inappropriate pain medication, progresses through
> the frequent use of tranquilizers and often ends with frankly puni-
> tive referrals to state institutions.[23]

Finally, "syndromes" have been created to categorize those who suffer from violence: rape trauma syndrome, battered woman's syndrome,
incest survivor's syndrome, self-defeating personality disorder. Thus,
women who experience violence are labeled, and their response to the
violence is categorized as an illness that requires treatment. The violence itself becomes invisible. While violence causes a great deal of
emotional as well as physical suffering, turning women's social experiences of suffering and violence at the hands of men into psychiatric
categories has its price. If a certain reaction to incest or rape or battering
is labeled a syndrome or disorder, the assumption seems to be that there
is a right and wrong way to react to these events, or at least a healthy and
unhealthy way to react. Psychiatric categories inherently describe abnormal or pathological symptoms or reactions.[24] This delegitimizes the
spectrum of personal reactions in these cases and makes the victim the
sick one rather than the attacker.

The labeling of these reactions to rape, battering, or incest as medical conditions that require treatment privatizes those reactions. Freud asked: "What do women want?" A good first step to answering this question is that women want men to stop driving them crazy. They want events like rape and battering and incest to be seen for what they are: violence inflicted on them by others and not violence that they themselves somehow attract; they want to stop having their suffering compounded by institutionalization and medication in a society where violence is the norm and the casualties are considered the social aberrations.

Women and Mental Health Treatment: The Need for Reform

Of course, a critique of the etiology of mental illness is no reason to attack the act of treatment. We may justly criticize a violent society without calling for emergency rooms to close or the wounded to go untreated. The foot, after all, must get treated. But what happens to the institutionalized woman in the name of treatment only exacerbates the problems that brought her to the attention of the mental health system in the first place. Institutions are not a treatment setting so much as the town dump for America's City on a Hill, the place for the wreckage of a violent, patriarchal society with no mercy for its injured or its poor. It is at the same time a painfully accurate and even intensified mirror of that society, so that those who have been injured in the process of getting there are hurt even more once they are there. Institutions are places where the price for a sexist and violent society are paid.

Institutions are hierarchical places with clear divisions of power. The key issue is control. In fact, control is transformed into treatment through the often heard platitude that "the patient needs structure." In the name of "structure," a patient's daily schedule is utterly predetermined, the rules are strict, and there is little choice left to the patient. For example, in one case in south Florida, patients were skipping out of their horticultural therapy and library therapy to take walks on the grounds in the springtime. The hospital responded by forbidding the patients to go outside at all for a week, and then instituted a system whereby patients "earned" what were called "grounds privileges."[25]

Institutions are also often violent places, from which no escape is possible. Dissent is diagnosed, criticism or resistance is a symptom, overt anger is severely punished, and attempts to exercise choice are met with hostility. Every behavior is medicalized and turned back on the patient. As one woman ex-patient wrote of her experience in an institution:

If I stay in my room they tell me I'm withdrawing and that's sick. If I join the girls in ward activities and start to have fun they tell me I'm being manic and that's sick. They want me to have friends but they say my relationship with Maggie [another girl on the ward] is sick . . . And when I get angry and tell them to mind their own fucking business they say I'm hostile. And you know, only sick people are hostile. Nobody takes you seriously, that's the worst part of it. And it's the most demoralizing experience in the world not to be taken seriously.[26]

One of the most pervasive aspects of institutional and community treatment of persons with mental illness — and the issue where feminist and ex-patient concerns seem to overlap most clearly — is the use of psychotropic medication to treat women labeled as mentally ill. Studies show that, overwhelmingly, women receive most of the psychotropic medication.[27] While the literature is somewhat problematic, because the definition of "psychotropic" drugs varies from study to study,[28] the figures are still staggering. For example, one study showed that 73 percent of psychotropic drug prescriptions written by doctors are written for women, and 27 percent are written for men.[29] Another noted that, although women made up 58 percent of all outpatient doctor visits, they received 78 percent of all psychotropic drug prescriptions.[30] Women also get the majority of electric shock treatments.[31] At least one psychiatric textbook recommends a higher voltage for women, and women tend to be subject to shock many more times in the course of treatment than men.[32]

One explanation is that ECT is used to treat depression, and a much greater proportion of those who suffer from depression are women. This may well be true, but it does not answer why the most intrusive therapies (such as ECT) are prescribed for conditions that are generally known to affect women. For example, the majority of psychosurgery is performed on women.[33] Although its use is much diminished, it has been suggested in extreme cases of anorexia, which is primarily a disorder affecting women.[34] Eating disorders themselves are another example of medicalizing what is in many ways a political and social issue.[35]

Not only are women subjected to most of the medication, ECT, and psychosurgery, they often receive these treatments as the result of a doctor or psychiatrist misdiagnosing a physical condition as a mental problem.[36] Women have a tremendous credibility problem, and it carriers over to their interaction with doctors.

Finally, the prescription of medication and other treatments often reinforces a woman's perception that something is the matter with her rather than with the situation in which she finds herself. The use of medication may also make it more difficult to solve the underlying problem that makes her anxious or depressed in the first place. With medication, women are placed in the all-too-familiar "sick role"; the goal of treatment is to reduce symptoms of anxiety or depression and help the patient cope by promoting a passive and disempowered stance. To summarize, in the words of one commentator, medication has

> been used frequently to silence the distress of women and to diminish the conscious pain they are suffering. If you believe anxiety and depression are signs of a problem that needs to be addressed, a diminution of such symptoms is not only not helpful but perhaps harmful. It is therefore important in the case of women and medications to look at when and why they are prescribed and whether they are being used to silence rightful complaints or anger about husband, job or family which others prefer not to hear.[37]

Current health care reform proposals appear to be tilted in favor of treatment through medication over other forms of treatment that are less biologically oriented. These coverage choices, apparently made because drugs are cheaper than other forms of therapy, are both short-sighted and, in the long run, damaging to women.

Health Care Reform of the Mental Health System: A New Feminist Perspective

While new attention is being focused on women's health needs, this has often been limited to an insistence on more research into breast cancer and osteoporosis, with no mention of mental illness at all. Even groups such as the Society for the Advancement of Women's Health Research, which does devote attention to women's mental health issues, primarily emphasizes increasing biological and drug-related aspects of research.[38]

I have tried to suggest that a mental health system responsive to the needs of women would require transformation — not more of the same research, based on the same assumptions and applied in the same framework. What would a mental health system look like if it were created by feminists with women's needs in mind?

Mental health reform from a feminist perspective means two basic things. First, it would create a system that recognizes and provides for women's specific gender-related issues, such as reproductive capacity, child custody, and the effects of living with the constant threat of sexual violence. Second, it would also be a system that functioned for all people, regardless of gender, on the basis of feminist principles.

Feminist principles suggest that the mental health system should replace hierarchy with participation and choice, enforced dependency with enhanced control, isolation with connection, models of pathology with models of recovery and strength, and objectification and a primarily biological model with an understanding of people as humans interacting with each other and operating in a social context that has a vast influence on their behavior and mental health.

These are more than simply overarching principles devoid of practical applications. Their effort on health care can be seen in the area of childbirth, which has been subject to a variety of feminist reforms encompassing these principles, resulting in significant changes in the use of anaesthesia, the presence of a supportive spouse, the environment of the delivery, and funding of alternatives such as midwifery. Such a perspective applied to mental health care could also radically transform the current mental health system in many ways. Feminist principles suggest change in a number of specific and concrete areas.

From Isolation to Connection
The current mental health system is predicated on a model of the mentally ill individual as an atomized, isolated, pathological individual suffering from an illness rooted in biology and principally responsive to biological forms of treatment, such as medication. Mental illness is conceptualized as a disease of brain disfunction or abnormality, which may be triggered by stressful situations, but which is essentially biological in origin and treatable through chemicals administered to the patient. The illness is located in the individual, which isolates the problem with the patient and takes little account of relationships or social context.

This means that individuals are isolated at every juncture. For example, state mental hospitals, especially in the Western states, are often located in remote rural areas, far from urban centers. People who are committed to these institutions are uprooted from whatever area is familiar to them and transported to places where it is extremely difficult for family members or friends to visit or take them out for a short time. Visitation is not only inconvenient; it is often discouraged. Even in institutions located in urban areas and even in private institutions, visitation is a "privilege," whose denial is often used as punishment for misbehavior.

Upon institutionalization, many women lose their children to the foster care system, cannot visit them, and ultimately may never regain custody. Within institutions, people are isolated from their communities and from the communities surrounding the institution. While most general hospitals are filled with family members and friends, and people can walk in at almost any time, psychiatric institutions are closed off and secretive, ostensibly for the protection of patients. Yet many of the patients long for contact with the outside world. If the isolation or denial of visitation or lack of access to the public makes the patients angry or frustrated or very depressed, they are isolated even further in seclusion rooms.

When discharged, individuals who are lucky enough to have community placements are often sent to the local version of a community residential facility — a halfway house or transitional housing or board-and-care or alternative community living facility. These are houses for four to twelve persons with mental disabilities, and are often located in industrial areas or poor neighborhoods that lacked the political clout to successfully oppose them. These facilities do not allow women to live with their children. The neighborhoods are often squalid, unsafe, and crime-ridden. Violence and the fear of violence is pervasive. Life in the community can be just as isolating as life in an institution.

Moreover, few state-funded mental health programs specifically address the needs of mothers.[39] In a 1990 survey of state hospital visitation practices, for example, "no state reported having a specific statewide policy regarding visitation between a hospitalized mentally ill mother and her children."[40] One of the few programs that does include children, the Elizabeth Stone House in Jamaica Plain, Massachusetts, is funded in large part by donations and private grants.[41]

Yet women are mothers and daughters, sisters and lovers. Over and over again, I have seen women who appear to be psychotic or severely disturbed pull themselves together to care for their children. The most motivated struggle for stability is that of the mother whose children require it. I have spoken with institutionalized women and ex-patients whose greatest rage or most profound depression arises from the fact that their journey through the mental health system deprived them of their children. Most institutions, however, are indifferent to the pain of women recently separated from their children.

Both women and men draw strength and identity from caring for and being cared for by others. A feminist mental health system would see the individual as connected in a variety of ways to a variety of people. It would conceptualize both the individual's distress and recovery as connected to the relational dynamics between the person and the people around them. Some forms of family therapy make this connection, but only as they pertain to an individual's family; rarely are the individual's ties to any larger community considered. Much of the psychosocial rehabilitation movement also recognizes this, but psychosocial rehabilitation is increasingly underfunded in an era where mental illness is located in an individual's biology.[42]

A feminist mental health system would see the individual's best hope for recovery in repairing and maintaining connections with those who could provide support and solace. It would seek to effectuate, encourage, and maintain connections that gave the individual strength while giving the individual support to transform or sever relationships that were causing pain and disfunction.

In concrete policy terms, this means an end to large state hospitals located in remote rural areas. Smaller acute-care units scattered throughout communities would enable those who need acute care to remain in places with which they are familiar. Such facilities and hospitals would have liberal visitation policies, especially for mothers and children. Visitation and open access would be the rule, not the exception. Mental health systems would take responsibility for coordinating such visitation with state foster care and child welfare agencies. There would no longer be the assumption that institutionalization is the first step down an inevitable road to loss of custody.

Community residential and programmatic alternatives would permit women to live with their infants and toddlers and to receive assistance in parenting and child care that is sensitive to cultural context. The Elizabeth Stone House in Massachusetts, for example, operates a therapeutic community for women and children, as well as a transitional housing program. In both programs women who are in emotional distress can live with their children and get support to improve their emotional and social circumstances.

In addition to alternative types of community programs, housing would be financed and housing subsidies such as Section 8 made more easy to negotiate. Many individuals could live on their own in the community with the help of visits from providers of home-based services or behavioral aide services. Current health care reform proposals include coverage only for aides for physically disabled people without recognizing the profound and cost-effective assistance that similar help for people with mental disabilities can provide.

Respite care programs would be supported so that parents who were living with their children could seek help before tensions escalate to violence or a total breakdown of family ties. These programs are also far more cost-effective than paying for institutionalization or even community residential programs. Home health care programs and support would be mandated if they provided a less expensive alternative for care. At present, for example, Medicaid waiver programs exist that would allow many physically disabled persons to receive home-based treatment with federal Medicaid funding (the so-called Katie Beckett waivers), but only twenty-six states have adopted the legislation necessary to take advantage of these programs, and of these, almost none are used to fund services for people with mental illness in their homes.[43]

Of course, not all personal relationships are supportive or give strength. As noted earlier, a feminist mental health system would recognize the damaging as well as the strengthening impact of relationships on people's mental health. In fact, one of the principal reasons that some institutions that otherwise follow a biological model of mental illness forbid or control visitation in general is that many family relationships can be the source of many women's disturbance and unhappiness; yet these institutions unhesitatingly discharge women back into these families.

The proposals for reform contained here are thus aimed primarily at supporting a mother's relationship with her child. Such support almost always correlates positively with increased stability and decreased craziness on the part of women diagnosed with mental illness.[44]

In a mental health system sensitive to women's concerns, agency directors who created and funded mental health services would be aware when their clients had been victims of sexual abuse, as well as sensitive to the stress of violence and fear of violence in every woman's life. Directors of institutions and professionals within institutional settings would take affirmative steps to prevent sexual abuse. This includes the provision of sex education in institutions as well as programs to help women gain skills to help prevent sexual assaults, including self-defense training and assertiveness training. It means having policies that do not permit male orderlies or attendants to be alone with women patients, particularly women who are medicated or in restraints. Sexual assault or advances by professionals on their patients would be taken as seriously as a physical attack by the professional on the patient and punished accordingly.

Furthermore, women would be assisted in terminating relationships of abuse and violence, rather than encouraged to return to them and work them out. Some community mental health programs have battered women's programs, where women are supported and encouraged to be independent and strong, rather than diagnosed to discover why they incite violence in their partners.

From Attributions of Disease to Examinations of Social Context
While a feminist mental health approach would pay more attention to the interrelationship between the individual and his or her family, a feminist mental health system would also respond to the interrelationship between social systems and the individual. This means, for example, understanding that the appropriate response to severe depression in an indigent woman who has children and lives in a crime-ridden neighborhood on inadequate social assistance or to the depression of a woman in a physically abusive relationship might not be medication or even individual psychotherapy, but a focus that supports the efforts of women to cope and works to help them gain the resources — economic as well as emotional — to change or leave the abusive situation.

It would mean understanding that violence on the part of someone who has been labeled mentally ill might be a sign of the remnants of health and self-regard rather than a particularly malignant symptom of an intractable disease. Hostility and anger are responses all of us feel when we are treated with condescension or arrogance, even more so when we are ignored altogether. In persons with diagnoses of mental illness, all reactions of hostility or frustration are simply chalked up as symptomatology. And yet voters and taxpayers who are angry with insensitive government bureaucracy and burdensome and incomprehensible regulations and endless forms rarely pause to envision the frustration of a person with a mental disability struggling to negotiate the complexity of applying for government disability benefits such as Supplemental Security Income (SSI) or Medicaid. These forms are so complicated, and many office workers so unhelpful and overloaded, that often the most severely disabled people simply give up.[45]

In concrete policy terms, recognizing social context means that community residential facilities and supported housing would be provided to women in safe neighborhoods. Community mental health centers would be easily accessible and would provide on-site child care for both the people who work in the centers and the clients.

In addition, police would receive training that would make it more likely that they would respond understandingly and promptly to calls for help from people they perceived as mentally ill, and would be far less likely to shoot them in moments of uncertainty about their intentions. The media regularly publishes stories of persons with mental illness — often women — shot and killed by police.[46]

At every governmental level — federal, state and local — the mental health system would streamline and redesign programs meant to provide assistance to people with disabilities. It would place a premium on treating a person with respect. This is being done in some places already. For example, one Florida Health and Rehabilitative Services administrator ordered the 4,500 employees she supervised to be courteous on the telephone and make eye contact with the citizens to whom they provide services. Four violations of these rules would be grounds for termination.[47]

Suggestions by some to place priority on matching clients and caseworkers by cultural and community backgrounds would be heeded over insistence on credentials.[48] A feminist recognition of the importance of experience over credentials is not necessary to see that a master's degree in psychology is unlikely to help the mental health worker who does not speak Spanish or Creole or Vietnamese if that is the primary language of his or her clients. Personal knowledge of the customs and culture of Puerto Rico may help with a Puerto Rican client more than hours of continuing education credit on cultural sensitivity.

From Denigration to Affirmation

Many women show remarkable strength and survival skills when confronted with draining and terrifying situations that last months or years. Women are expected to provide nurturance and support to family members who are sick or disabled or elderly. Women take care of grandchildren, nieces, and nephews whose parents are sick, in jail, or dead. This adds tremendous strain to their lives, and yet many women struggle with multiple demands, live in poverty, and face crime and harassment from men on the street as well as police or welfare workers or others who are employed to protect and serve their needs.

However, when such women seek support because of the enormous stresses under which they function, the mental health system, oriented to deficiencies and impairments, sees deficits rather than strengths, symptoms rather than coping strategies.[49] Often women who are rightly angry and frustrated have their anger and frustration labeled as symptoms of a mental illness. Once labeled as mentally ill, these women find that all their emotional reactions — anger, tears, frustration — are seen as further evidence of mental illness. And the parts of their lives that give them strength and encouragement — children, jobs, and friends — are at risk if they are diagnosed as suffering from severe mental illness, particularly in an institutional setting.

This search for deficiency and impairment is a product both of deeply ingrained theories of the mental health profession and of practical requirements of insurance and governmental reimbursement. Time spent preventing a crisis or giving support is not reimbursable. In order to be compensated, a professional must diagnose the client. No diagnosis, no reimbursement, no help. Out of this fact many diagnoses are born. But diagnoses carry a great many consequences for the people diagnosed. This is because a diagnosis is by definition "the process of identifying specific mental or physical disorders."[50] There is no such thing as a diagnosis that the *situation* in which an individual finds herself is irrational, pathological, or disordered. Either the person herself is diseased, and thus entitled to help, or she is not. If she is not diseased, she receives nothing. In addition, because women tend to be more likely than men to seek treatment when they are under heavy strain, the weight of the problem of stigmatizing diagnoses rests more heavily upon them.

Given the emphasis on prevention in other areas of health care — such as prenatal and well-baby care, diet counseling, etc. — the failure to permit people to seek help unless they are diagnosed as disordered seems imprudent and cost-inefficient. Prevention is the centerpiece of many plans for health care reform, both because it is more humane to prevent people from suffering than to heal them after they are already ill and because it is much less expensive to do so. Promotion of good eating habits is less expensive than coronary bypass surgery, even if the promotion ends up helping people who would never have had heart problems in the first place. The same is true of mammograms in women over 50; we do not require a diagnosis before these forms of health care are funded.

Furthermore, there is an increasing emphasis on transferring care from expensive hospital and nursing home settings into the person's home, in the form of subsidizing home health care and aides for people with physical disabilities. The obvious parallels in mental health care are to promote care in the home and the community over the more expensive institutional alternatives.

The psychosocial rehabilitation model of mental health treatment already emphasizes housing, providing the support necessary to maintain or resume meaningful employment, and helping to establish a supportive community. It does so, however, from the perspective of re-habilitating a disabled individual rather than helping a person cope with almost insuperable real, external causes of pain and misery. What the psychosocial model has failed to do is provide assistance with children, child care and parenting skills training, self-defense training, and other skills needed primarily by women.

When the Elizabeth Stone House was founded in 1974, it was de-signed specifically to meet these needs. As a former resident of the House stated:

> I needed a place where I was safe from violence and where I could be myself and be cared for, for who I am, rather than for what others wanted me to be . . . if I have to say what's the most important thing I've gotten at the Elizabeth Stone House, I'd say it's the chance to have an ordinary life and to be a strong woman.[51]

The emphasis on promoting women's own strength appears throughout the Elizabeth Stone House's materials, which discuss women in emo-tional distress and not diagnoses or stereotypes. As Jean Baker Miller, a board member, put it: "There are few places in the world which convey the basic thought: We want you to be a strong woman. The Elizabeth Stone House is one of those places." There can be others.

From Objectification and Coercion to Participation and Choice

Perhaps the single most distasteful and controversial aspect of the men-tal health system is that it infantilizes its clients (just as men infantilize women) in the name of benevolent treatment, denies them both cred-ibility and choice (just as women were for many years relegated to the home, and disbelieved if their stories contradicted the official dogma), and operates on overt and covert coercion and force. The fact that the mental health system replicates a patriarchal system suggests its own reform: including the client in creation of the system that ostensibly exists to serve her needs.

This means more than having "patient councils" in institutions. It means, as has already begun to happen, client representation at every level of decision making. This does not mean one "consumer," defined as either an ex-patient or family member, on every fifteen- to-twenty-member board. Family members have their own legitimate concerns, and should be included as part of the policy-making process, since they are often de facto service providers and case managers of last resort. But they are not "consumers" in the mental health system. One token representative cannot be a meaningful influence. In addition, health care reform should diversify the options available to individuals in the mental health system, including client-run alternatives and peer support groups, many of which are less expensive and more effective than more traditional models.

Reform of the Mental Health System in the Context of Health Care Reform

Many of the issues addressed above are not part of the current health care debate over mental health treatment, which centers for the most part on parity and insurance reform. Some aspects of the debate — such as whether treatment should be funded in institutional settings or in the community, whether drugs should be funded preferentially over psychotherapy, and whether involuntary treatment should be funded — *are* relevant to the concepts discussed above.

Emphasis on inpatient hospitalization rather than in-home alternatives such as respite care or home health care assistants encourages isolation and disrupts the maintenance of parental and community bonds. No funding should be available for coerced and involuntary treatment; this would encourage respite care, preventive or "wellness" counseling, and programs in the community to respond to the true needs of people the programs seek to help. Funding would not be restricted to drugs and biological treatments, but would include room not only for psychotherapy but for alternative approaches run by ex-patients Still, all current proposals assume the retention of many of the most problematic aspects of an individual medical and diagnostic focus rather than a public health, preventive, and environmentally sensitive approach.

The benefits of current proposals go almost entirely to the upper- and upper-middle-class economic brackets, by forcing private insurers to cover people with preexisting health conditions. This issue is one of the banes of people with private insurance coverage who have children or dependents with mental illness, but it has little impact on the very poor, who are covered by Medicaid, or on the lower middle class, who have no coverage at all. People on Medicaid in many states — such as New York, Massachusetts, Wisconsin, and Vermont — are better off now in terms of coverage of innovative community mental health services than they would be under most current health care reform proposals.

Conclusion

Mental health treatment is already the disfavored stepchild in health care reform. It is the only kind of health care frequently denied to those who want it and forced on those who do not. Health care reform promises a unique opportunity to reform the entire structure of mental health care. In mental health, some of the crucial questions of health care reform take on an added poignance: for many people, preserving patient choice and maximizing options does not mean maintaining the current system, but introducing a whole new approach to care and treatment.

Notes

1　In 1986, the most recent year for which comprehensive national data are available, 730,557 women were admitted to inpatient treatment. Department of Health and Human Services (DHHS), Public Health Service, Center for Mental Health Services, and the National Institute of Mental Health, *Mental Health, United States, 1992* (Washington, D.C.: DHHS, 1992), 284, Table 2.3: "Inpatient Admissions." (The 1986 data were first published in *Mental Health, United States, 1990.* The data reported here are taken from the 1992 edition, which contains an errata sheet for the 1990 edition.)

2　In 1986, 721,287 women underwent outpatient mental health care; 69,730 women were in inpatient facilities. Ibid., 289 (Table 2.9) and 283 (Table 2.2).

3　Symposium issue entitled "Relationships: Friendship, Intimacy and Sex," *Journal of the California Alliance for the Mentally Ill* 5, no. 2 (1994).

4　In fact, several state statutes specifically provide that mental disability is a sufficient reason in and of itself to remove a child from a parent's custody. Robert Hayman, "Presumptions of Justice: Law, Politics and the Mentally Retarded Parent," *Harvard Law Review* 103 (1990): 1235–1236.

5　One early exception was Phyllis Chesler, whose book *Women and Madness*, first published in 1972, explored mental health issues from a feminist perspective and remains a classic to this day.

6　Thomas Szasz, *Ideology and Insanity* (Garden City, N.Y.: Anchor Books, 1970); Peter Breggin, *Toxic Psychiatry* (New York: St. Martin's, 1991); Jeffrey Masson, *Against Therapy: Emotional Tyranny and the Myth of Psychological Healing* (New York: Atheneum, 1988).

7　Judi Chamberlin, *On Our Own* (New York: McGraw-Hill, 1978); Kate Millet, *The Loony Bin Trip* (New York: Simon and Schuster, 1990); Janet and Paul Gotkin, *Too Much Anger, Too Many Tears* (New York: Quadrangle Books, 1975; reprint, New York: Harper Perennials, 1992).

8　American Psychiatric Association (APA), *Diagnostic and Statistical Manual IV* (Washington, D.C.: APA, 1994), 708–709 (abbreviated DSM-IV).

9　There is some precedent for forcing medical treatment on objecting prisoners, based on the unique situation of their imprisonment; see *Commissioner of Correction v. Myers*, 399 N.E.2d 452 (Mass. 1979), *State ex rel. White v. Narick*, 292 S.E.2d 54 (W. Va.

1982). However, more recently courts have been permitting prisoners to refuse medical treatment; see *Thor v. Superior Court of Solano County*, 5 Cal. 4th 725, 21 Cal. Rptr 2d 357, 855 P.2d 375 (1993). People being forcibly medicated in state institutions have not committed any crimes and may not be punished; see *Youngberg v. Romeo*, 457 U.S. 307 (1982).

10   Thomas Szasz, *Law, Liberty and Psychiatry* (New York: Macmillan, 1963). See also citations in notes 6 and 7.

11   Juan E. Mezzich, Arthur Kleinman, Horacio Fabrega Jr., Delores Parron, Byron J. Good, Gloria Johnson-Powell, Keh-Ming Lin, and Spero Manson, "Revised Cultural Proposals for *DSM-IV*," (Washington, D.C.: American Psychiatric Association, 1993).

12   Helen Gremillion, "Psychiatry as Social Ordering: Anorexia Nervosa, A Paradigm," *Social Science and Medicine* 35 (1992): 57–71.

13   Michael Perlin, *The Jurisprudence of the Insanity Defense* (Durham, N.C.: Carolina Academic Press, 1993), discussing sanism in general.

14   E. Shur, *Labelling Women Deviant: Gender, Stigma and Social Control* (1983) (Philadelphia: Temple University Press, 1983), 199, quoting Joel Kovel, "The American Mental Health Industry," in *Critical Psychiatry*, ed. David Ingleby (New York: Pantheon, 1980), 86.

15   Teresa Bernardez, "Prevalent Disorders of Women: An Attempt Toward a Different Understanding and Treatment," in *Women and Mental Health: New Directions for Change*, ed. Carol T. Mowbray, Susan Lanir, and Marilyn Hulce (New York: Haworth, 1984), 19–20.

16   Hearing Before the Select Committee on Children, Youth, and Families, "Women, Violence, and the Law," 100th Cong., 1st Sess., September 16, 1987, 2 (opening statement by Honorable George Miller).

17   Jeffrey B. Bryer et al., "Childhood Sexual Abuse as Factors in Adult Psychiatric Illness," *American Journal of Psychiatry* 144 (1987): 1426, 1427.

18   James C. Beck and Bessel Van der Kolk, "Reports of Childhood Incest and Current Behavior of Chronically Hospitalized Women," *American Journal of Psychiatry* 144 (1987): 1474.

19   Evan Stark and Anne Flitcraft, "Personal Power and Institutional Victimization: Treating the Dual Trauma of Woman Battering," in *Post-Traumatic Therapy and Victims of Violence*, ed. Frank Ochberg (New York: Brunner/Mazel, 1988), 119–120. See generally Susan Stefan, "The Protection Racket: Rape Trauma Syndrome, Psychiatric Labeling, and Law," *Northwestern Law Review* 88 (1994): 1271, 1284–1285, 1312–1313.

20   See, e.g., Andrea Jacobson and Bonnie Richardson, "Assault Experiences of 100 Psychiatric Inpatients: Evidence of the Need for Routine Inquiry," *American Journal of Psychiatry* 144 (1987): 908–913; Andrea Jacobson, Jill Kohler, and Curley Jones-Brown, "The Failure of Routine Assessments to Detect Histories of Assault Experienced by Psychiatric Patients," *Hospital and Community Psychiatry* 38 (1987): 386–389, and articles cited therein.

21   As psychiatrist Jean Baker Miller wrote, referring to the recent research on violence against women: "Prior to this research, most mental health professionals did not 'know' that such sexual and physical violence existed. I can offer myself as an example." Jean Baker Miller, *Women's Psychological Development: Theory and Application*,

(Rockville, Md.: National Institute of Mental Health, Office of the Associate Director for Special Populations [sic], 1986), 7.

22   Evan Stark and Anne Flitcraft, "Personal Power and Institutional Victimization: Treating the Dual Trauma of Woman Battering," in *Post-Traumatic Therapy and Victims of Violence*, ed. Frank M. Ochberg (New York: Brunner/Mazel, 1988), 124.

23   Ibid.

24   The word "syndrome" means "a group of symptoms that occur together and that constitute a recognizable condition." (A "symptom" is "a manifestation of a pathological condition.") A syndrome is "less specific than 'disorder' or 'disease.'" Definitions are taken from the glossary of the APA's *Diagnostic and Statistical Manual III-R* (Washington, D.C.: APA, 1987), which serves as the official diagnostic manual of the American Psychiatric Association (hereafter DSM-IIIR Glossary).

25   *Johnson v. Insley*, Case No. 85-644-CA (Cir. Ct. De Soto County, Fla. 1986), later known as *Johnson v. Bradley*, No. 87-369-CIV-T-10A (M.D. Fla. 1987) (pleadings on file with the author at the University of Miami School of Law).

26   Gotkin and Gotkin, *Too Much Anger, Too Many Tears, supra* note 7, 98.

27   Anita Eichler and Delores L. Parron, eds., *Women's Mental Health: Agenda for Research* (Rockville, Md.: National Institute of Mental Health, 1987), 8.

28   For example, in some studies benzodiazepines (milder tranquilizers such as Valium) are included in the definition of psychotropic drugs. In other studies only the stronger tranquilizers and neuroleptics are included.

29   Nancy Felipe Russo, ed., *A Women's Mental Health Agenda* (Washington, D.C.: APA, 1987), 20; see also Gena Corea, *The Hidden Malpractice* (New York: Harper, 1985), 84–86.

30   "Women and their Physicians: The Evidence," in *Women and Mental Health*, ed. Mowbray et al., *supra* note 15, 121–141.

31   Jane Ussher, *Women's Madness: Misogyny or Mental Illness* (Amherst: University of Massachusetts Press, 1991), 108 (in patients diagnosed as depressed, women receive ECT two to three times as often as men); Richard Parker, "Sex Bias in the Administration of California's Mental Health Law," *Golden Gate University Law Review—Women's Law Forum* 8 (1979): 515, 530 (citing national statistics).

32   Parker, "Sex Bias," *supra* note 31, 515, 530 (citing national statistics).

33   Ibid.

34   Ninety-five percent of diagnoses of anorexia are given to women. APA, DSM III-R Glossary, *supra* note 24, 66.

35   See Ellyn Kaschak, *Engendered Lives* (New York: Basic, 1992), 190–209; Eichler and Parron, *Women's Mental Health, supra* note 27, 33–34.

36   Corea, *The Hidden Malpractice, supra* note 29, 83–86; Leona Bachrach, "Chronically Mentally Ill Women: Emergence and Legitimation of Program Issues," *Hospital and Community Psychiatry* 35 (1985): 1063 (a mentally ill woman who sought help for abdominal pain at a general hospital was referred to a community mental health center, where she bled to death from a ruptured ectopic pregnancy over a two-day period during which she was in seclusion).

37   Teresa Bernardez, "Sex Differences in Women's Mental Health Problems and Their Causes," in *Women and Mental Health*, ed. Mowbray et al., *supra* note 15, 23.

38   Susan J. Blumenthal and Tracy Johnson, *Women's Health Research: Perspectives and*

Priorities in the 1990s (Washington, D.C.: Society for the Advancement of Women's Health Research, n.d.).

39 Almost every state-funded program of this nature has been created specifically to protect the child or children of a mother with mental disabilities. These programs largely focus on the child; benefits to the mother almost seem incidental to program administrators, most of whom do not hesitate to testify against the mothers who are ostensibly their clients at custody hearings when they deem it necessary.

40 Joanne Nicholson, Jeffrey Geller, William Fisher, and George Dion, "State Policies and Programs that Address the Needs of Mentally Ill Mothers in the Public Sector," *Hospital and Community Psychiatry* 44 (May 1993): 486.

41 Women, including ex-patients, founded this organization in 1974, because they felt that traditional services were not meeting their needs. In the years since it was established, it has lost some of the radical and political orientation of its earlier years, as funding pressures increased and the program nearly failed altogether. The program that remains is still a model program, from which state mental health systems could learn a great deal.

42 See, e.g., Office of Technology Assessment, *The Biology of Mental Disorders* (Washington, D.C.: Government Printing Office, 1992).

43 Conversation with Joseph Manes, policy analyst, Bazelon Mental Health Law Center, January 25, 1994.

44 The National Association of Social Workers has published an important document called *Helping the Strong: An Exploration of the Needs of Families Headed by Women*, by Dorothy C. Miller, which reports the results of a project that explored the needs of families headed by women by asking both the women themselves and the professionals who served them about their strengths, stresses, and needs. Throughout their responses, the women stressed the centrality of their children and the importance of services that supported that relationship. Dorothy Miller, *Helping the Strong* (Washington, D.C.: National Association of Social Workers, 1987).

45 *J.L. and K.P. v. Social Security Administration*, 971 F.2d 260, 262 (9th Cir. 1992) (challenging forms and procedures required to apply for benefits based on mental disability as difficult or impossible for a mentally disabled person to fill out and therefore discriminatory; the court ordered plaintiffs to try to work with the Social Security Administration to develop more accessible forms and procedures before it would consider the legal claim).

46 Examples include Eleanor Bumpurs, a 66-year-old black woman, who was killed by a policeman in New York City who claimed that his second, fatal shot was necessary to protect himself from a knife she was wielding, despite the fact that his first shot blew off the hand holding the knife. "Court Rules that Bumpurs Case Should Be Tried," *New York Times*, November 30, 1986, sec. 4, p. 6, col. 1; and another case in which police trying to serve a warrant on a mentally ill man set fire to his cottage and fatally shot him when he ran out. "Ex-patient Killed by Officers," *New York Times*, August 15, 1982, sec. 1, part 1, p. 16, col. 6.

47 Oscar Musiby and Donna Gehrke, "Boss Orders HRS Workers to be Nice or Else," *Miami Herald*, October 31, 1993, sec. B, p. 1. One of the recommendations of single mothers in *Helping the Strong* was "improved training of income maintenance workers that stresses respect, compassion and efficiency." Miller, *Helping the Strong, supra* note 44.

48 Joel A. Dvoskin and Henry J. Steadman, "Using Intensive Case Management to Reduce Violence by Mentally Ill Persons in the Community," *Hospital and Community Psychiatry* 45, no. 7 (July 1994): 679–684.

49 Interestingly, in *Helping the Strong*, Miller found that single mothers saw themselves as far stronger individuals than did the professionals who provided services to families headed by single mothers.

50 DSM-IIIR Glossary, *supra* note 24, 397. (Note that the term "diagnosis" has been removed entirely from the Glossary of Technical Terms in DSM-IV [1994].)

51 Pamphlet issued by the Elizabeth Stone House, Jamaica Plain, MA 02130.

10

ABORTION, LAW, AND PUBLIC HEALTH

. . . .

Ann Scales
with Wendy Chavkin, M.D.

The Public Health Background

by Wendy Chavkin, M.D.

The debate over abortion generally centers on women's rights to autonomy, bodily integrity, and privacy versus the legal and moral status of the fetus. A parallel line of argument underscores the medical and public health impact of abortion.

Because of the heated controversy surrounding it, abortion has been one of the most closely scrutinized surgical procedures. Therefore, when we report that it is one of the safest, and that the benefits to women's health are incontrovertible, we do so with the confidence resulting from critical review of a large database.[1]

Abortion related deaths in the United States dropped precipitously after abortion was legalized in 1973.[2] In 1973 the death rate was 3.3 per 100,000 legal abortions; by 1985 the rate had dropped to 0.4, more than a fivefold decline.[3] This decline has been attributed, in part, to increased physician proficiency.[4] The number of residency programs offering training in abortion increased after the *Roe v. Wade* decision.[5] Changes in methods employed also played a role in the decline in deaths, as suction curettage became the accepted, routinely employed technique for first-trimester procedures and dilatation and evacuation replaced instillation procedures for second-trimester terminations.[6]

The third major contributor to the drop in the death rate was the improved access that attended legalization, and the resultant shift in the gestational age profile; most abortions were performed in the first trimester, the safest stage.[7] Gestational age remains the most important risk factor for abortion-associated death and morbidity.[8] Maternal age, race, medical history, and method used are still risk factors for both mortality and complications.[9] Maternal mortality in general, and abortion mortality specifically, had begun to decline prior to the legalization of abortion. The introduction of antibiotics and of effective contraceptives (oral contraceptives and intrauterine devices) each contributed significantly to this decline; the former enabled the treatment of infection and the latter reduced the number of unwanted pregnancies. In the mid-1960s legal abortions began to substitute for illegal ones, as individual states relaxed restrictive laws. However, the steepest decline in mortality occurred in the mid-1970s as the benefits associated with legalization became widespread. The risks associated with both abortion and childbirth declined in the 1970s, but the slope of the decline of abortion-associated risks was much steeper (89 percent).

The risk of death associated with abortion is significantly lower than that associated with carrying a pregnancy to term, and the gap between the two widens once age, race, preexisting medical conditions, and gestational age are accounted for. A 1982 study reported that the mortality rate for pregnancy-associated maternal mortality was approximately twelve times higher than for abortion-related mortality.[10]

Reduction in infant mortality is also associated with access to legal abortion and is thought to reflect reductions in both unwanted and high-risk pregnancies. According to one group of analysts, this reduction was most pronounced for those at highest risk: poor African-Americans.[11]

About three-quarters of women having abortions intended to have children in the future, according to a 1987 survey.[12] The Centers for Disease Control reviewed the risk of abortion for future childbearing and concluded that suction curettage (vacuum aspiration) in the first trimester does not impair future childbearing capacity, nor is it associated with later adverse birth outcomes. Dilatation and evacuation, however, is associated with increased risk of later preterm delivery and low birthweight, although the independent contributions of the procedure and the late gestational age at which this procedure is performed have not been disentangled.[13] Although refinements of technique, such as the introduction of absorbent nontraumatic cervical dilators (laminaria, dilapan), have certainly contributed to enhanced safety, much of the decreased risk is also attributed to improved surgical proficiency resulting from experience. A decline in the routine provision of abortion training in OB-GYN residencies thus has implications for technical proficiency, as well as for access.

Despite this, after an initial burst, there has been marked reduction in the number of obstetric gynecology residencies that routinely include training in abortion. Between 1976 and 1985, there was a 22 percent decline in the number of OB-GYN residency programs offering training in first-trimester procedures.[14] Half of these programs offered such training as an option, and half reported that 50 percent of residents did not participate. Simultaneously, the proportion of programs not offering even optional training increased to 25 percent.

In a 1992 survey of chief residents in OB-GYN training programs, 29 percent reported not having received instruction in the performance of first-trimester induced abortions and 47 percent reported having no clinical experience. Thirty-one percent stated that they had not received instruction in second-trimester dilatation and evacuation.[15]

This decline in formal training paralleled a move of the procedure out of the hospital. This trend resulted from complex forces: generalized movement toward outpatient ambulatory surgery, cost reduction, initial association between some freestanding clinics' efforts to provide counseling and support, and lack of interest and commitment on the part of hospitals and academic medicine. In 1988, 64 percent of abortions were performed in "abortion clinics."[16] Thus the clinical and technical advances accruing from experience have evolved outside of the hospital and medical educational establishment.

Fear of harassment and pressure from community and peers have clearly contributed to the reluctance of many physicians to perform abortions. The freestanding, specialized abortion clinic is visible and vulnerable as a target. Eighty-five percent of these clinics reported anti-abortion harassment in 1988.[17] Such a setup not only demands heroism on the part of the physician but also requires that physician to repetitively perform the same procedure without the opportunity to develop ongoing relationships with patients.

These converging factors have all led to a severe provider shortage, particularly outside of major metropolitan areas. Eighty-three percent of United States counties lack abortion providers, and 27 percent of women seeking abortions had to travel more than fifty miles to reach services.[18] State restrictions, such as waiting periods and parental requirements, significantly compound the difficulties of obtaining an abortion for women who have to travel.[19]

The impediments to access resulting from shortage and maldistribution are significantly compounded by restriction of public funds. The Alan Guttmacher Institute estimated that 20 percent of Medicaid-eligible women who want abortions do not have them when funding is not available and that another 22 percent of such women delay their abortions until the second trimester.[20] The public health implication is that some women will carry an unwanted pregnancy to term and that some will have an abortion but at a later stage of gestation because of these delays. As described earlier, gestational age remains the most important risk factor for abortion-associated complications.

One response to medical recognition of provider shortage and vulnerability has been to try to reintegrate abortion training and provision into the medical mainstream. Planned Parenthood in New York City has arranged a training program in abortion that local OB-GYN residency programs are permitting their residents to take electively.[21] Some family practice, pediatric, and internal medicine residents are also participating. Simultaneously, a group of medical students in New York have circulated petitions to their schools demanding that abortion training be routinely incorporated into the curriculum.[22] The American Medical Women's Association (AMWA) has initiated a project to develop model curricula in reproductive health, including abortion, for medical school and residency training.[23] AMWA has also inaugurated the Reproductive Health awards to honor courageous abortion providers. The National Abortion Federation and the American College of Obstetricians and Gynecologists held a symposium in 1990 to investigate the shortage of abortion practitioners and jointly developed a series of specific recommendations to reintegrate such training into medical education and to support providers.[24]

The murder of Dr. David Gunn in 1993 galvanized pro-choice supporters throughout the country, including the medical establishment to some extent. Organized medicine — particularly, of course, OB-GYN — has recently (belatedly) become more assertive in defense of abortion and its providers. While there is certainly no pro-choice consensus among clinicians, organized medicine has become aware of the many issues at stake. Restrictions on abortion not only impede patients' access to the procedure but also threaten the autonomy of the physician, medical judgment, and the doctor-patient relationship.[25] After the 1994 murders of employees in a Massachusetts Planned Parenthood Clinic, many prominent medical associations held a press conference to decry the violence and uphold their medical commitment to addressing patient needs.

Lack of training in abortion techniques deprives physicians of a realm of technical competence. Medicaid prohibitions on abortions force physicians to forgo payment or to collude with local government in imposing health risks on the most vulnerable women. All of these threaten the integrity and power of the medical profession. Reevaluation of this latter point provides a public-health/medical argument for including abortion in any medical benefits package.

Legal abortion has been demonstrated to be safe, and its availability is associated with improvements in various important reproductive health parameters. These public health benefits accrue when abortion is not only legally available but accessible without financial, geographic, or other constraints. The dramatic and rapid improvements in technology and skill that have been demonstrated since legalization underscore the necessity for maintaining clinical training and research in this area. New developments, such as the discovery that certain oral medications can successfully cause termination of early pregnancy, herald a new era with profound implications for practice and for public health.

The most widely known of these "medical abortifacients" is mifepristone, or RU 486, a synthetic steroid that competes with progesterone for receptor sites in the uterus and thus prevents it from binding and performing its pregnancy-sustaining function. Since its synthesis in 1981, mifepristone has been tested in about twenty countries, including both highly developed and developing nations.[26] More than 150,000 women have used it as an abortifacient. When followed by a prostaglandin, which augments uterine contractions, it has demonstrated an efficacy rate of 96 percent.

Although there are extensive data from French, British, and Swedish trials, the Food and Drug Administration (FDA) has asked for additional U.S. trials prior to use in this country.[27] A multisite trial, expected to enroll 2,000 women, has recently been initiated under the auspices of the Population Council, to whom the French manufacturer Rousell-Uclaf has transferred U.S. patent rights.

The introduction of mifepristone led to recognition of the promise that other medications might also successfully interrupt pregnancy. Misoprostol, a prostaglandin administered orally as a treatment for ulcers, has reportedly been used by women to induce abortion in Brazil, where abortion is illegal.[28] Methotrexate, an antimetabolite used for diverse treatments, including those for certain cancers and psoriasis, has been successfully used for termination of ectopic pregnancies during the past few years.[29] Recently, individual clinicians have used methotrexate, followed by oral or vaginal misoprostol, for the termination of early intrauterine pregnancies and have reported 94 percent efficacy and only minor side effects.[30] Both methotrexate and misoprostol are available on the U.S. market and thus not subject to the kind of obstacles that have slowed the introduction of mifepristone.

The medical abortifacients currently known appear useful for terminating pregnancies of up to nine weeks gestation. This limitation means that they cannot totally replace surgical abortion, which will continue to be necessary for pregnancies of gestational age beyond this. On the other hand, these agents can be used earlier in gestation than the surgical procedure. Most importantly, the introduction of these agents heralds a new age of privacy for the abortion patient and provider, as no special facilities are required. These drugs could be administered by a wide range of medical providers, in diverse settings, with surgical abortion facilities and providers available as backup. The possibility of widening the pool of providers and reducing their visibility, and thus vulnerability, is significant.

There are several reasons why the inclusion of abortion coverage under any health care financing plan is critical. The first is obvious — to ensure equitable access to this service and to remove the financial barriers currently in place. It is also important to reintegrate abortion provision into the mainstream of reproductive health services and primary care. Such a move would diminish both patient and provider vulnerability to harassment. It would also increase the likelihood that training of physicians and other clinicians in abortion techniques could be routinely incorporated into clinical education. The impact of such integration extends beyond abortion alone. It would indicate an understanding that primary care includes the full range of reproductive health services and that the furtherance of women's health is a public health and social goal.

Abortion and the Law

by Ann Scales

Should the definitive history of women's status in the United States ever be written, the year 1973 will figure saliently. That was when the U.S. Supreme Court declared abortion a constitutional right. In many ways, *Roe v. Wade*[31] was the beginning of a public reconceptualization of women as real legal/political *persons*. In addition, after 1973, there were demonstrable improvements in women's health. However, the reconceptualization of womanhood has been incomplete, and the health benefits have not been as great as they could have been, due to the ferocity of ongoing legal, political, and medical struggles around the issue of abortion.

Access to safe abortion is only one aspect of women's reproductive health, and an aspect that tends (or is manipulated) to overshadow the larger issues of women's well-being. That fact notwithstanding, abortion deserves a great deal of time and attention. The right to abortion — at least for now — is a critical part of the struggle for women's health, equality, and very lives.

With respect to abortion, the women's health agenda needs to pursue four strategies: (1) protect abortion providers, (2) reinstate abortion funding for low-income women, (3) reduce the number of unwanted and/or dangerous pregnancies, and (4) redescribe abortion as a constitutional equality right, rather than as a privacy right, so that its role in the lives of women is clarified.

Law After Roe v. Wade

Women's struggle for reproductive freedom did not begin with *Roe v. Wade* and surely has not ended there. The massiveness of the controversy has been due in large part to the tireless efforts by state legislatures to find ways to circumvent and undermine *Roe*. Just since 1989,[32] state legislatures have introduced more than 500 bills intended to restrict or ban access to abortions.[33] Of these, only about a dozen have passed. Defeating the other bills, however, has required a mobilization of effort that is unmatched since the tireless campaigns for women's right to vote. And the bills that did pass (along with other abortion-related legal issues, such as remedies against Operation Rescue) have tied up enormous energies in the courts.

Given the personnel changes on the Supreme Court wrought by the Reagan and Bush administrations, it was widely believed as of 1989[34] that *Roe v. Wade* was going to be overruled outright. The outcome of the case in which that was supposed to happen, *Planned Parenthood of Southeastern Pennsylvania v. Casey*,[35] was not as bad as it could have been. True, a majority of the Court voted to uphold almost all of Pennsylvania's draconian restrictions on abortion.[36] True, the Court found that abortion no longer had the status of a "fundamental right," such that restrictions would be upheld unless they constituted an "undue burden" on the now less-than-fundamental right to abortion. And true, four Justices — William Rehnquist, Antonin Scalia, Clarence Thomas, and Byron White — voted to overrule *Roe* altogether. But there was no fifth vote to trash *Roe*.[37] Nor does it presently appear that there will be: Ruth Bader Ginsburg, an abortion advocate, has replaced Byron White, a longtime opponent of abortion rights. Stephen Breyer has replaced abortion-rights defender Harry Blackmun. It remains to be seen whether Justice Breyer will help those who support abortion rights. Conventional wisdom is that he will not harm us.

Thus, the legal line has shakily held. Yet, the right to abortion is in more jeopardy than at any time since before 1973. What is going on, and what strategies can shore up the abortion right?

Protection of Providers

In the "civil war" metaphor that has become common in describing the abortion rights battle, it might be said that the abortion front shifted away from the judicial arena to the streets, in the form of organized violence against abortion clinics and abortion providers. As one commentator has noted about right-wing forces, this was a shift from a legal strategy to a "supply-side strategy: to prevail by severely reducing the number of doctors willing to perform abortions. The strategy depends on public disclosure and scorn."[38] It also depends upon arson, torture, and murder. In mid-August of 1993, the leader of Operation Rescue, Randall Terry, told his followers in Fort Wayne, Indiana, to "let a wave of intolerance wash over you. I want you to let a wave of hatred wash over you."[39]

This campaign has been far more effective than the legislative and judicial struggles. As of 1992, abortion was unavailable in 83 percent of counties in the United States,[40] as the number of providers steadily decreased. In the past fifteen years, anti-abortion terrorists have bombed or set fire to more than 100 clinics, invaded more than 300, and vandalized more than 400.[41] The violence is characterized by gruesome escalation in recent years. In 1990, approximately 100 abortion-related acts of violence — from bombings to arson to death threats — were reported to police. By 1992, that number had risen almost 600 percent, to 667 reported incidents. The incidence of reported clinic vandalism rose 100 percent from 1991 to 1992. Arson rose from 4 cases in 1990 to 12 in 1992.[42] These figures are probably low, due to providers' hesitation to report threats out of fear of increased violence.[43]

The violence and harassment have demonstrated sickening creativity. Clinics are sprayed with foul-smelling butyric acid, forcing them to close for weeks at a time in order to replace carpets and scrub walls.[44] A flyer circulated in Charleston, South Carolina, advertised how much cash the Charleston Women's Medical Clinic would have on hand at any time, a veritable "invitation to rob the place."[45] At least one clinic experienced a drive-by shooting.[46] Clinics have been forced to add expensive security systems, the costs of which divert already limited funds from medical services.[47] The clinics least able to prevent attacks tend to be in rural areas, at facilities that may be the only source for other women's health services, such as pelvic exams, pap tests, prenatal care, and breast cancer screening.[48]

Recently, the violence and intimidation have shifted from the clinics that provide abortions to the individuals, homes, and family lives of the medical personnel who perform or facilitate them. This campaign, de-nominated "No Place to Hide" by Operation Rescue,[49] has no end in sight.[50] Randall Terry of Operation Rescue said, "We've found the weak link is the doctor. We're going to expose them. We're going to humiliate them."[51]

Doctors, nurses, and other personnel are routinely followed;[52] their homes picketed around the clock; their names, addresses, and faces put on "wanted" posters in their communities; their families and friends publicly and privately harassed.[53] Death threats have become common,[54] and clinic personnel have taken routinely to wearing bulletproof vests and arming themselves.[55] And it has come to serial murder.

On March 10, 1993, Dr. David Gunn of the Pensacola (Florida) Women's Medical Services Clinic was assassinated as he walked into work. A "wanted poster" of Dr. Gunn, including his picture and home telephone number, had been distributed the summer before at a rally in Alabama.[56] After the murder, Houston-based "Rescue America" imme-diately established a fund for the legal defense of the killer, Michael Griffin.[57] A phone message was left at a Florida clinic: "One down — how many more?"[58]

On August 19, 1993, Dr. George Tiller was shot twice as he drove away from work in Wichita, Kansas. The shooter, Rachelle Shannon, wrote a letter to Michael Griffin (the killer of Dr. Gunn), stating that her shooting of Tiller was "the most holy thing . . . I've ever done."[59] The wounds were superficial, and Dr. Tiller was able to come to work the next morning. This was not his first brush with the violence of the anti-choice forces. His clinic had been one of three under siege in Wichita by Operation Rescue in the summer of 1991, during which 2,700 "res-cuers" were arrested.[60]

A third abortion provider, Dr. George Wayne Patterson of Mobile, Alabama, was murdered on August 21, 1993, only two days after the shooting of Dr. Tiller. The authorities have concluded that the killing was unrelated to the abortion issue. However, the provision of abortion services in the Gulf Coast region was dramatically affected. Dr. Patterson had been regularly flown in to the Florida clinic as a substitute for the assassinated Dr. Gunn. The clinic then had to bring in another doctor from hundreds of miles away.[61] That doctor, John Britton, was murdered outside the Pensacola clinic on July 29, 1994, by a former Presbyterian minister named Paul Hill. Also murdered was Dr. Britton's volunteer escort, Mr. James H. Barrett, a retired Air Force lieutenant colonel. Wounded was Mr. Barrett's wife, June.[62]

Previously, just days after the murder of Dr. Gunn, Paul Hill had appeared on the television shows *Donahue* and *Nightline*, saying that deadly force was entirely justifiable to protect the unborn.[63] After taking over from Dr. Gunn, Dr. Britton had received many threats, including a message taped to his office door that read, "What would you do if you had five minutes left to live?"[64] Dr. Britton had complained to his escorts that his bulletproof vest was too short: "I'd like it so they can't get me in the gut."[65] Dr. Britton and Mr. Barrett were killed by shotgun blasts to their heads.[66]

In response to the escalation in violence, some emphasis in the struggle has appropriately shifted back to legal institutions. With the strong backing of Attorney General Janet Reno[67] and under the leadership of Senator Edward Kennedy, the United States Congress in 1993 passed the Freedom of Access to Clinic Entrances Act (FACE), which became law early in 1994.[68] Under this measure, those who commit violence against women seeking abortion or against abortion providers can face three years in jail or fines up to $250,000. If the violence results in bodily harm, the Act provides for a ten-year jail sentence, for life imprisonment when death is caused. Even "nonviolent" protests that block abortions or obstruct clinics can result in eighteen-month jail terms and fines up to $25,000. FACE allows clinic operators to seek injunctions in order to stop clinic harassment and allows public officials to instigate civil proceedings against anti-abortion harassers.[69]

Governmental agencies, as well, are taking significant measures to curb the violence. For example, on November 16, 1993, the Bureau of Alcohol, Tobacco, and Firearms announced the establishment of a citizen reward system that will provide up to $100,000 for information leading to arrests and convictions of those committing violence at abortion clinics. A million dollars to fund this program was provided by an anonymous donor.[70] The Bureau has set up a 24-hour-a-day, toll-free number to receive such information.[71]

Finally, there is new momentum in the federal courts to apply existing laws to anti-abortion harassers. Among these efforts, the press has given most attention to *National Organization for Women v. Schiedler.*[72] In that case, the United States Supreme Court unanimously ruled that anti-abortion harassment is subject to the federal "racketeering" law (RICO),[73] which provides criminal penalties and allows the courts to triple the amounts awarded to those damaged by such sets of behaviors. It is hard to say how much deterrence value this ruling will provide, as harassment forces have tended not to pay judgments already rendered against them under different laws. However, there is symbolic value in public recognition that anti-abortion harassment is a version of *organized crime.*

This recognition, though valuable, must be pressed further. The actions at issue in the abortion context are not just the crimes that constitute the usual turf of traditional organized crimes: crimes against taxation authorities, crimes against property, and even crimes against particular persons and vulnerable groups. The organized actions against abortion are, precisely, *crimes of hatred against women as women.* Randall Terry was right: the doctors are the "weak link," because there are so few of them and they are so visible. But the real target is women's control over their own reproductive capacities. Vigilance in the protection of providers is vigilance in protection of women in general.

Reinstating Funding for Low-Income Women
When attention was focused on the possibility that *Roe v. Wade* would be overruled, many lost sight of the fact that the right to abortion was already long-lost for most low-income women. As of 1980, upholding ever more restrictive versions of the Hyde Amendment, the U.S. Supreme Court had ruled that the federal government and states could, consistent with the U.S. Constitution, refuse Medicaid funding for abortion.[74]

Beginning in 1977, and engineered by anti-abortion crusader Representative Henry Hyde of Illinois, Congress passed a series of laws (known as the Hyde Amendments) which prohibit the expenditure of federal Medicaid funds for abortions. Medicaid, which is a joint federal/state program that provides medical assistance to eligible low-income persons, requires the federal government to pay the bulk of costs for "covered services"; the states pay the balance. The Hyde Amendments prohibit any federal matching funds to be used to fund most abortions.[75]

Of course, this denial of funding is the grossest sort of discrimination against low-income women. This is particularly so when, as is usually the case, state Medicaid laws fund every other "medically necessary" procedure for all Medicaid eligible people, both men and women.

The states are free to fund otherwise excluded abortions if they choose. Of course, without federal help, there is little incentive for the states to do so. Nonetheless, in response to the constitutional lapse on the federal level, some states have voluntarily funded abortions for low-income women.[76] In the meantime, feminist lawyers around the country have looked beyond the federal scene, and in reliance on state constitutional and/or state statutory law, have already secured decisions commanding twelve states to pay for abortion services for Medicaid-eligible women on the same terms as other pregnancy-related and general health services are funded.[77]

These state efforts have political significance beyond their immediate boundaries. Many disenfranchised peoples have for too long depended on the federal courts to protect them *in pater familias*. As great a defender as Harry Blackmun was on the Court,[78] women's reproductive freedom could not hinge solely on him. These more recent efforts are teaching abortion defenders new strategies. Of greatest importance, these state efforts have actually delivered abortion funding in those states for low-income women in medical need.

From a medical point of view, the need for abortion funding for low-income women could not be more clear. Recent scholarship demonstrates that denial of abortion funding presents severe public health consequences. As Wendy Chavkin reports in the first section of this chapter, a fifth of Medicaid eligible women who want or need abortions forgo them, and another fifth delay them, inviting dangerous health risks. Therefore, funding abortions for low-income women can substantially increase the health and political well-being of women and children. Funding abortion actually tends to decrease by 26 percent the number of women who receive late or no prenatal care.[79] Such an increase in prenatal care means healthier babies, healthier mothers, and substantial cost savings in terms of decreased hospitalization, postpartum care, and other public assistance expenditures.

Of most startling consequence, a state that funds abortion may reduce the teenage birth rate by as much as 67 percent.[80] In the country with the highest teenage pregnancy rate in the industrialized world, the benefits of such a reduction cannot be overestimated. Again, there are substantial calculable savings to the public coffers. As teenage mothers are least likely to have prenatal care and most likely eventually to depend on public assistance to support themselves and their children, to fund abortion reduces expenditures for hospitalization, extended postnatal care,

Aid to Families with Dependent Children (AFDC), nutritional assistance to women on Medicaid, and other public assistance programs.

Over the longer term, such a reduction in the teenage birth rate can have profound impacts on the lives of young women and their future children. Both they and the society in which they live benefit from sparing them the agonies of education truncated, aspirations dashed, and years of dependency on public assistance. If so much unwanted teen pregnancy could be so simply avoided, how might these young women be liberated to decide their own and society's futures? How might the antiquated expectation of women as breeders be transformed?

Decreasing the Need for Abortion

The best means to quell the violence surrounding the abortion issue is to reduce the need for abortions. There will always be a need for some means of pregnancy termination, even if only in situations involving medical complications during desired pregnancies. I would not presume to suggest, however, that abortions be available only in such circumstances. Ultimately and always, the choice of whether or not and why to have an abortion must be the prerogative solely of the pregnant woman. Nonetheless, there are measures that could dramatically reduce the number of *unwanted* pregnancies, which, it seems obvious, would decrease the need for abortion.[81]

Though simple to state, the goal of reducing unwanted pregnancies requires multiple strategies and lots of hard work. These strategies fall roughly into three overlapping categories: economic issues, health care issues, and sexual access issues.

1. Economic independence for women. Some women who choose abortion might carry their pregnancies to term if they could care for the children they brought into the world. For single mothers, that would require serious and systematic enforcement of child-support obligations. As it is, nationwide, 49 percent of court-ordered child-support obligations go fully or partially unenforced.[82]

For every woman, economic independence would require an absolute end to sex discrimination in employment. It is a national disgrace that, almost a quarter century after the enactment of the Equal Pay Act,[83] women still earn only 75 percent of what men do.[84] Insofar as that statistic results from discrimination against women *because* they bear children, it is already illegal, pursuant to the Pregnancy Discrimination Act of 1978.[85] That act must not only be rigorously enforced, its parameters must be expanded. Although the federal Family and Medical Leave Act of 1993 allows that both men and women can get limited time off work to care for children without losing their jobs,[86] that law provides no compensation for those activities, leaving the U.S. alone among "industrialized" countries without some guarantee that the tasks of child-*rearing* will not be economically devastating. For single women and for working families, being able to care for children will also require the provision of affordable and reliable day care.

2. *Health care.* The failure of national health care reform in 1994 was a tragedy for women.[87] President Clinton's original Health Security bill would have included universal coverage for pelvic exams (including pap tests for cancer screening), treatment of gynecological disorders and sexually transmitted diseases, contraception, abortion (while allowing specific doctors and hospitals to opt out of performing this service), pregnancy testing, fertility treatment (excluding *in vitro* fertilization), prenatal care, obstetrics, and postnatal care. Each of these covered areas either would have contributed to the prevention of unwanted or medically dangerous pregnancies or would have assured women that any pregnancy carried to term would result in as risk-free a labor/delivery and as healthy an infant as can reasonably be expected with otherwise competent medical care. The Clinton bill would also have provided coverage for drug- and alcohol-dependency treatments. When women are addicted and cannot recover from their addictions, for whatever reasons, they have less incentive either to prevent pregnancy or to carry a pregnancy to term. It thus seems likely that a national dependency-treatment guarantee would also decrease the need for abortion.

As it is, confidence in health care is the province of only the most fortunate women. The rest are left to the economic self-interests of private insurance companies or to the ever-diminishing generosity of public medical assistance. Until the imperative of national health care can be realized, the goal of reducing unwanted and/or dangerous pregnancies will depend upon local initiative. Supporters will have to stay on the backs of state legislatures and administrative units to guarantee the funding and safety of all procedures necessary to women's reproductive health. We will have to do whatever is necessary to make safe contraceptives available to all women. That will include the necessity to fight furiously for meaningful sex education in public schools.

3. *Control of sexual access.* The allegation that "double standards" are deployed is thrown around like confetti — particularly by white people when denied anything at all. But nowhere does the double-standards

charge have more realistic application than in the sexual lives of women. Sexual access to women is at once publicly deplored and privately expected. This is true even for grown, supposedly self-possessed women. Professor Catharine MacKinnon encapsulated the problem in her description of the legalistic concept of "consent" to intercourse: given statutory rape laws, young women *cannot* consent; given the practical interpretation of the consent defense in rape law (and the existence in some states of marital exemptions for rape) mature women *cannot withhold* consent.[88]

The sexual access problem is particularly acute for adolescent women, whose lives are defined by sexual schizophrenia. The world of adults insists upon sexual abstinence; the world of peers insists upon "putting out." Contemporary sex education debates focus clearly on the former of these imperatives, but take too little account of the *immense* power of the latter.[89]

The summary of the cultural lesson for women is that their value is in their sexual availability. What would it take for young women's self-worth to comprise more than clothes, dates, and calories? The first avenue must be genuine and broad-ranging sexual education, which must be made democratically available, meaning that it must happen in public schools.

Meaningful sex education would include not only how babies get made and how, technically, to prevent that from happening. It would include a realistic appraisal of the consequences, particularly for young women, of teenage pregnancy. It would include a tough, perhaps traumatizing, interrogation of the processes of sexual socialization for both young men and young women. Thus, social discourse might shift from argument about the tired refrain of "abortion on demand" to consciousness of the realities of "sex on demand." Meaningful sex education would include a study of *sexism*, from the economic dependence of females in domestic settings to the accepted, supposedly inevitable social institutions — such as pornography[90] and prostitution[91] — that in fact perpetually reinscribe the meaning of femaleness as *expendability*. Meaningful sex education might even have to include a critical discussion of the institutions — such as sports and militarism — through which young men too often achieve false senses of entitlement to women.

In addition, the issues of sexual access require getting deadly serious about sex crime. All forms of rape — from marital rape to "date rape" to stranger rape — not only result in unwanted pregnancies. Given the constant threat of such invasions, they also encourage women to become dependent on men and to convince ourselves, in some circumstances, that we really want "it," even when we really don't.[92] This incentive to "desire adjustment" itself perpetuates the vicious cycle of sexual access and unwanted pregnancy. To take sex crimes seriously will require reconceptualization of the idea of "forced" intercourse. Force does not mean only having a knife at one's throat and generally fearing for one's physical safety. It also includes economic coercion, social conventions (e.g., "putting out" after X number of dates), and the devastating psychological threats of ostracization and/or verbal degradation should a woman dare to say "no."

As the flip side to reconceptualizing "force," we must reconsider the notion of "consent." Is there consent to intercourse in any case when a woman's existence — from the maintenance of "mere" self-esteem to being allowed to live — requires being available for sex and/or the bearing of children? As Robin West has noted, "[w]omen — somewhat uniquely — consent to their misery."[93] The legalistic concept of consent — that bright line that little girls have no choice but to cross in the process of becoming big girls — has no absolute meaning in this world where women are perpetually engaged (consciously or not) in finding ways to avoid sexual predation. Both in courts of law and in daily life, consent must be always contextualized, framed in the matrix of societal gender inequality, and deemed to exist only in situations where interpersonal equality can also be proven.

My recent undertaking is to talk to "the other side" in the abortion controversy about how to decrease the need for abortion. The results to date, though by no means dispositive, are rather predictable. There are some among the anti-abortion camp who find each and every one of my suggestions way too radical, particularly when the discussions come around to universal and publicly funded contraception, the criminalization of marital rape, and the deconstruction of sports and the military. Upon pressing the matter, I find that many of these people, both men and women, believe that woman fulfills her destiny only when she breeds: the institutions that coerce that "choice" are by definition good institutions.

On the other hand, some anti-abortion activists — stuck on the moral/theological issue of when life begins — genuinely hadn't thought about whether or not we could find common ground. After agreeing to disagree about whether some abortions (or less intrusive means of pregnancy termination) will always be necessary, there is at least some room to talk about how to reduce the number of unwanted pregnancies. The more I explain about, say, the social contexts of pregnancy, the more they listen. Interestingly, some of the most avid listeners are older, ex-military men; they seem to know, if only subconsciously, that masculine institutions create inequality by the very ways that they celebrate male entitlements. Obviously, other good listeners are often male single parents. Several anti-abortion activists have said that they would stand shoulder to shoulder with me in promoting legislation, including sex education programs, that might decrease the number of unwanted pregnancies.

This must be the wave of the immediate future. No one otherwise inclined will accept feminist accounts of the need for abortion; we will never achieve consensus about when life begins, or about why that isn't the question. But when we keep talking about all the ways that women get pregnant against their will or in derogation of their health, we will find an audience of people who will listen, whether that be a function of democratic instinct, liberal philosophy, or Christian morality.

The success of any of those discussions depends on demonstrating the connection between unwanted pregnancy and *women's inequality*. But before the discussions with "the other side" can produce good results, we must assure ourselves that "the equality route" is the only way to go.

Abortion as an Equality Right

After the nomination of Ruth Bader Ginsburg to the U.S. Supreme Court in June of 1993, some feminists expressed skepticism and fear over then-Judge Ginsburg's criticism of *Roe v. Wade*. Listening to the mainstream media, one could almost have concluded that Justice Ginsburg was anti-abortion. It is crucial to recognize, however, that Ginsburg was just one of many legal commentators who disagreed not with the right to abortion itself but with the constitutional basis on which the right was grounded.

In *Roe*, the Supreme Court extrapolated the right to abortion from the right to privacy. Neither abortion nor civil privacy are expressly mentioned in the Constitution. Rather, the right to privacy was itself first extrapolated from the guarantee of "liberty" expressed in the due process clause of the Fourteenth Amendment, as well as the Third Amendment guarantee against quartering soldiers, the Fourth Amendment prohibition on unreasonable searches, the Fifth Amendment right to avoid self-incrimination, and the Ninth Amendment reservation of all unenumerated rights to the people.[94]

There are at least four overlapping problems with this approach. First, given the strange pedigree of the privacy right, it rests on shifting constitutional sands.[95] Second, the concepts of privacy and "choice" are located entirely within liberalist discourse that preconceives each of us as *citizen-blanks:* as equally autonomous vessels of potential self-determination, undetermined and uninfluenced by social context. The rhetoric of choice, though valuable in the past, does not nearly encompass the meaning of access to abortion for real women living through real crises.

Third, the language of privacy and choice also has the effect of *privatizing* the injury of unwanted pregnancy and subsequent decision making. Pregnancy and abortion become personal problems, and the rest of society can ignore them. The set of concrete, tragic conundra become merely mental events. It all happens, in Andrea Dworkin's words, "in the head, a vast cavern somewhere north of the eyes."[96] Thereby, antiabortion forces get enormous mileage out of the phrase "abortion on demand," as if women were having abortions for fun, just for the hell of it, as a way of exercising their constitutional rights just for the sake of exercising them.[97]

Fourth, the choice approach obscures the history of what constitutional equality has meant for women, and what it should mean. It is only in the past thirty years that any federal authority has considered women worthy of guarantees of equality.[98] In both law and social rhetoric, however, women's equality has depended on showing that they are *like* men before they can be allowed rights *equal* to men's. Equality so premised has fallen off the edge of the legal world in the obvious cases where women are not like men — that is, in situations involving women's reproductive capacities,[99] with very few exceptions.[100]

As now seems obvious, it took a long time to demonstrate how the requirement that women be *like* men in order to achieve equality assumed *maleness as the norm.*[101] The relationship between mother and fetus is paradigmatic of this problem. There was no way for law or political discourses even to talk about that relationship:

> the fetus . . . must be like something men have or are: a body part to the Left, a person to the Right . . . Had women participated equally in designing laws, we might now be trying to compare other relationships — employer and employee, partners in a business, oil in the ground, termites in a building, tumors in a body, ailing famous violinists and abducted hostages forced to sustain them — to the maternal/fetus relationship rather than the reverse.[102]

Justice Ginsburg's point was simply that we could avoid more general jurisprudential pitfalls about "privacy" and give stronger meaning to equality by relocating the abortion right within the context of equality doctrine.[103] Such a reassignment of constitutional authority not only would give stronger legal legs to the right (by relying on an explicit constitutional guarantee), but would speak more accurately to the role of abortion in women's lives. The question is not simply women's "autonomy" in the abstract. The question also fundamentally implicates social constructions of women's — as opposed to men's — place in the world.

> The conflict . . . is not simply one between a fetus' interests and a woman's interests, narrowly conceived, nor is the overriding issue state versus private control of a woman's body for a span of nine months. Also in the balance is a woman's autonomous charge of her *full life's course* . . . her ability to stand in relation to man, society, and state as an independent, self-sustaining, *equal* citizen.[104]

Abortion stories are never about women's frivolity, bullheadedness, or murderousness. No woman has ever had an abortion for fun. It is always a morally difficult decision, but one that happens in a concrete context rather than in that vast cavern north of the eyes. To relocate the right to abortion in equality doctrine is to acknowledge the reality of women's circumstances, and to honor the differential boundaries for women and men between choice and choicelessness. It is also to reclaim the moral high ground from the radical right. It could be a way actually to improve the reproductive lives of women.

Conclusion

In identifying the overly narrow focus of pro-choice advocates, I have not in this chapter meant to castigate our foremothers and coworkers in the struggle for full reproductive rights. I recognize the utility of that approach within past and present political discourses. Thus, the first two of these four agenda items devolve fully on ways to protect our advances and/or regain lost ground.

The last two of my suggestions, however, involve reconceptualizing strategies about abortion and women's health generally. In requiring all of us to take equality seriously, they also demand attention to myriad forms of violence against women, whether perpetrated by teenaged peers, political institutions, or military organizations. Putting abortion in perspective demands that. If the equality guarantee cannot devolve attention to the roles of reproduction in real women's lives, that guarantee is not really worth much.

Notes

1   C. Tietze, "The Public Health Effects of Legal Abortion in the United States," *Family Planning Perspectives* 26 (1984): 26–27; W. Cates Jr., "Legal Abortion: The Public Health Record 1982," *Science* 215 (1982): 1586–1587; Council on Scientific Affairs, American Medical Association (AMA), "Induced Termination of Pregnancy Before and After *Roe v. Wade:* Trends in the Mortality and Morbidity of Women," *Journal of the American Medical Association* 268, no. 22 (1992): 3231–3239.

2   H. K. Atrash, H. T. MacKay, N. J. Binkin, and C. J. R. Hogue, "Legal Abortion Mortality in the United States: 1972 to 1982," *American Journal of Obstetrics Gynecology* 156 (1987): 605–612.

3   H. W. Lawson, H. K. Atrash, A. F. Saftlas, L. M. Koonin, M. Ramick, and J. C. Smith, "Abortion Surveillance, United States, 1984–1985," *Morbidity and Mortality Weekly Report* 38 (1989): 1–45; S. K. Henshaw and J. Van Vort, *Abortion Factbook, 1992 Edition: Readings, Trends and State and Local Data to 1988* (New York: Alan Guttmacher Institute, 1992).

4   Tietze, "Public Health Effects of Legal Abortion," *supra* note 1; Cates, "Legal Abortion," *supra* note 1; Council on Scientific Affairs, AMA, "Induced Termination of Pregnancy Before and After *Roe v. Wade,*" *supra* note 1; Atrash et al., "Legal Abortion Mortality," *supra* note 2.

5   R. T. Burkman, T. M. King, L. S. Burnett, and M. F. Atienza, "University Abortion Programs: One Year Later," *American Journal of Obstetrics Gynecology* 119 (1974): 131–136; P. D. Darney, U. Landy, S. MacPherson, and R. L. Sweet, "Abortion Training in U.S. Obstetrics" *Family Planning Perspectives* 19 (1987): 158–162.

6   N. Binkin, "Trends in Induced Legal Abortion Morbidity and Mortality," *Clinical Obstetrics Gynecology* 13 (1986): 83–93; H. K. Atrash, H. W. Lawson, and J. C. Smith, "Legal Abortion in the U.S.: Trends and Mortality," *Contemporary OB/GYN* 35 (1990): 58–69.

7   S. K. Henshaw and J. Van Vort, "Abortion Services in the United States: 1984–1985," *Family Planning Perspectives* 19 (1987): 63–70; S. K. Henshaw and J. Van Vort, "Abortion Services in the United States, 1987 and 1988," *Family Planning Perspectives* 22 (1990): 102–108.

8   S. K. Henshaw and J. Silverman, "The Characteristics and Prior Contraceptive Use of U.S. Abortion Patients," *Family Planning Perspectives* 20 (1988): 158–168.

9   Medical Students for Choice, Executive Director P. Anderson, 1436 U St., N.W., Washington, DC 20009.

10 W. Cates Jr., R. W. Rochat, D. A. Grimes, and C. W. Tyler Jr., "Legalized Abortion: Effect on National Trends of Maternal and Abortion-Related Mortality (1940–1976)," *American Journal of Obstetrics Gynecology* 132 (1978): 211–214; W. Cates Jr., J. C. Smith, R. W. Rochat, and D. A. Grimes, "Mortality from Abortion and Childbirth: Are the Statistics Biased?" *Morbidity and Mortality Weekly Report* 248 (1982): 192–196; C. Tietze, "The Effect of Legalization of Abortion on Population Growth and Public Health," *Family Planning Perspectives* 7 (1975): 110–113; H. K. Atrash, L. H. Koonin, H. W. Lawson, A. L. Franks, and J. C. Smith, "Maternal Mortality in the United States, 1979–1986," *Obstetrics Gynecology* 76 (1990): 1055–1060; W. Cates Jr. and C. Tietze, "Standardized Mortality Rates Associated with Legal Abortion: United States, 1972–1975," *Family Planning Perspectives* 10 (1978): 109–

112; S. A. LeBolt, D. A. Grimes, and W. Cates Jr., "Mortality from Abortion and Childbirth: Are the Populations Comparable?" *Morbidity and Mortality Weekly Report* 248 (1982): 188–191.

11 H. Corman and M. Grossman, *Determinants of Neonatal Mortality Rates in the United States*, National Bureau of Economic Resources (NBER) working paper series no. 1387, (Cambridge, Mass.: NBER, 1984).

12 Henshaw and Silverman, "Characteristics and Prior Contraceptive Use of U.S. Abortion Patients," *supra* note 8.

13 C. J. R. Hogue, W. Cates, and C. Tietze, "The Effects of Induced Abortion on Subsequent Reproduction," *Epidemiology Review* 4 (1982): 66–94; C. J. R. Hogue, "Impact of Abortion on Subsequent Fecundity," *Clinical Obstetrics Gynecology* 13 (1986): 95–103; H. K. Atrash and C. J. Hogue, "The Effect of Pregnancy Termination on Future Reproduction," *Baillieres Clinical Obstetrics Gynecology* 4 (1990): 391–405; P. I. Frank, "Sequelae of Induced Abortion," *Ciba Foundation Symposium* 115 (1985): 67–82.

14 Darney et al., "Abortion Training in U.S. Obstetrics," *supra* note 5.

15 C. Westhoff, F. Marx, and A. Rosenfield, "Residency Training in Contraception, Sterilization and Abortion," *Journal of Obstetrics and Gynecology* 81, no. 2 (February 1993): 311–314.

16 Henshaw and Van Vort, "Abortion Services in the United States," *supra* note 7.

17 S. K. Henshaw, "The Accessibility of Abortion Services in the United States," *Family Planning Perspectives* 23, no. 6 (1991): 246–263.

18 Though many restrictive bills were introduced prior to that time, 1989 is significant because it was the year the U.S. Supreme Court decided *Webster v. Reproductive Health Services*, 492 U.S. 490 (1989). Because *Webster* suggested the imminent demise of *Roe*, it was a veritable invitation to states to introduce more legislation that might be the vehicle for *Roe's* final ride. That is, in at least six cases prior to 1989, the Court had consistently struck down state restrictions on abortion, including mandatory waiting periods, hospitalization requirements, and parental and/or spousal consent laws. In addition, as recently as 1986, the Court had strongly reaffirmed *Roe* and its commitment to abortion rights, in *Thornburgh v. American College of Obstetricians and Gynecologists*, 476 U.S. 747 (1986). In *Webster*, however, the Court upheld the Missouri restrictions at issue, including restrictions on the use of public hospitals for performing abortions, a ban on performance of abortions by public employees, and requirements of testing to determine fetal viability. Most significantly, for the first time a majority of the Supreme Court suggested that *Roe* should be diluted or abandoned altogether. That dilution, though not the complete abandonment, came to pass three years later in *Planned Parenthood of Southeastern Pennsylvania v. Casey*, 505 U.S. 883, 112 S. Ct. 2791 (1992).

19 J. L. Rogers, R. F. Boruch, G. B. Stoms, and D. DeMoya, "Impact of the Minnesota Parental Notification Law on Abortion and Birth," *American Journal of Public Health* 81 (1991): 294–298; B. Nestor, "Public Financing of Contraceptive Services, 1980–1982," *Family Planning Perspectives* 14 (1982): 198–203.

20 Alan Guttmacher Institute, 120 Wall Street, 21st Floor, New York, NY 10005.

21 Planned Parenthood, New York City, Inc., Clinical Training Initiative (1993).

22 Medical Students for Choice (1993), *supra* note 9.

23　American Medical Women's Association, The Reproductive Health Initiative (1993), Executive Director E. McGrath, 801 N. Fairfax St., Alexandria, VA 22314.

24　National Abortion Federation (NAF), *Who Will Provide Abortions? Ensuring the Availability of Qualified Practitioners* (Washington, D.C.: NAF, 1991), 1–27.

25　W. Chavkin, "A Chill Wind Blows: Webster, Obstetrics, and the Health of Women," *American Journal of Obstetrics Gynecology* 163, no. 2 (1990): 450–452; G. J. Annas, L. H. Glantz, and W. K. Mariner, "The Right of Privacy Protects the Doctor-Patient Relationship," *Journal of the American Medical Association* 263 (1990): 858–861.

26　D. Grimes, D. Mishell, and H. David, "A Randomized Clinical Trial of Mifepristone (RU 486) for Introduction of Delayed Menses: Efficacy and Acceptability," *Contraception* 46, no. 1 (1992); J. Norman, K. Thong, and D. Baird, "Uterine Contractibility and Induction of Abortion in Early Pregnancy by Misoprostol and Mifepristone," *Lancet* 338 (1991): 1233–1236; G. Tang, "A Pilot Study of Acceptability of RU 486 and ONO802 in a Chinese Population," *Contraception* 44 (1991): 523–533.

27　A. Ulmann, L. Silvestre, et al., "Medical Termination of Early Pregnancy with Mifepristone (RU 486) Followed by a Prostaglandin Analogue: Study of 16,369 Women," *Acta Obstet. Gynecol. Scand.* 71 (1992): 278–283; U.K. Multicentre Trial, "The Efficacy and Tolerance of Fopristone and Prostaglandin in the First Trimester Termination of Pregnancy," *British Journal of Obstetrics and Gynaecology* 97 (1990): 480–486.

28　R. Barbosa and M. Arilha, "The Brazilian Experience with Cytotec," *Studies in Family Planning* 24 (1993): 236–240.

29　H. Fernandez, J. Benifia, C. Lelaidler, et al., "Methotrexate Treatment of Ectopic Pregnancy: 100 Cases Treated by Primary Transvaginal Injection Under Sonographic Control," *Fertility and Sterility* 59 (1993): 773–777.

30　M. Creinin and E. Vittinghoff, "Methotrexate and Misoprostol vs. Misoprostol Alone for Early Abortion: A Randomized Controlled Trial," 272 (1994): 1190–1195; R. Hausknecht, personal communication, New York City, 1994.

31　410 U.S. 113, *rehearing denied*, 410 U.S. 959 (1973), establishing a limited constitutional right to abortion. In describing *Roe*, the key word is "limited." By a 7–2 vote, the *Roe* Court constructed an unprecedented constitutional scheme whereby women's rights disappear over time. As of 1973, a woman's right to choose abortion was most nearly absolute only during the first trimester of pregnancy. In the second trimester, the states could regulate abortion for the sake of the health of the mother. In the third trimester, states could prohibit abortion altogether, for the sake of preserving the government's interest in "potential life." Since *Roe*, the trimester scheme has been abandoned, and all state restrictions on the "quasi"-right to abortion are measured by whether they place an "undue burden" on the woman's choice. See *Planned Parenthood of Southeastern Pennsylvania v. Casey*, 505 U.S. 883, 112 S. Ct. 2791 (1992).

32　See note 18 *supra*.

33　R. Pine and S. Law, "Envisioning a Future for Reproductive Liberty: Strategies for Making the Rights Real," *Harvard Civil Rights–Civil Liberties Law Review* 27 (1992): 407, 446 note 168.

34　See note 18 *supra*.

35　505 U.S. 883, 112 S. Ct. 2791 (1992).

36 The restrictions upheld were: (1) a narrow exception for "emergency" situations; (2) the provision of certain discouraging information to the patient (denominated "informed consent") at least twenty-four hours prior to the abortion; (3) a requirement of parental consent of one parent for a minor's abortion, with an option for judicial "bypass" of the parent; (4) and the imposition of reporting requirements on facilities performing abortions. The Court struck down the provision that required a married woman to notify her husband.

37 It was no surprise, of course, when Clarence Thomas voted to overrule *Roe*. When Thomas replaced Thurgood Marshall, who had been a stalwart supporter of women's rights, it was clear that vote was lost. The surprises were that Sandra Day O'Connor, Anthony Kennedy, and David Souter did not vote to overrule *Roe*. O'Connor and Kennedy had voted with the majority in *Webster*, so at least one of them was expected to go along with overruling *Roe* in *Casey*. Souter had replaced William Brennan. Brennan had been a reliable abortion supporter, but Souter, a Bush appointee, was expected to vote the other way.

38 "Lawmakers Target Anti-Abortion Tactic," *Los Angeles Times*, May 10, 1993, A3.

39 "The War on Abortion Clinics," *New York Times*, September 9, 1993, A25. This hatred is nonetheless continually exercised in the name of God. The people arrested for three clinic bombings in Pensacola, Florida, on Christmas day in 1984 stated that the bombings were "a gift to Jesus on his birthday." "Two Men, Two Views on Abortion," *St. Petersburg (Fla.) Times*, November 5, 1993, 1A.

40 "Abortion Foes Strike at Doctors' Home Lives: Illegal Intimidation or Protected Protest?" *Washington Post*, April 8, 1993, A1.

41 "The Death of Dr. Gunn," *New York Times*, March 12, 1993, A28.

42 "Abortion Clinics Said to Be in Peril," *New York Times*, March 6, 1993, A6.

43 "Abortion Foes Strike," *supra* note 40.

44 "Abortion Clinics in Peril," *supra* note 42.

45 Lorraine Maguire, director of Charleston Women's Medical Clinic, quoted in "Abortion Foes Strike," *supra* note 40.

46 "Abortion Clinics in Peril," *supra* note 42, reporting drive-by shooting in Grand Rapids, Michigan

47 "Security Is Stringent at Clinic's Opening," *Los Angeles Times*, October 25, 1993, B1.

48 "Half of Abortion Clinics in Survey Report Hostile Acts," *Boston Globe*, November 5, 1993, 6.

49 "Lawmakers Target Anti-Abortion Tactic," *supra* note 38.

50 Though the national anti-choice groups decry the murders of Dr. Gunn, Dr. Britton, and Mr. Barrett, and the attempted murder of Dr. Tiller, their strategies are increasingly severe. Joseph Scheidler, director of Pro-Life Action in Chicago (and defendant along with Randall Terry in the U.S. Supreme Court "racketeering" case [*see* note 72, infra]), is the architect of the "No Place to Hide" campaign. In 1985, he wrote a book called *Closed: 99 Ways to Stop Abortion*. Now he is writing a manual instructing the faithful how to circumvent abortion laws and picketing restrictions. "Lawmakers Target Anti-Abortion Tactic," *supra* note 38. Operation Rescue has now begun "No Place to Hide: Phase II," targeting the homes of OB-GYN's who provide abortions as part of their overall practices. Later phases may include picketing of the few medical schools that still train students to do any abortions (*supra* note 14 and accompanying text) and picketing at the homes of people employed by

companies that remove or analyze fetal remains. "Lawmakers Target Anti-Abortion Tactic," *supra* note 38.

51 "Protect the People Who Patronize Abortion Clinics," *Phoenix Gazette*, November 16, 1993, B12.

52 "Abortion Foes Strike," *supra* note 40; "U.S. Seeking Curbs on Clinic Attacks," *New York Times*, September 12, 1993, A31. Personnel at 14 percent of clinics surveyed by the Fund for the Feminist Majority in 1993 reported having been stalked. "50% of Abortion Clinics Violence Targets," *Houston Chronicle*, November 5, 1993, 18. See also "Abortion Foe Puts Florida Law to Test in Nurse-Stalking Case," *Houston Chronicle*, April 25, 1993, A12. In Fort Walton Beach, Florida, anti-choice activist Jack Randy Hinesley was charged with stalking a particular nurse for more than a year. He threatened to kill her, repeatedly blocked her path, used flashbulbs to blind her while she was driving, took her picture in a bank and put it on a "wanted poster." The prosecution of Hinesley was the first under the Florida anti-stalking law, which carries maximum penalties of a $1,000 fine or one year in jail.

53 "Abortion Foes Strike," *supra* note 40. This article features an interview with Joseph Scheidler, the architect of the "No Place to Hide" strategy:

> Residential picketing, Scheidler said, is "very effective because it brings their trade right into their families and their neighborhoods" and often creates a rift among neighbors. Targeting spouses is acceptable, he said, "if you've tried to deal with the wife and she's for abortion, well, she's part of the team." Scheidler opposes "going after kids." But he said he believes it is permissible to try to talk with adolescents about what their parents do.

Private harassment has been indiscriminately vicious. The same article reports that someone called the 80-year-old mother of abortion provider Dr. Frank Sedley at 3:00 A.M., claiming to be a Florida Highway Patrol officer, and told her that her son had been killed in an auto crash. Mrs. Sedley, who had a heart condition, was dangerously distraught until she learned several hours later that her son was safe.

54 Twenty percent of the clinics surveyed by the Feminist Majority in 1993 reported death threats to personnel. "50% of Abortion Clinics Violence Targets," *supra* note 52, 18. Betty Hoover, a clinic director in El Paso, Texas, reported the following phone call to the receptionist:

> You tell Betty Hoover I'm watching her. I know where she goes, what she does, when she does it, and I'm going to cut her up into little pieces like all the babies she's killed.

"Abortion Clinics in Peril," *supra* note 42.

55 These protective measures are often taken on the advice of local police, who are otherwise unable to deal with the violence. "Reno Urges Senate to Curb Anti-Abortion Violence," *New York Times*, May 13, 1992, A21. About these measures, Dr. Brian Finkel of the Metro Phoenix Women's Center has said: "I don't believe as a physician, I should have to wear a bulletproof vest. I am a gynecologist in Arizona, not a Ranger in Mogadishu." Quoted in "Abortion Providers Seek More Protection," *Orlando (Fla.) Sentinel*, October 19, 1993, B1.

56 "Abortion Clinics in Peril," *supra* note 42.

57 "Legal Barricade Staked Before Abortion Foes; Judge Prohibits Stalking of Doc-

tors," *Houston Chronicle*, June 25, 1993, A29. Michael Griffin was convicted of first-degree murder and sentenced to life in prison on March 5, 1994. "Antiabortion Activist Is Convicted, Sentenced to Life in Killing at Clinic," *Washington Post*, March 6, 1994, A22.

58 "Abortion Under Fire in U.S.," *Newsday*, November 5, 1993, 37.

59 "Judge Asked to Keep Chicago Schools Open," *USA Today*, October 4, 1993, 9A. Ms. Shannon was convicted of attempted murder and given a prison sentence by a Kansas state court on April 26, 1994. "Woman Who Shot Doctor Gets Nearly 11 Years," *Washington Post*, April 27, 1994, A24.

60 "Woman Charged After Abortion Doctor is Shot," *Los Angeles Times*, August 21, 1993, A1.

61 "U.S. Seeking Curbs on Clinic Attacks," *supra* note 52.

62 "Doctor, Escort Slain Near Abortion Clinic," *Sacramento Bee*, July 30, 1994, A1.

63 " 'Deadly Force Should Be Used,' " *Sacramento Bee*, July 30, 1994, A26.

64 "2 Slain at Abortion Clinic; Ex-Minister Is Arrested in Shootings," *St. Louis Post-Dispatch*, July 30, 1994, 1A.

65 " 'Deadly Force,' " *supra* note 63.

66 Paul Hill was convicted of two counts of first-degree murder in a Florida state court on November 10, 1994. Although Mr. Hill had not been sentenced as of this writing, the jury in his case had unanimously recommended to the court that he receive the death penalty. "Jury Urges Death Sentence in Abortion Clinic Murders," *Washington Post*, November 14, 1994, A1. Previously, Paul Hill was the first person convicted by a federal court of criminal activity under the new federal Freedom of Access to Clinics Entrances Act. He was found guilty of three violations of that act, and was to be sentenced on December 9, 1994. "Hill Guilty in Abortion Access Case," *Washington Post*, October 5, 1994, A3. On the recent passage and meaning of the Freedom of Access to Clinic Entrances Act, see notes 67–69.

67 So concerned has the Attorney General been with clinic violence that at an October 29, 1993, meeting with women's rights groups on the issue, she gave them her home phone number! "Reno Meets with Groups on Both Sides of Abortion Issue," *Los Angeles Times*, October 30, 1993, A21.

68 The Freedom of Access to Clinic Entrances Act (FACE) became law in 1994. 18 U.S.C. § 248 *et seq*. FACE provides civil and criminal penalties against anyone who

> by force or threat of force or by physical obstruction, intentionally injures, intimidates or interferes with or attempts to injure, intimidate or interfere with any person because that person is or has been, or in order to intimidate such person or any other person or any class of persons from, obtaining or providing reproductive health services.

Ibid. § 248(a)(1). Since its enactment, FACE has been repeatedly challenged in various federal courts as an unconstitutional infringement on the guarantee of freedom of speech. Every court to address the issue has rejected the challenge, and the United States Supreme Court has twice declined to review these decisions. *American Life League v. Reno*, 47 F.3d 642 (4th Cir.), *cert. denied*, — U.S. —, 116 S. Ct. 55, 133 L. Ed. 2d 19 (1995); *Woodall v. Reno* 47 F.3d 656 (4th Cir.), *cert. denied* — U.S. —, 115 S. Ct. 2577, 132 L. Ed. 2d 827 (1995); *Council for Life Coalition v. Reno*, 856 F. Supp. 1422 (S.D. Cal. 1994); *Cheffer v. Reno*, — F. Supp. —, 1994 WL 644873 (M.D. Fla.

1994), *appeal pending*, No. 94-2976 (11th Cir. 1994); *Cook v. Reno*, 859 F. Supp. 1008 (W.D. La. 1994); *Riely v. Reno*, 860 F. Supp. 693 (D. Ariz. 1994); *United States v. Brock*, 863 F. Supp. 851 (E.D. Wis. 1994), *appeal docketed sub nom. United States v. Hatch*, No. 95-1494 (7th Cir. 1995). One federal district court has held FACE unconstitutional, not as violative of freedom of expression, but on federal Commerce Clause grounds. *United States. v. Wilson*, 880 F. Supp. 621 (E.D. Wis.), *appeal docketed*, No. 95-1494 (7th Cir. 1995).

69   18 U.S.C. § 248(a)(1–3), (b)(1–3), (c)(1)(B), (c)(2)(A).

70   "Senate OK's Bill Aimed at Anti-Abortion Tactics," *Houston Chronicle*, November 17, 1993, A1.

71   The toll-free number for reporting information about violence committed at abortion clinics is 1-800-ATF-4867.

72   *National Organization for Women v. Scheidler*, — U.S. —, 114 S. Ct. 798, 127 L. Ed. 2d 99, *rehearing denied* — U.S. —, 114 S. Ct. 1340 (1994).

73   RICO is the Racketeer Influenced and Corrupt Organizations Act. 18 U.S.C.A. §§ 1961–1968. Under § 1962(c) thereof, it is unlawful

> for any person employed by or associated with any enterprise engaged in, or the activities of which affect, interstate or foreign commerce, to conduct or participate, directly or indirectly, in the conduct of such enterprise's affairs through a pattern of racketeering activity.

> RICO was originally enacted as a broad net in which to catch "traditional" organized crime, but it is not a big conceptual stretch to apply RICO to anti-abortion protestors. Traditional organized crime thrives on the pimping of women into prostitution and pornography. Forced childbearing is just another aspect of the control and consumption of women.

> Two legal factors are crucial to the application of RICO to anti-abortion groups. First, 18 U.S.C. § 1961(1) defines "racketeering activity" as, among other things, any act or threat involving murder or arson. Second, while RICO's primary targets are the profit-motivated activities of organized crime, the U.S. Supreme Court in *Scheidler* interpreted RICO *not* to require any economic profit motive in defendants.

74   *Maher v. Roe*, 432 U.S. 464 (1977), allowing denial of Medicaid funding for "nontherapeutic" abortions; *Harris v. McRae*, 448 U.S. 297 (1980), allowing denial of Medicaid funding for "therapeutic" abortions, that is, even for abortions necessary to a woman's health.

75   Since 1977, the Hyde Amendments have allowed for various exceptions. In all of its versions, the Amendments have provided federal funds for abortion where the mother's life would be endangered if the fetus were carried to term. This exception is itself mandated by *Roe v. Wade* and was acknowledged even by the dissenters, Justices Rehnquist and White, in that case. In fiscal years 1978 and 1979, the Hyde Amendments had an exception that allowed federal abortion funding to be provided when two physicians certified that "severe and long-lasting physical health damage" to the mother would result if the pregnancy were carried to term. See *Harris v. McRae*, 448 U.S. 297, 302–303 (1980). The most recent version of the Hyde Amendment, like some previous incarnations, contains an additional exception allowing funding for abortions of pregnancies resulting from rape or incest. Health and Human Services Appropriation Act, Pub. L. No. 102-112, § 509, 107 Stat. 1082, 1113 (1993).

76 As of this writing, four states voluntarily fund medically necessary abortions under Medicaid pursuant to state statute or regulation: Alaska, Hawaii, New York, and Washington.

77 Eleven of these orders — those in Minnesota, New Mexico, Montana, Illinois, Idaho, West Virginia, Connecticut, Vermont, New Jersey, California, and Massachusetts — rest on independent state constitutional grounds: *Women of Minn. v. Gomez*, No. CX-94-1442 (Minn. Dec. 15, 1995); *New Mexico Right to Choose, et al. v. Danfelser*, No. SF 95-867(C) (N.M. Dist. Ct., July 26, 1995) (appeal pending); *Jeannette R. et al. v. Ellery et al.*, No. BDV-94-811 (Mont. Dist. Ct., May 22, 1995); *Doe v. Wright*, No. 91 CH 1958 (Cook Cnty. Cir. Ct. Dec. 2, 1994); *Roe v. Harris*, No. 96977 (Idaho Dist. Ct. Feb. 1, 1994); *Women's Health Center v. Panepinto*, Nos. 21924–21925 (W. Va. Dec. 17, 1993); *Doe v. Maher*, 515 A.2d 134 (Conn. Super. Ct. 1986); *Doe v. Celani*, No. S81-84CnC (Vt. Super. Ct. 1986); *Right to Choose v. Byrne*, 450 A.2d 925 (N.J. 1982); *Committee to Defend Reproductive Rights v. Myers*, 625 P.2d 779 (Cal. 1981); *Moe v. Secretary of Admin. & Fin.*, 417 N.E.2d 387 (Mass. 1981). The Oregon Supreme Court ordered funding on state statutory grounds. *Planned Parenthood Ass'n v. Department of Human Resources*, 687 P.2d 785 (Or. 1984). Only three state courts, Kentucky, Michigan, and Pennsylvania, have refused state constitutional challenges to restore Medicaid abortion funding. *Doe v. Childers*, No. 94CIO2183 (Ky. Dist. Ct. Aug. 3, 1995); *Doe v. Department of Social Services*, 487 N.W.2d 166 (Mich. 1992); *Fischer v. Department of Public Welfare*, 502 A.2d 114 (Pa. 1985).

78 Justice Blackmun was, of course, the author of the *Roe v. Wade* decision. He has spoken publicly and often of the ways that decision changed his life. History is replete with reports of thousands of pieces of hate mail delivered to him, numerous death threats, and the showering of his home with bullets. His judicial record speaks eloquently to his commitment, at least since 1973, to full and equal personhood for women. Among the most moving statements in all of U.S. constitutional law appears in Justice Blackmun's dissent in *Webster*, 492 U.S. at 538–560 (1989):

> I fear for the future. I fear for the liberty and equality of the millions of women who have lived and come of age in the 16 years since Roe was decided. I fear for the integrity of, and public esteem for, this Court. . . . For today, at least, the law of abortion stands undisturbed. For today, the women of this Nation still retain the liberty to control their destinies. But the signs are evident and very ominous, and a chill wind blows.

Then again, dissenting in *Casey* in 1992, 505 U.S. at —, 112 S. Ct. at 2854–2855, Blackmun wrote:

> I am 83 years old. I cannot remain on this Court forever, and when I do step down, the confirmation process for my successor well may focus on the issue before us today. That, I regret, may be exactly where the choice between . . . two worlds will be made.

79 K. J. Meier and D. R. McFarlane, "State Family Planning and Abortion Expenditures: Their Effect on Public Health," *American Journal of Public Health* 84, no. 9 (September 1994): 1470.

80 Ibid. Put more scientifically, funded abortions are associated with a drop in births to

teen mothers of as many as 0.67 for every abortion funded per 1,000 women of childbearing age.

81 To its credit, the National Abortion Rights Action League (NARAL) has recently decided to change its strategy away from focusing solely on abortion to focusing on both women's and men's reproductive health. NARAL President Kate Michelman has said: "We think abortion is a bad thing. No woman wants to have an abortion." As of January 1994, the name of the organization will be changed to the National Abortion and Reproductive Rights Action League, and much more attention will be given to preventing teen pregnancy, improving prenatal care, and promoting sex education, contraceptive research, and infant care. "Abortion-Rights Groups Ready to Change Course," *Albuquerque Journal*, December 13, 1993, A4.

82 1990 U.S. Dept. of Health and Human Services, Office of Child Support Enforcement, Annual Report 5.

83 29 U.S.C. § 206(d)(1), prohibiting discrimination in wages for "equal work" on the basis of sex.

84 U.S. Department of Labor, Women's Bureau, No. 93-2, *Twenty Facts on Working Women* 2 (June 1993).

85 42 U.S.C. § 2000e-2 (1978). The Pregnancy Discrimination Act amended Title VII of the Civil Rights Act of 1964 in an effort to reverse a decision of the U.S. Supreme Court which had held that job discrimination on the basis of pregnancy was not sex discrimination. *General Electric Co. v. Gilbert*, 429 U.S. 125 (1976). The Pregnancy Discrimination Act simply amended the definitions section of Title VII to say that discrimination on the basis of pregnancy *was* sex discrimination; it did not require any *particular* treatment of pregnant women—that is, that they be given leave or medical/disability/maternity benefits—it required only that pregnant women be treated the same as other workers on the basis of "their ability or inability to work." See H.R. Rep. No. 948, 95th Cong., 2d Sess. 7, 4, reprinted in 1978 U.S. Code Cong. and Ad. News 4749.

86 29 U.S.C.A. §§ 2601–2654 (1993). Section 2612 of the Family and Medical Leave Act provides in part that qualifying employees are entitled to a total of twelve weeks of unpaid leave per year whenever they are attending to the birth of a child, the adoption of a child, the illness of a child, or serious medical conditions among their immediate family, including parents.

87 H.R. 3600 was introduced in the House on November 20, 1993, by then-House Majority Leader Richard Gephardt. S. 1757 was introduced in the Senate, also on November 20, 1993, by then-Senate Majority Leader George Mitchell. After less than one year of debate, the 103rd Congress recessed after deciding that nothing would be done with either bill. "Health Care Reform: The Collapse of a Quest," *Washington Post*, October 11, 1994, A6.

88 On this point, MacKinnon writes:

The law of rape divides women into spheres of consent according to indices of relationship to men. . . . The paradigm categories are the virginal daughter and other young girls, with whom all sex is proscribed, and the whorelike wives and prostitutes, with whom no sex is proscribed. Daughters may not consent; wives and prostitutes are assumed to, and cannot but. Actual consent or nonconsent, far less actual desire, is comparatively irrelevant.

Catharine A. MacKinnon, *Toward a Feminist Theory of the State* (Cambridge: Harvard University Press, 1989), 175.

89 For a moving description of the experience of adolescent women, see Robin West, "The Difference in Women's Hedonic Lives: A Phenomenological Critique of Feminist Legal Theory," *Wisconsin Women's Law Journal* 3 (1987): 81, 101–103.

90 See, e.g., Andrea Dworkin, *Pornography: Men Possessing Women* (New York: Perigee, 1981).

91 See, e.g., Margaret A. Baldwin, "Split at the Root: Prostitution and Feminist Discourses of Law Reform," *Yale Journal of Law and Feminism* 5 (1992).

92 West, "Difference in Women's Hedonic Lives," *supra* note 89, 103–106.

93 Ibid., 93.

94 This "constitutional stew" was the basis of the 1965 decision which found that the resulting "penumbral" right of privacy ensured the right to use contraceptives. *Griswold v. Connecticut*, 381 U.S. 479 (1965). That decision was fundamental to the Supreme Court's decision in *Roe v. Wade*, though the latter case determined the relevant privacy right to be derived entirely from the Fourteenth Amendment's guarantee that "liberty" could not be deprived without due process of law. 410 U.S. 113, 153 (1973).

95 See, e.g., John Hart Ely, "The Wages of Crying Wolf: A Comment on Roe v. Wade," *Yale Law Journal* 82 (1973). See also *Thornburgh v. American College of Obstetricians and Gynecologists*, 476 U.S. 747, 828 (1986) (O'Connor, J., dissenting); *City of Akron v. Akron Center for Reproductive Health*, 462 U.S. 416, 453, 461–463 (1983) (O'Connor, J., dissenting).

96 Andrea Dworkin, "Against the Male Flood: Censorship, Pornography, and Equality," *Harvard Women's Law Journal* 8 (1985): 3.

97 In all of this, women are also portrayed as senseless murderers, as *amoral* annihilators of what is right and good. Instead, we should be asking, with Adrienne Rich:

> who indeed hates whom, who is killing whom, whose interest is served, and whose fantasies expressed, by representing abortion as the selfish, wilful, morally contagious expression of *woman's* predilection for violence?

A. Rich, *On Lies, Secrets, and Silence: Selected Prose, 1966–1978* (New York: W. W. Norton, 1979), 17 (emphasis in original).

98 Title VII of the Civil Rights Act of 1964, for example, prohibits discrimination on the basis of sex (along with discrimination on the basis of race, national origin, and religion) in employment. 42 U.S.C. 2000e *et seq.* (1964). As a telling example of women's tenuous claim to legal equality, however, it must be noted that during congressional wrangling over this historic bill, "sex" was added as a prohibited basis of discrimination at the very last minute as a strategy for defeating the entire Civil Rights Act. The act passed anyway. 100 Cong. Rec. 2577 (1964). In the constitutional realm, it was not until 1971 (under the tutelage of then-advocate Ruth Bader Ginsburg) that the U.S. Supreme Court allowed women meaningful recourse under the Equal Protection Clause. *Reed v. Reed*, 404 U.S. 71 (1971). That and other ground-breaking Equal Protection cases involved situations where women really are just like men. *Reed*, for example, required the state of Idaho to consider women as eligible administrators of estates on the same basis as it did men, because women are just as likely to be able to read the intestate succession statute and to do the math.

99   See, e.g., *Geduldig v. Aiello*, 417 U.S. 484 (1974), which held that discrimination on
      the basis of pregnancy is not sex discrimination within the meaning of the Equal
      Protection Clause; *cf. Bray v. Alexandria Women's Clinic*, 506 U.S. 263, 113 S. Ct. 753
      (1993). In this decision, holding that Operation Rescue could not be found guilty of
      a conspiracy to deprive women of their constitutional rights under a Civil War–era
      federal statute, Justice Scalia explained how discrimination against abortion was not
      sex discrimination:

> Whatever one thinks of abortion, it cannot be denied that there are common and
> respectable reasons for opposing it, other than hatred of or condescension to-
> ward (or indeed any view at all concerning) women as a class — as is evident from
> the fact that men and women are on both sides of the issue.

      506 U.S. 263, —, 113 S. Ct. 753, 760 (1993).
100   To date, the most exceptional decision of the United States Supreme Court has been
      California Federal Sav. and Loan Ass'n v. Guerra, 479 U.S. 272 (1987). That case
      upheld a California law that required employers to hold jobs open for pregnant
      workers who take pregnancy-related leaves of absence. That is, the Court held that it
      is not sex discrimination for a state to recognize the actual reproductive circum-
      stances of women.
101   See, e.g., Ann Scales, "Towards a Feminist Jurisprudence," *Indiana Law Journal* 56
      (1981): 375; *cf.* Ann Scales, "The Emergence of Feminist Jurisprudence," *Yale Law
      Journal* 95 (1986): 373.
102   Catharine A. MacKinnon, "Reflections on Sex Equality under Law," *Yale Law Jour-
      nal* 100 (1991): 1281, 1314.
103   See, e.g., Ruth Bader Ginsburg, "Some Thoughts on Autonomy and Equality in
      Relation to *Roe v. Wade*," *North Carolina Law Review* 63 (1985): 375. In fairness to
      Ginsburg's critics, it should be noted that she also stated that the Supreme Court
      may have gone too far too fast in deciding *Roe*. According to Ginsburg, by declaring a
      sweeping constitutional right to abortion, the Supreme Court virtually guaranteed
      the very social upheaval that has come to pass. The Court could have achieved the
      same legal result (i.e., invalidation of the Texas criminal abortion law at issue in *Roe*)
      but on a narrower ground. As it was, she argues, the "line in the sand" drawn by the
      Court may have halted a trend toward state liberalization of abortion-restrictive
      laws. *Id.* at 379–381. It is surely debatable whether Ginsburg was right about state
      law liberalization — whether it was really happening or would have continued. How-
      ever, Ginsburg's argument here is *not* an anti-abortion position but only a reflection
      of her incrementalist philosophy of federal judicial decision making. And we must
      recognize that it was that reticent judiciousness that allowed her to be confirmed to
      the high Court. I have no doubt that, at the end of the day, Justice Ginsburg will be
      there for women, whether the right to abortion is founded on due process or equal
      protection or any other constitutional basis whatsoever.
104   Ibid., 383 (citations omitted, emphasis added). Particularly in the discussions of
      equality cited in this chapter, now-Justice Ginsburg relied heavily on Kenneth Karst,
      "Forward: Equal Citizenship Under the Fourteenth Amendment," *Harvard Law
      Review* 91 (1977): 1.

11

WOMEN PRISONERS AND HEALTH CARE

Locked Up and Locked Out

. . . .

Ellen M. Barry

Jane B.[1] was a 36-year-old mother of two who was serving two years at a large state women's prison for forging checks worth about $1,000. She suffered from a severe gastrointestinal disorder. In spite of her requests for assistance, she was given neither effective medical or psychological care for her condition. She slowly starved to death, and the county coroner's report indicated starvation as the cause of death. She left two young daughters and an elderly, disabled mother.

■

Mary H. was a 40-year-old woman serving a three-year sentence for possession of drugs. She had a serious heart condition for which she received very little effective treatment or care. On the day she died, she requested to be seen by medical staff at the infirmary on two separate occasions but was denied treatment both times. Later that day, she had a heart attack and died on the way to the outside hospital.

■

Angela H. was a 20-year-old woman from a large county in Southern California. She was serving time on a parole violation for possession and sale of marijuana and she was almost five months pregnant at the time she entered the state prison. Soon after she was incarcerated, she began to experience vaginal bleeding, cramping, and severe pain. She requested medical assistance numerous times over a period of three weeks, but was not seen by an OB-GYN, since there was no OB on contract with the institution. She was finally seen by the chief medical officer, an orthopedist, who diagnosed her as having a vaginal infection without examining her physically or running any laboratory tests and prescribed Flagyl, a drug that should be avoided during pregnancy because it can induce premature labor. The next day, Angela went into labor and delivered on the way to the outside hospital. Her infant son lived approximately two hours.

Introduction

There is a critical need for national policymakers to address the serious deficiencies in medical care received by women in prisons and jails nationwide. While a few national agencies have addressed the question of comprehensive standards for institutional medical care, women's health concerns are largely ignored.[2] By the same token, although medical advocacy groups such as the American College for Obstetricians and Gynecologists (ACOG) promulgates standards for OB-GYN care generally, these standards have yet to be adapted to the correctional setting.[3]

Profile of Women Prisoners

While the health care available to low-income women in the United States is generally poor, medical conditions for women in United States prisons and jails are appallingly bad. There are few correctional systems that provide adequate or good care. Those that do usually are compelled to do so under court order or do so because they have unusually good medical staff. However, these systems are the rare exceptions. Based on information gleaned through class-action litigation, research, investigative journalism, and legislative studies, a picture has emerged that reflects a systematic pattern of neglect and, sometimes, abuse of women prisoners in need of medical care.

At the end of 1994, almost 95,000 women were incarcerated in state prisons and federal institutions and jails nationwide. This figure represents an increase of more than 275 percent, compared with a percentage increase of 160 percent of male prisoners in the period between 1980 and 1992.[4] While women prisoners comprise less than 6 percent of the population of the prisoners in United States prisons[5] and less than 10 percent of the county jail population,[6] their role in the correctional process is certainly important in terms of determining ethical public policy. As in all areas of our society, women prisoners suffer adversely from the effects of gender bias and unequal treatment. These women have less access to programs and services than their male counterparts, and this inequity is reflected in reduced access to medical care. In addition, a significant percentage of women prisoners are pregnant (10 percent) or have been pregnant in the previous twelve months (postpartum) period (15 percent), and incarcerated pregnant women face unique problems.[7]

The inadequacy of medical care has had severe repercussions for women prisoners, leading in many cases to late-term miscarriages, untreated cancer and other life-threatening diseases, increased disability as a consequence of poor or nonexistent care and, in some instances, death. This pattern of inadequate care has a significant racial component since nationwide more than 60 percent of women in prison are women of color. African-American women are most dramatically overrepresented in the criminal justice system, comprising 46 percent of women prisoners in 1992 while African-Americans represented only 12 percent of the population nationwide. Hispanic women and Latinas are 12 percent of the population of women in prison as compared with 9 percent of California's statewide population. In addition, Native American women, although a small overall percentage of the population of women in prison, are also dramatically overrepresented in comparison with their percentage in the national population. Finally, in the past decade, there is a small but growing number of Asian–Pacific Islander women entering the criminal justice system in the United States.[8]

Thus, a great number of women who will suffer the consequences of inadequate medical care while incarcerated will be women of color. In addition, since certain forms of cancer, high blood pressure, diabetes, lupus, and other serious medical conditions have been found to affect African-American women and other women of color at greater rates than Caucasian women, incarcerated women of color statistically will be at greater risk for having these conditions and thus will be at even greater risk if they are unable to receive appropriate or adequate treatment for these conditions.

Barbara F. was an African-American woman in her forties who was serving a lengthy sentence for killing her abusive partner. While incarcerated, she was diagnosed with cancer of the esophagus. Because of the length of her sentence, it was unlikely that she would be released before she died. Through aggressive legal intervention, Barbara was granted clemency and released into the community. Four days later, after saying good-bye to her mother, sister, and son, she died. Although she was only out for a short period before she died, she was able to die in freedom.

Summary of Women Prisoners' Health Concerns

Women generally feel discounted and disenfranchised by a medical care system that historically has ignored their needs. Incarcerated women are even further isolated and disempowered, lacking any semblance of choice or control over their medical care.

In most systems, women in prison and jail are completely dependent on correctional staff to obtain any form of medical care. Although several courts have held that nonmedical correctional staff cannot act as gate-keepers, deciding which prisoners see medical personnel,[9] this procedure is often the reality in most women's prisons. Regardless of whether non-medical correctional staff are part of the formal medical screening process, in many systems they can effectively prevent or deter women from seeing medical personnel for their medical complaints. In addition, women prisoners routinely have difficulty obtaining a second medical opinion, even in life-threatening or critical medical situations.

Yvonne H. was in her late twenties, serving time for fraud at a federal correctional institution. She was diagnosed with fibroid uterine tumors and told by the chief medical officer at the prison that she was being scheduled for a hysterectomy. She requested a second opinion, but the warden denied her request. After extensive legal intervention, she was able to see a second, noncorrectional OB–GYN. She remarked that finally a medical person had talked to her as if she were a human being and explained to her clearly what was going on with her body and what her options were.

Training of nonmedical staff in basic emergency procedures is often a critical problem. Most correctional institutions are not equipped to handle the delivery of infants. Yet because prisoners are often not believed when they advise staff that they are in labor, and because staff (medical and nonmedical) are not always aware of correct emergency responses to medical situations, staff are sometimes called upon to respond to emergency deliveries of infants even though they lack the basic training to do so.

Loreena Y. advised correctional staff that she was in labor at approximately 9:00 p.m. on a Friday evening. She was told that no medical personnel would be on duty until early the next morning and that she would have to wait until then to deliver. She labored throughout the night, and returned to the jail clinic early the next morning, where she gave birth on the floor outside of the medical clinic with only the assistance of an untrained guard. The baby suffered meconium ingestion and oxygen loss during the birth process and died several months later.

Women are seen as "complainers" by medical personnel, and their serious symptoms are often labeled as "psychosomatic" and fabricated. Women in prison face this same attitude, but in a much more dangerous and frightening context. If women on the outside are disbelieved, they at least have the theoretical option of seeing another physician (although, in reality, these women often lack the economic means and psychological framework to seek another opinion). However, incarcerated women have no other option. Through nineteen years of experience interviewing women prisoners about their medical care, and countless conversations with other attorneys, doctors, and prisoners' advocates, I am aware of hundreds and hundreds of examples — from gynecological problems, to incorrectly set bones, to incorrect medications, to misdiagnosed fatal illnesses — where women in prison have received thoughtless, careless, deliberately malicious, and sometimes barbaric treatment.

Estella C. was a young, undocumented woman from Mexico who entered the prison system when she was almost four months pregnant. Over the next five months, she was never once seen by an OB, even though she suspected that she was having a problem with her pregnancy. As a result of legal intervention when she was almost full term, she was finally seen by a noncorrectional OB who did a sonogram and determined that there was a live fetus but realized that the fetus was experiencing developmental problems. Estella was ordered to return to the outside hospital the following week, but she was never brought to this appointment. The following week, at full term, the fetus died in utero. The chief medical officer told Estella, and her attorney, that she had lost the baby before she was incarcerated and that she had been carrying a dead fetus in her body for over five months.

■

Nicole J. was an African-American woman in her late twenties serving time at an urban county jail. When she was about three months pregnant, she experienced a miscarriage, not unlike thousands of women on the outside. But, as she lay on the gurney in the jail clinic, bleeding from the loss of her pregnancy, the head nurse, experienced in OB–GYN care, told her that she would be better off, and so would the baby, if she lost this baby.

While the provision of adequate, responsive, and appropriate medical care is a complex challenge in any context, it is particularly challenging in a correctional setting. Prisons and jails are severely stressful environments — they are often dramatically overcrowded (a number of women in a large rural jail reported having to sleep on thin mats on the floor during late stages of pregnancy in cells designed to hold sixteen which routinely held twenty-four or twenty-five women). They are often unsanitary and intolerably loud. (Many women reported having to wade through sewerage several inches deep to use toilets; others reported being restricted to one pair of underwear per week which they had to wash out in water coolers.) Nutrition is almost always a low priority, even for pregnant women, who report receiving sour milk, food contaminated with roaches, mold, and other uninviting elements, and generally inadequate diets. (One pregnant woman joked about enjoying her assignment at the honor farm of a large women's jail; as she picked string beans, she would put one in the basket and pop another in her mouth — the only fresh vegetable in her diet that week.)

However, as difficult as it might be to overcome the factors of overcrowding, sanitation, noise, nutrition, and patients who have had a history of poor medical care, the most discouraging and pernicious factor — the factor that cannot be legislated or changed by court order but which *must* be changed if the quality of medical treatment care is to be improved for women prisoners — is the attitude of correctional staff, both medical and nonmedical.

The Status of Legal Protections

The current constitutional standard for determining whether or not a prison system has failed to provide adequate medical care for prisoners was established in the United States Supreme Court decision in the case of *Estelle v. Gamble*.[10] The Court found that "a prisoner must allege acts or omissions sufficiently harmful to evidence deliberate indifference to serious medical needs" in order to establish a valid claim of cruel and unusual punishment under the Eighth Amendment.[11] In defining "deliberate indifference," the Court held that the pattern or practice challenged would have to amount to the " 'unnecessary and wanton infliction of pain' proscribed by the Eighth Amendment."[12]

Following *Estelle*, a number of appellate courts further clarified the definition of "deliberate indifference" in the context of providing medical care to prisoners. Thus, in cases where prisoners were denied access to medical care,[13] where correctional staff prevented prisoners from receiving treatment prescribed by medical personnel,[14] and where correctional medical personnel have specifically ignored the medical needs of prisoners,[15] courts in several federal circuits have held that such conduct amounted to a violation of prisoners' constitutional rights under the Eighth Amendment. In another significant decision, the Tenth Circuit held that deliberate indifference to prisoners' serious medical needs could be established in a situation where there were "repeated examples of negligent acts which disclose a pattern of conduct by the prison medical staff."[16]

Todaro v. Ward was the first major lawsuit brought on behalf of women prisoners that raised the issue of inadequate medical care and clarified the Supreme Court's definition of deliberate indifference.[17] Women prisoners confined in the New York state prison, Bedford Hills, sued on behalf of all prisoners, alleging a systematic pattern of inadequate medical care. The plaintiffs raised a number of issues, including inadequacy of dental and psychiatric care as well as standard medical care. The district court found a number of specific practices to be unconstitutional, including the inadequate access of prisoners to medical staff, the use of a "lobby clinic" for screening medical complaints, and several medical and record-keeping procedures that caused substantial delays in prisoners receiving medical care. The court held that

> [w]hile a single instance of medical care, denied or delayed, viewed in isolation, may appear to be the product of mere negligence, repeated examples of such treatment bespeak a deliberate indifference by prison authorities to the agony engendered by haphazard and ill-conceived procedures.[18]

Throughout the 1980s a number of lawsuits were filed on behalf of women prisoners who alleged that they had been denied adequate medical, dental, and psychiatric care. These suits raised significant concerns and resulted, in many cases, in strong decisions and consent decrees mandating better medical treatment.[19] While the standard established in *Estelle* and further clarified in *Todaro, Ramos,* and other appellate cases is still current, there has been a recent trend in Supreme Court opinions to significantly narrow the constitutional rights of prisoners.[20] It is likely that this trend will continue unless the composition of the Supreme Court changes considerably.

Although litigation filed in the 1980s on behalf of women prisoners resulted in significant improvements in the provision of medical care for a certain period of time in a number of prisons and jails throughout the country, both prisoners and advocates have determined that the provision of adequate medical care remains one of the most serious problems for women prisoners in the 1990s. Thus, in April of 1995, women prisoners confined at two large California prisons, the Central California Women's Facility (CCWF) in Chowchilla and the California Institution for Women (CIW) in Frontera, filed a federal class-action lawsuit, *Shumate et al. v. Wilson,* in U.S. District Court in Sacramento. The suit charged that the prisons' dramatically deficient medical care for chronically and terminally ill women has caused needless pain and suffering and threatened their health and lives.

The plaintiffs include incarcerated women with cancer, heart disease, sickle cell anemia, AIDS, tuberculosis, and other illnesses. They are suing Governor of California Pete Wilson and the California Department of Corrections (CDC) for systematic deprivation of essential care for their medical needs.

The lawsuit describes case after case of shockingly deficient treatment:

–A seizure patient at CCWF who is paralyzed on her left side has never been given occupational or physical therapy.
–A 68-year-old woman at CIW who has asthma and cardiac problems was placed in a locked room for approximately twelve hours without oxygen, necessary medication, or treatment.
–A woman at CCWF who suffered burns over 54 percent of her body has gradually lost mobility because she was denied the special bandages that would prevent her burned skin from tightening.
–A prisoner at CCWF was confined naked in a filthy cell where she ingested her own bodily waste. She died of untreated pancreatitis that went undiagnosed until she was terminally ill.
–A woman at CCWF unsuccessfully begged staff for months to allow her to see a doctor. She was finally diagnosed with cancer. Though in enormous pain, she received almost no pain medication. Because of swelling in her legs, she could barely walk, yet she was required to walk to the dining hall if she wanted to eat. She died approximately nine months after the diagnosis.

Plaintiffs allege that the CDC lacks basic, standardized systems for the delivery of health care, so that women with chronic health problems come to expect disruptions in their treatment and chaotic follow-up. For example, many women with serious high-risk factors for breast and cervical cancer have been denied necessary mammograms and pap smears. HIV-positive women at both prisons also have been denied necessary specialized care, pain medication, and hospice treatment.

The suit also alleges that women are routinely forced to wait for long periods of time to obtain necessary medications and frequently experience interruptions of medications. Plaintiffs with diabetes, heart conditions, and AIDS are denied medically necessary diets. These conditions amount to cruel and unusual punishment and therefore, the prisoners argue, violate the Eighth Amendment of the Constitution.[21] The case is pending.

Treatment of Pregnant Women Prisoners

Bernida J. was a 25-year-old African-American woman from San Bernardino, California. She was experiencing breakthrough bleeding and cramping late in her pregnancy but, in spite of these symptoms, was assigned to clean institutional floors by pushing a heavy floor buffer. She experienced repeated episodes of bleeding, and at eight months gestation, began hemorrhaging. The fetus died in utero and she came close to death. She was given an emergency hysterectomy.

There is perhaps no other situation more shocking to the conscience in the correctional context than the deliberate and callous disregard shown by some correctional personnel — medical and nonmedical — to pregnant women experiencing serious medical complications. However, practitioners in a number of jurisdictions have documented repeated examples of cases where pregnant women prisoners have been treated in a manner that is nothing short of barbaric.

Although I have many years of experience working with women prisoners, prior to initiating litigation on behalf of women prisoners I was unprepared for the shocking disregard of basic humanity that I saw reflected in the treatment to which pregnant women are subjected. There is a unique form of misogyny that certain correctional personnel — both medical and nonmedical — exhibit in connection with the abusive treatment of pregnant women.

Substantial litigation has been brought on behalf of pregnant and parenting women prisoners to challenge the inadequate quality of medical care provided to them during and after pregnancy and to expand alternatives to incarceration and programs for incarcerated mothers and their children. In one landmark case, *West v. Manson*,[22] women prisoners confined to a Connecticut state prison challenged the lack of medical care and social services for pregnant and parenting women. In one instance, a class member was forced to deliver while her legs were shackled together, leading to the deaths of her infant twins. Plaintiffs entered into a wide-reaching settlement agreement that not only addressed remedies to correct inadequate medical care but also expanded social services programs for incarcerated mothers and their children and required the establishment of a statewide task force, which continued to address the concerns faced by incarcerated mothers and their children.

Women prisoners in California jails and prisons have filed several lawsuits within the past decade challenging grossly inadequate medical conditions in several California correctional facilities. In *Harris v. McCarthy*,[23] a large class of pregnant and postpartum women prisoners filed suit challenging a widespread pattern of deficient medical care. Angela H. (see case summary at beginning of chapter) served as lead plaintiff in this lawsuit, which resulted in a comprehensive settlement agreement mandating substantial changes in the provision of care for pregnant and postpartum women prisoners.

Pregnant women prisoners in county jail systems have also been subjected to seriously deficient medical care. Several lawsuits have been filed in California challenging inadequate care in a variety of different jail systems — large and small, urban and rural. In one large urban jail, plaintiffs not only challenged the quality of care provided to pregnant women generally, they also addressed the question of inadequate care provided to pregnant, substance-dependent women (see case summary of Dolores M. in section on treatment of women with substance dependency problems). The lawsuit *Jones v. Dyer*[24] was filed in Alameda County Superior Court in 1986 and settled in 1989. The settlement addressed all of the issues raised by plaintiffs in their initial complaint and resulted in a settlement agreement that required defendants to provide immediate treatment to pregnant women at the time of booking; immediate pregnancy testing, if desired; and treatment protocols and requirements for pregnant drug- and alcohol-dependent women. In addition, the agreement contained restrictions on the use of shackles and leg irons on pregnant women; requirements concerning pregnancy diets, vitamins, exercise, availability of pregnancy care materials; grievance procedures to address circumstances of miscarriage and infant death; and notification of prisoners concerning their rights under this agreement. The agreement required defendants to increase medical staffing, training of staff, and staffing hours for existing staff, and to use all means available to place pregnant women in alternative community-based programs. Finally, the defendants agreed to explore the establishment of a parenting program at the jail and a Contact Visitation Program for prisoners with children.

In *Yeager v. Smith*,[25] plaintiffs in a large rural county jail challenged severely inadequate conditions of confinement for pregnant women, raising issues of sanitation, overcrowding, and segregation policies as well as overall medical care and treatment of pregnant, substance-dependent women. The lawsuit was filed in federal district court in 1987 and settled in 1989. Again, plaintiffs entered into an extensive and comprehensive settlement agreement that addressed all aspects of pregnancy and postpartum care. One of the strongest elements of the agreement was the selection of a monitor, a former public defender and respected local attorney in private practice. Because of her ability to negotiate and communicate effectively with both plaintiffs and defendants and their attorneys, the monitor was a tremendous asset in insuring full implementation of the settlement agreement.

In an equally effective but different way, the monitor in *Jones v. Dyer* has been highly effective in working with plaintiffs, defendants, and the settlement judge to insure that the terms of the agreement are fully implemented. The monitor in *Jones* was a doctor who had extensive experience in correctional health care, obstetrics, and medical accreditation issues. She was highly accessible to women prisoners at the jail while maintaining an excellent working relationship with plaintiffs' attorneys and defendants' attorneys, the sheriff, and sheriff's department personnel. When the court-ordered monitoring period came to a close, she agreed to continue to act in an advisory capacity under an independent contract with the sheriff's department.

Although class-action litigation can be an effective tool for correcting limitations in prison and jail medical care, it is by no means the permanent cure.[26] Long-term remedies to the provision of substandard medical care involve constant surveillance and monitoring, not only by attorneys but also by health professionals, public officials, and policymakers.

AIDS and HIV Seropositivity

Judy T. was diagnosed with the AIDS virus and was serving a sentence of sufficient length that it was unlikely she would be released before she died. She requested that she be allowed to see her 14-year-old son for a Family Living Unit (FLU) visit, where she would be able to spend two days and nights with her son in a home-like setting in a trailer beside the prison grounds. But for her HIV-positive status, she was otherwise eligible for the FLU visit. Correctional authorities denied her request.

■

Plaintiff Jane Doe II is HIV-positive. She lives in Walker A, the unit at CIW designated for prisoners who are HIV-positive. Her confinement in Walker A automatically discloses her HIV status. She cannot move to any other housing without specifically informing any prospective cellmate of her HIV status. In 1993 she tested positive for tuberculosis infection. Despite her known HIV status, she was taken off tuberculosis medications after she became pregnant. As a result, she developed active tuberculosis. She was denied proper treatment during her pregnancy, including treatment for a vaginal infection, appropriate follow-up at a high-risk pregnancy clinic, evaluation of possible injuries from a fall, and provision of a special diet. During her pregnancy, CIW medical staff failed to diagnose or treat her lung problems, with the result that her pneumonia was not diagnosed or treated until she was sent to a hospital to deliver her baby. Although she bled heavily during and after delivery, she was returned to CIW after one day and not given follow-up examinations for a significant period of time. After her return to CIW, she was locked overnight in the Out Patient Housing unit in a cold and drafty room that lacked a call button, even though she was unable to use the bathroom by herself.[27]

Although exact figures on the percentage of women who are HIV-positive are difficult to obtain, one recent study of New York state prisoners found that 19 percent of women and 17 percent of men were HIV-positive.[28] Official figures are lower in California and other Western states, but most medical experts agree that the percentage of HIV-positive prisoners will continue to rise in the foreseeable future.[29]

Generally, women prisoners are routinely subjected to outbreaks of contagious diseases, from tuberculosis to hepatitis to measles and German measles. These outbreaks can lead to serious and sometimes fatal consequences for HIV-positive women and pregnant prisoners. While outbreaks of such contagious diseases can be damaging to all women who are susceptible, they have particularly dire consequences for women who are incarcerated and unable to leave the environment in which they are confined.

In *Shumate v. Wilson* (see above), HIV-positive women at the Central California Women's Facility and the California Institution for Women are alleging that complicating medical conditions such as meningitis, herpes, tuberculosis, pregnancy, and pneumonia have not been treated until they have led to a medical crisis. On several occasions, women dying of AIDS have been denied pain medication to relieve their suffering. And, women who are HIV-positive are systematically denied privacy by virtue of prison practices in housing and dispensing of medications.

Until recently, very few of the clinical drug trials for new AIDS treatments have included women. Even fewer of the trials have included pregnant women who are HIV-positive. However, women prisoners should be afforded access to current medications and treatment and should be given the option to freely and voluntarily participate in clinical trials when available.

As with medical staff outside the correctional environment, doctors, nurses, and other institutional staff who work with women prisoners who are HIV-positive must be trained in the proper medical procedures for dealing with AIDS awareness. For example, one woman prisoner with AIDS was recently transferred to an outside medical facility for tests and treatment. The nursing staff at the prison had refused to enter her room or bathe her.

Finally, women prisoners with AIDS and HIV are dealing with complex, painful, and difficult issues concerning their children and families. Many such women are reluctant to tell their family members about their illness because they fear rejection from their families or they are afraid of subjecting their children and family members to ostracism. Women who are public about their HIV-positive status often have to deal with rejection and stigma from institutional staff, other prisoners, and sometimes their own families. These families need access to contact visiting programs and, where available, overnight visiting programs, in order to deal with the very painful reality of AIDS and HIV. Family support is critical to all women dealing with life-threatening illnesses, let alone incarcerated women with AIDS. When women with AIDS are released from prison or jail, there must also be viable pre-release and discharge plans that make provisions for linking them with medical and social services once they are released. Making such provisions will greatly reduce the likelihood that these women will return to custody.

The vast majority of women prisoners—including women who have AIDS or are HIV-positive—are serving time for nonviolent, property, and drug-related charges. Compassionate release should be considered for women with life-threatening diseases—including AIDS, cancer, advanced sickle-cell anemia, and advanced diabetes. Incarcerating these women is not only prohibitively expensive for the taxpayer, it serves no penological purpose, since these women are, by and large, not a threat to society.[30] In addition, humane and cost-effective hospice programs should be developed outside of the institutional setting to allow prisoners who are living with AIDS to reenter the community when they are released from prison.

Reproductive Choice and Abortion

Terry B. and Sabina T., prisoners confined to a federal institution, both got pregnant through consensual sexual interactions with male prisoners in the prison. They were both placed in solitary confinement once their pregnancies were discovered, and were initially prohibited from contacting attorneys. They were told that, while they could obtain an abortion, they would be required to pay between two and three times the normal rate to the contract doctor, who would perform the medical procedure as a private physician. Sabina was finally able to obtain permission to go to an outside clinic with legal intervention and family support. In spite of aggressive legal intervention, Terry B. was unable to raise the money for the procedure or obtain permission to visit the outside clinic until the end of the second trimester. The outside clinic was unable to perform the abortion because Terry was too far along due to the delays of the correctional officials, and was forced to carry the pregnancy to term. Sabina is Caucasian; Terry, African-American.[31]

Women prisoners are consistently denied effective access to reproductive choice, either because of anti-choice attitudes on behalf of correctional staff, prohibitive financial restrictions, sloppy medical procedures and testing (which prevent women from getting accurate pregnancy testing), or a general disregard of women prisoners' needs and concerns. On some occasions, correctional officials, both medical and nonmedical, have denied women prisoners reproductive choice by coercing them to have abortions when they prefer to carry the pregnancy to term. However, the ethical concern — that women be allowed complete freedom to choose whether or not to terminate their pregnancies — is the same in either case. Restrictions on the reproductive freedom of pregnant women prisoners extend beyond the active interference with women's right to choose to have an abortion or to carry a pregnancy to term. Women prisoners report unauthorized hysterectomies or tubal ligations, or circumstances where they believe they were not fully informed of the consequences of such medical procedures. Other prisoners talk about the inherent coercion that they feel not to carry their pregnancies to term in an environment that is so damaging, or the consequences to carrying their pregnancies to term in an environment that is so severely stressful and inappropriate.

In only a few instances have courts dealt with the question of women prisoners' right to abortion services while incarcerated. In *Monmouth County Correctional Institution Inmates v. Lanzaro*,[32] women prisoners challenged several county policies that directly interfered with their ability to obtain abortions: (1) a requirement that women receive a court order in order to obtain an abortion outside of the correctional institution; (2) the refusal of the county to pay for abortion services, and (3) the county's refusal to provide abortion services to women who, for security reasons, would not be able to have an abortion outside of the institution. Plaintiffs obtained injunctive relief prohibiting the county from requiring women to obtain a court order in order to get an abortion, requiring the county to pay for all abortion services, even elective abortions, and requiring the county to take the necessary steps to insure that women had access to abortion, including providing transportation for women who requested abortions. In *Reproductive Health Services v. Webster*,[33] plaintiffs challenged state statutory provisions that prohibited the use of state funds for the purpose of providing staff and transportation for women prisoners to obtain abortion services. Through court order, and later through a consent decree, the state was barred from placing such restrictions on women prisoners' access to abortion.

The issue of access to abortion services continues to be one of the most controversial issues surrounding women prisoners' health care, in spite of the clear authority establishing the right of women prisoners to reproductive choice. Some states, such as California, even have statutory language clarifying the right of women prisoners to have abortions. However, the issue continues to arise in the county jail context, where women have been (1) refused all access to abortion services by administrative officials who do not approve of abortion ; (2) advised that they could have an abortion only if they paid for the procedure themselves and, in some cases, for the time of the sheriff's deputies accompanying them to the outside medical clinic; or (3) discouraged from having abortions in more subtle ways by staff who disapprove of abortion. As long as the issue of reproductive choice remains a controversial one, women prisoners and their advocates will need to be vigilant about preserving an effective right to choose for incarcerated women. When effective access to reproductive choice is threatened, it is usually low-income women who suffer first. Because they are not only low-income but also incarcerated, women prisoners are even more vulnerable to assaults on their right to choose.

Treatment of Women with Substance Dependency Problems

Dolores M. was sentenced to serve six months in a large urban county jail when she was seven months pregnant. Ordinarily, she would likely have received a lighter sentence for a minor probation violation, but the sentencing judge apparently wanted to ensure that she remained in custody for the duration of her pregnancy. Dolores was addicted to heroin and, prior to her sentencing, had sought methadone treatment at a local community-based program. Instead of receiving the treatment she needed, she was forced to withdraw from heroin "cold turkey" when she entered the county jail. She suffered severe withdrawal, with vomiting, headaches, abdominal pain, diarrhea, and other traumatic symptoms. She was not examined by an obstetrician for almost six weeks and received no follow-up appointment or medical treatment. When she was approximately eight and one-half months pregnant, she had severe uterine pain and felt no fetal movement. Three days later, her stillborn daughter was removed by cesarean section.

The vast majority of women in prisons and jails have substance dependency problems — addiction to drugs, alcohol, or, most commonly, poly-drug use. Research indicates that as many as 70 percent of incarcerated women have a history of substance dependency. The issue of addiction is a critical factor in determining the health care needs of women in prisons and jails.

One major factor that appears to be related to the high incidence of substance dependency problems for incarcerated women is the equally high prevalence of women in prison who are victims of childhood sexual or physical abuse or battering as adult women. Although research in this area is still fairly limited, it appears that a significant percentage of adult survivors of physical and sexual abuse turn to alcohol and drugs as a means of coping with the severe trauma of abuse. In a similar fashion, many battered women use drugs and alcohol to deal with the reality of physical, sexual, and emotional abuse. Often, the batterer is an addict or alcoholic, and the battered woman is initially forced to participate in the addictive behavior. In other instances, battered women are coerced by their abusers — either directly or indirectly — into taking part in criminal activity.[34]

Over the past decades, in part because of increasing drug penalties, an increase in women's involvement with crack cocaine, and an increase in the role of women as "drug mules" (minor players in drug trafficking activity), the number of women who have been incarcerated for drug possession and sales has risen dramatically. However, few correctional systems have made any serious attempt to address the issue of drug/alcohol addiction among women as a health issue. While model programs do exist,[35] they are available to only a small percentage of addicted women, and their funding sources remain unstable. Drug and alcohol addiction is one of the major issues confronting women in prison. In-depth, long-range planning must be done by correctional officials, judges, advocates and other policymakers. This is a health and social services issue, not merely a criminal justice issue.

The problems facing pregnant, substance-dependent women are especially difficult. As of 1995, experts had identified more than 200 instances where women who were pregnant and substance dependent had been charged with criminal violations of laws that related to child abuse and drug transportation and trafficking solely because they were alcohol- or drug-dependent and pregnant. In most instances, prosecutors who pursued these indictments relied on interpretations of these statutes that greatly distorted the original intent and language of the laws. In one case that received significant national attention, *State of Florida v. Johnson*,[36] Jennifer Johnson, a pregnant woman struggling to deal with an addiction to cocaine, was arrested shortly after she gave birth. She was charged with, and ultimately convicted of, delivery of an illegal substance to a minor. In a completely distorted interpretation of the statutory language and intent, the prosecutor argued that Ms. Johnson was guilty of "delivery" of the cocaine to her infant because the illicit drug passed through the umbilical cord during the birth process.

The *Johnson* case is not an isolated one. Prosecutions have occurred in a number of states and the District of Columbia in the last ten years, and certain states (such as South Carolina) have been particularly punitive toward pregnant, substance-dependent women. In some instances, the "charges" lodged against the pregnant woman are less criminal in nature than moralistic.[37] In the case of Pamela Rae Stewart, a pregnant woman was charged with "failing to follow her doctor's advice" to stay off her feet, to avoid street drugs and sexual intercourse, and to seek immediate medical attention if she experienced difficulties with her pregnancy.[38]

In one case, a judge in a Michigan probate court removed an infant from his mother based on her alleged use of "illegal drugs." The petition claimed that several weeks prior to delivery, the mother took non-prescription Valium four times to relieve pain that she was experiencing as a result of an automobile accident. Although the infant evidenced some effects from the drugs, he did not suffer from drug withdrawal after birth. Even though the mother had no previous history of drug addiction or child neglect, it took her over a year to regain custody of her son.[39]

In the debate over whether or not to incarcerate pregnant women who are drug or alcohol dependent, one factor that receives little attention is the quality of medical care available to pregnant, substance-dependent women who *are* incarcerated. While some of the judges who incarcerate pregnant, substance-dependent women appear to do so simply to punish these women, many judges are genuinely concerned about insuring that these women receive adequate prenatal care and do not continue to use drugs or alcohol during their pregnancies.[40]

However, many jail and prison systems do not have medical protocols or procedures specifically designed to address the safe detoxification of pregnant women addicted to drugs or alcohol. Few jails and prisons have an OB–GYN on staff, let alone medical personnel with expertise in the appropriate treatment of pregnant women addicted to heroin, cocaine, methamphetamines, or alcohol. The experience of Dolores M., described above, is the reality for most pregnant, substance-dependent women who are sentenced to jail "for their own protection" or "for the protection of the fetus." Detoxification through "cold turkey" withdrawal can have serious — often fatal — consequences for pregnant, substance-dependent women, yet this method is often the only kind of treatment that addicted women receive once they are sentenced to jail.[41]

Once an addicted, pregnant woman enters the jail or prison system, she experiences the same type of poor medical care received by nonaddicted, pregnant women. Thus, sentencing pregnant, substance-dependent women to serve time for the duration of their pregnancies in order to insure that they receive adequate medical care is rarely an effective means of accomplishing this goal.

Finally, incarceration does not prevent pregnant, drug- or alcohol-dependent women from having access to drugs or alcohol — drugs and alcohol are readily available in all prisons and jails, for a price, and if a pregnant woman is addicted and given no opportunity to participate in an effective recovery program, she will in all likelihood continue to use.

While most prisons and jails have Narcotics Anonymous and Alcoholics Anonymous groups, pregnant, substance-dependent women require more intensive and comprehensive treatment programs to increase the likelihood of successful recovery. Programs like Mandela House in Oakland, California, and the Neil J. Houston House in Boston, Massachusetts, offer an effective alternative to incarcerating pregnant, substance-dependent women.[42] However, these programs, and programs like them, must be assured sufficient funding and be utilized by sentencing judges, probation departments, and other arms of the criminal justice system if they are to be part of a comprehensive solution to the treatment of pregnant, substance-dependent women. Unfortunately, one recent study of sentencing judges indicated that judges often lack knowledge about the *availability* of such effective alternatives to incarceration, as well as accurate *information* about the medical consequences of drug and alcohol addiction.[43] Judicial education must be part of the overall effort to educate the public about the need for a more compassionate response to the treatment of pregnant, substance-dependent women.

As with many women in the general population, incarcerated women are either medically underinsured or uninsured prior to their incarceration. The lack of adequate health insurance plays a major role in the inability of many women to obtain treatment for drug and alcohol dependency, placing them further at risk for criminal involvement. Thus, health insurance programs that cover drug and alcohol treatment, psychological counseling for recovery from physical and sexual abuse, and basic medical services are an integral part of a long-term solution for reducing the number of women who become enmeshed in the criminal justice system.

Recommended Policy Reforms for Women Prisoners Denied Access to Adequate Medical Care

In the current public debate over correctional policy, there is very little discussion of compassionate or humane approaches to the treatment of prisoners. In spite of the numerous documented instances of women prisoners being denied adequate medical care, many policymakers and members of the general public assume that prisoners receive "Cadillac care," care that is better than that received by many people in the general population. In fact, the inadequate care or lack of care on many occasions is nothing short of barbaric. Policy reforms that would begin to address these concerns are very much needed. Specifically,

1. Basic Standards of Care promulgated by general medical associations (American Public Health Association, American Medical Association, etc.) and correctional medical associations should be extended to include care for incarcerated women.
2. Pregnant women prisoners should be receiving the same basic care that is recommended for pregnant women generally through the American College of Obstetricians and Gynecologists.
3. Pregnant, substance-dependent women should not be sentenced for

longer periods of incarceration solely because they are pregnant, and they should receive adequate prenatal care, including appropriate treatment for drug and alcohol dependency. Wherever possible, they should be placed in effective alternative treatment programs in lieu of incarceration.

4. Women prisoners with AIDS, terminal cancer, and other serious and chronic disease should receive humane and appropriate care while ill and compassionate treatment while dying. Wherever appropriate, women prisoners who are terminally ill should be released through compassionate release and commutation of sentences.

Conclusion

Universal access to adequate health care for *all* women is clearly a major priority for any comprehensive agenda on behalf of women. Women prisoners and their children must be included in this agenda. Women who are incarcerated today will, in most cases, reenter society in another capacity tomorrow — often as low-income, single mothers with all the same critical health concerns as nonincarcerated, low-income women. Certain groups of women prisoners — pregnant women, HIV-positive women, drug-dependent women, women suffering from life-threatening illnesses, elderly women, disabled women, immigrant women, battered women — face even greater obstacles to obtaining adequate medical care while incarcerated than do incarcerated women in general.

While litigation can address and rectify certain of the more egregious conditions faced by women prisoners who are denied adequate medical care,[44] the courts cannot legislate change in the attitudes of correctional staff and medical personnel. Nor can they legislate change in the growth of an increasingly hostile climate toward prisoners — women prisoners included. This attitude has been fostered, in part, by a legitimate concern and fear about violent crime. But, the rising rate of opposition toward prisoners and defendants *cannot* be attributed to an equivalent rise in crime statistics. According to FBI statistics, there has only been a slight increase in crime over the past decade.[45] Yet, there has been a staggering increase in the number of people incarcerated, particularly people of color. Women of color — especially African-American women and Latinas — are most disproportionately represented in this move to incarcerate more people. Race has been a primary factor in the increase in incarceration rates over the past decade, and by extension, race, class bias, and misogyny are significant factors in the incarceration of more women of color.

Health care reform for women prisoners must be done with an understanding and appreciation of these complex social factors. An effort to increase health care access for women with breast cancer, for example, should include advocacy on behalf of incarcerated women who suffer from this disease as well as nonincarcerated women, with special concern for the fact that African-American women have a higher rate of breast cancer than women of other specific ethnic groups and are disproportionately represented in the prison and jail population. An effort to improve the quality of maternal and child health issues should address the concerns of pregnant prisoners as well. Advocacy on behalf of HIV-positive women would, of necessity, include advocacy on behalf of women prisoners with AIDS. Until the health care issues of women prisoners are addressed in conjunction with health care issues for women generally, incarcerated women will continue to suffer the abuses of an isolated and largely uncaring system.

Notes

The author would like to acknowledge the assistance of Kirby Randolph, Judy Greenspan, Virginia Villegas, Stephanie Godt, and Karen Shain in the preparation of this article, and would like to dedicate this article to the incarcerated women who have come forward to challenge inadequate medical conditions in California prisons and jails, particularly Annette, Doris, Louwanna, and Charisse.

1   All names of women prisoners in this article have been changed to protect confidentiality, but all cases are factual portrayals of actual clients in several California prisons and jails. The women described throughout the article are or were plaintiffs or class members in the following lawsuits: Jane B. (*Shumate v. Wilson*), Mary H. (*Shumate v. Wilson*), Angela H. (*Harris v. McCarthy*), Barbara F. (Petition for Commutation, 1991), Yvonne H. (no litigation), Loreena Y. (*Yeager v. Smith*), Estella C. (*Harris v. McCarthy*), Nicole J. (*Jones v. Dyer*), Berrida J. (*Harris v. McCarthy*), Judy T. (no litigation), Terry B. and Sabina T. (no litigation), Jane Doe (*Shumate v. Wilson*), Dolores M. (*Jones v. Dyer*). Full citations of all these cases appear below, in notes 19 and 21.

2   See National Commission on Correctional Health Care, *Standards for Health Services in Jails* (1987); see also American Public Health Association, *Standards for Health Services in Correctional Institutions*, 2d ed. (Washington, D.C.: American Public Health Association, 1986).

3   See generally American College of Obstetricians and Gynecologists (ACOG), *Standards for Obstetric-Gynecologic Services* (Washington, D.C.: ACOG, 1992).

4   See National Women's Law Center (NWLC), "Incarcerated Women: Facts and Figures, 1992" (Washington, D.C.: NWLC, 1992), citing Bureau of Justice Statistics, *Prisoners in 1992* (Washington, D.C.: U.S. Department of Justice, 1992), 1.

5   Bureau of Justice Statistics, *Special Report: Women in Prison,* March 1991, 1 (1989 population figure).

6   Bureau of Justice Statistics, *Special Report: Women in Jail, 1989,* March 1992, 2.

7   C. McCall, J. Casteel, and N. Shaw, "Pregnancy in Prison: A Needs Assessment of Prenatal Outcome in Three California Penal Institutions," Report to the State of California Department of Health Services, Maternal and Child Health Branch, Contract No. 84-84085 A-1 (1985).

8   Figures for breakdown of incarcerated women by race are from NWLC, "Incarcerated Women," *supra* note 4; figures for general population are from U.S. Census Bureau (Washington, D.C.: GAO, 1992).

9   *Todaro v. Ward,* 431 F. Supp. 1129 (S.D.N.Y. 1977), *affirmed,* 565 F.2d 48 (2d Cir. 1977).

10   *Estelle v. Gamble,* 429 U.S. 97 (1976), *rehearing denied,* 429 U.S. 1066 (1977).

11   *Estelle v. Gamble* 429 U.S., 106.

12   Ibid., 104 (citing *Gregg v. Georgia,* 428 U.S. 153, 173 (1976).

13   See *Newman v. Alabama,* 503 F.2d 1320, 1331 (5th Cir. 1974), *rehearing denied,* 506 F.2d 1056 (1975), *certiorari denied,* 421 U.S. 948 (1975).

14   See *Martinez v. Mancusi,* 443 F.2d 921, 922–923 (2d Cir. 1970), *certiorari denied,* 401 U.S. 983 (1971).

15   See *Williams v. Vincent,* 508 F.2d 541, 543–544 (2d Cir. 1974).

16   *Ramos v. Lamm,* 639 F.2d 559, 575 (10th Cir. 1980), *certiorari denied,* 450 U.S. 1041 (1981).

17   *Todaro v. Ward, supra* note 9.

18   Ibid., 52.

19   See *West v. Manson,* No. N83-366 (D. Conn. filed May 9, 1983; settled June 14, 1984) (general medical care, psychiatric, substance abuse, prenatal and postnatal care); *Canterino v. Wilson,* 456 F. Supp. 174 (W.D. Ky. 1982) (general medical and dental care); *Wright v. McCarthy,* No. OCV 33880 (Cal. Super. Court, San Bernardino Cty., filed August 29, 1984) (general medical/licensure); *Witke v. Crowl,* C.A. No. 82-3078 (D. Idaho, filed Sept. 9, 1982; settled Jan. 22, 1985) (medical, dental, psychiatric); *Klatt v. King,* Civ. No. 80-971-JB (D. N.M. Consent Order, 1983) (medical, psychiatric, substance abuse); *Beehler v. Jeffes,* No. CVV-83-1024 (M.D. Pa. filed July 1983) (psychiatric); *Spear v. Ariyoshi,* Civ. No. 84-1104 (D. Hawaii, settled June 1985) (medical, psychiatric); *Harris v. McCarthy,* No. 85-6002 (C.D. Cal., filed Sept. 11, 1985; settled April 1987) (prenatal and postpartum care); *Jones v. Dyer* (Cal. Super. Court, Alameda Cty., filed Feb. 25, 1986; settled Nov. 1989) (prenatal and postnatal care, county jail); *Yeager v. Smith,* No. CV-F-87-493-REC (E.D. Cal., filed Sept. 2, 1987; settled Dec. 1989) (prenatal and postnatal care, county jail).

20   While recent Supreme Court decisions such as *Wilson v. Seiter,* 501 U.S. 294 (1991) have significantly reduced the scope of prisoners' rights to be free from cruel and unusual punishment under the Eighth Amendment of the Constitution, the *Estelle* decision and its many progeny still define the standard of adequate medical care for prisoners.

21   *Shumate v. Wilson,* No. CIV-S-95-619 WBS PAN (U.S. D. Ct., E.D. Cal. filed Apr. 4, 1995). Plaintiffs are represented by the National Prison Project of the American Civil Liberties Union (ACLU); Legal Services for Prisoners with Children (LSPC); the law firm of Heller, Ehrman, White & McAuliffe; law offices of Catherine Campbell; the ACLUs of Northern and Southern California; Central California Legal Services; and

the USC (University of Southern California) Post Conviction Justice Project. For further information, contact LSPC at 100 McAllister St., San Francisco, CA 94102.

22 *Supra* note 19.

23 *Supra* note 19.

24 *Supra* note 19.

25 *Supra* note 19.

26 If a case is brought to trial and a decision is rendered by a judge, that decision (and subsequent decisions issued on appeal) will have precedental value — that is, it will be binding on future cases that raise similar issues. If a case is settled and a consent decree or settlement agreement is agreed to by the parties and approved by the Court, the consent decree does not have binding authority over future cases. However, many prisoners' rights attorneys are opting to settle cases as opposed to bringing cases to trial because consent decrees may, in many instances, create remedies that are more far-reaching and comprehensive than court opinions.

27 This statement was included because Jane Doe II is one of the plaintiffs in *Shumate* and the case has not yet been resolved. The language is taken from the complaint.

28 Cathy Potler, *AIDS in Prison: A Crisis in New York State Corrections*, monograph (New York: Correctional Association of New York, 1987).

29 National Commission on AIDS, *Report: HIV Disease in Correctional Facilities* (Washington, D.C.: National Commission on AIDS, March 1991), 2–3.

30 A number of states have provisions for the release of prisoners in extraordinary circumstances such as serious or terminal medical conditions. In California and in a number of other states the process is known as "compassionate release." Often, prisoners are required to have a doctor's confirmation that they are terminally ill and the recommendation of the warden or chief medical officer at the prison that they be released. In some instances, sentencing judges may be involved. Although very few prisoners are actually released under the provisions, such policies make a great deal of sense since they result in enormous savings to the taxpayer as well as a humane and compassionate result for the prisoner and her family. (See story of "Barbara F." in "Profile of Women Prisoners.")

31 In early 1995, after a prolonged period of time, the Federal Bureau of Prisons finally proposed and adopted regulations that expand access to abortion services for women prisoners in the federal prison system.

32 834 F.2d 326 (3d Cir. 1987).

33 655 F. Supp. 1300 (W.D. Mo. 1987, settled June 23, 1987).

34 See generally Minouche Kandel, "Clemency for Battered Women in Prison," in *Women and the Law*, ed. Carol Lefcourt and Adria Hillman (New York: Clark, Boardman, 1992).

35 For example, the Forever Free program, California Department of Corrections (state prison) and Berkeley Addition Treatment Services program, Santa Rita County Jail, Alameda County, California (county jail).

36 *State of Florida v. Johnson*, No. E89-890-CFA (Fla. Cir. Ct. July 13, 1989), appeal docketed, No. 89-1765 (Fla. Dist. Ct. App. Aug. 31, 1989); see also Kary L. Moss, "Recent Update: Substance Abuse During Pregnancy," *Harvard Women's Law Journal* 13 (1990): 278–299.

37 See analysis of this trend in Lynn M. Paltrow, "When Becoming Pregnant Is a Crime," *Criminal Justice Ethics* 9, no. 1 (Winter/Spring 1990).

38 *State v. Stewart*, No. M508197 (San Diego Muni. Ct., 1987).

39 *In Re J. Jeffrey*, No. 99851 (Mich. Ct. of App. filed April 9, 1987).

40 Barrie Becker and Hon. Peggy Hora, "The Legal Community's Response to Drug Use during Pregnancy in the Criminal Sentencing and Dependency Context: A Survey of Judges, Prosecuting Attorneys and Defense Attorneys in Ten California Counties," *Southern California Review of Law and Women's Studies* (Spring 1993): 527.

41 See E. M. Barry, "Pregnant, Addicted and Sentenced: Debunking the Myths of Medical Treatment in Prison," *ABA Criminal Justice Journal* (winter 1991): 23–27.

42 For more information on Mandela House, contact Minnie Thomas, Executive Director, Solid Foundation, Administrative Offices, 3723 Hillview, Oakland, CA 94621.

43 See Becker and Hora, "The Legal Community's Response to Drug Use during Pregnancy," *supra* note 40.

44 Most litigation filed on behalf of women prisoners who are experiencing seriously inadequate health care in prisons and jails has resulted in judicial rulings, consent decrees, or settlement agreements that have improved the quality of and access to medical care. See citations in note 19; see also Shelly Geballe and Martha Stone, "The New Focus on Medical Care Issues in Women's Prison Cases," *National Prison Project Journal* no. 15 (spring 1988): 1–7, and Ellen M. Barry, "Pregnant Prisoners," *Harvard Women's Law Journal* 12 (1989): 189–205, for analyses of case law involving medical care issues affecting women prisoners.

45 Federal Bureau of Investigation (FBI), *Uniform Crime Report, 1993* (Washington, D.C.: FBI, 1993).

Notes on Contributors

Ellen M. Barry is Director and Managing Attorney of Legal Services for Prisoners with Children (LSPC). She founded LSPC with a grant from the Berkeley Law Foundation in November 1978, and has been Director since then. She received a B.A. from Swarthmore College in 1975, and a J.D. from New York University Law School in 1978. She served as interim director of the Ex-Offender Employment Project for the Employment Law Center from 1981–1982 and has been lead counsel or co-counsel on a number of lawsuits brought on behalf of incarcerated women, pregnant women prisoners, prisoners, and parolees. She has written widely on issues affecting incarcerated parents and their children, pregnant prisoners, special problems of women prisoners, and prisoners' rights in general, and has spoken extensively on these same issues. Ms. Barry is the recipient of the 1990 Annual Legal Services Section, chairs the California State Bar Committee on Legal Services for Prisoners, is a commissioner on the California Commission on Female Inmates and Parolees, and is Co-Chair of the National Legal Aid and Defenders Association's (NLADA) Section on Institutions and Alternatives.

Laurie R. Beck is Director of Education Policy at the Community Service Society of New York. She holds a law degree from City University of New York Law School at Queens College and a master's degree in sociology from Columbia University. She completed additional graduate study at Brandeis University. Her areas of interest include education law and policy and medical sociology.

Joan E. Bertin is Clinical Professor of Public Health at Columbia University and Director of the Program on Gender, Science, and Law, a women's health policy program. During the 1995–1996 academic year, she held the Joanne Woodward Chair at Sarah Lawrence College. Previously, she was Associate Director of the Women's Rights Projects of the American Civil Liberties Union, where she represented women with regard to employment rights, pregnancy discrimination, and other issues. She writes and speaks frequently on women's rights and women's health.

Janet M. Calvo is on the faculty of the City University School of Law where she has taught in the areas of immigration and health law. Her publications have focused on health care access, public benefits, and the impact of immigration on women immigrants. She has also worked on cases that have sought to broaden the access of the foreign-born to health services and on legislation that has addressed the problems of abused immigrant women and children.

Wendy Chavkin, M.D., has been active on a host of reproductive health issues. Her clinical training is in obstetrics and gynecology. She holds a Master's of Public Health (M.P.H.) in reproductive epidemiology, and is board certified in public health and preventive medicine. She has worked as a public health official, researcher, and academic. She is currently a senior research associate at the Beth Israel Medical Center and is also an Associate Professor of Clinical Public Health and Obstetrics and Gynecology at the Columbia University's School of Public Health and College of Physicians and Surgeons. She has written extensively about women's reproductive public health issues, including her 1984 book, *Double Exposure: Women's Health Hazards at the Job and at Home.* She has recently become Editor-in-Chief of the *Journal of the American Medical Women's Association.*

Kay Dickersin received her master's degree in cell biology from the University of California at Berkeley and her Ph.D. in epidemiology from the Johns Hopkins University School of Hygiene and Public Health. She is Assistant Professor in the Department of Epidemiology and Preventive Medicine at the University of Maryland School of Medicine and Director of the Baltimore Cochrane Center. Her major research interests are related to clinical trials of new treatments, meta-analysis, and dissemination of available medical knowledge to the medical community. She has been a member of the Board of Directors of the National Breast Cancer Coalition, the Maryland Women's Health Coalition, and the National Cancer Advisory Board. In addition, she has been a member of the Institute of Medicine's Committee to Advise the Department of Defense on its FY-1993 Breast Cancer Program, the National Cancer Institute's Breast Cancer Working Group, the Department of the Army's Breast Cancer Research Program Integration Panel, and the Department of Health and Human Services' National Action Plan on Breast Cancer Steering and Executive Committees.

Abigail English is Project Director of the Adolescent Health Care Project and staff attorney at the National Center for Youth Law in its Chapel Hill, N.C., office. She has participated in major litigation affecting the legal rights of children and adolescents, authored numerous publications, and lectured widely to youth-serving professionals. She has also taught courses on children and the law at the University of California at Berkeley's Boalt Hall School of Law. Ms. English was honored by the Society for Adolescent Medicine in 1987 as a Gallagher Lecturer on legal and ethical aspects of AIDS in adolescents. Her article, "The HIV-AIDS Epidemic and the Child Welfare System: Protecting the Rights of Infants, Young Children, and Adolescents," appeared in a special symposium issue of the *Iowa Law Review* in 1992. She serves as Chair of the Board of Advocates for Youth and was a member of the advisory panel for the Office of Technology Assessment's 1991 study of adolescent health. She is currently undertaking a two-year project, "Adolescent Health Care in Transition: Medicaid, Managed Care, and Health Care Reform."

Elizabeth Fee is the Chief of the History of Medicine Division, National Library of Medicine, at the National Institutes of Health. She is also Adjunct Professor of History and Health Policy at the Johns Hopkins School of Hygiene and Public Health and holds a joint appointment in the Department of History of Science, Medicine, and Technology of the Johns Hopkins School of Medicine. She is the author of *Disease and Discovery* (1987), and editor or coeditor of eight other books, including *AIDS: The Burdens of History* (1988), *AIDS: The Making of a Chronic Disease* (1992), and *Making Medical History: The Life and Times of Henry E. Sigerist* (1996). She has published many articles on the history of public health, health policy, and women's health, and serves as contributing editor for the *American Journal of Public Health*. She is currently conducting research on the history of public health and social medicine since 1940.

Carol J. Gill is a clinical and research psychologist specializing in health and disability. She received her Ph.D. in psychology from the University of Illinois at Chicago in 1979. She has served as Director of Rehabilitation Psychology at Glendale Adventist Medical Center in Los Angeles, Acting Director of the Program in Disability and Society at the University of Southern California, and Commissioner for Mental Health on the Los Angeles County Commission on Disabilities. Her articles on disability issues have appeared in professional and academic journals, books, and the popular disability press. She is currently President of the Chicago Institute of Disability Research, Adjunct Professor of Physical Medicine and Rehabilitation at Northwestern University Medical School, and serves on the Board of the Health Resource Center for Women with Disabilities in Chicago. Dr. Gill uses a wheelchair as the result of childhood polio.

Nancy Krieger is Assistant Professor in the Department of Health and Social Behavior at the Harvard School of Public Health and Adjunct Professor at the Division of Research of the Kaiser Foundation Research Institute, Oakland, California. Her research focuses on issues of race/ethnicity, class, gender, and health, particularly as it relates to breast cancer; other work concerns the history and theoretical underpinnings of epidemiology. She is coauthor of *The Politics of AIDS* (1986) and coeditor of *AIDS: The Politics of Survival* (1994) and *Women's Health, Politics and Power: Essays on Sex/Gender, Medicine and Public Health* (1994).

Joyce E. McConnell is Associate Professor of Law at the University of West Virginia College of Law. She received her J.D. in 1982 from Antioch School of Law and an L.L.M. from Georgetown Law School. From 1982 to 1984 she clerked for the chief judge and other administrative law judges at the National Labor Relations Board. She received a fellowship at Georgetown University Law Center to teach in the Center for Applied Legal Studies. Professor McConnell teaches and writes in the areas of constitutional law, criminal law, torts, and feminist legal theory.

Kary L. Moss is an attorney specializing in civil rights law and public health. While a staff attorney at the American Civil Liberties Union (A.C.L.U.) Women's Rights Project, from 1989 to 1991, she worked to defend the rights of women arrested or who had lost custody of their children for using alcohol or drugs while pregnant. She received a master's degree in international affairs from Columbia University and a law degree from City University of New York Law School at Queens College. She is coauthor of *The Rights of Women*, with Susan Deller Ross, Isabelle Katz Pinzler, and Deborah Ellis (1993) and author of numerous law review articles on the subject of social control of women. She is currently the Executive Director of the Maurice and Jane Sugar Law Center for Economic and Social Justice, located in Detroit.

Judy Norsigian is a coauthor of *Our Bodies, Ourselves* and *The New Our Bodies, Ourselves* as well as a member and codirector of the Boston Women's Health Book Collective. She has served on the Board of the National Women's Health Network for more than ten years and speaks frequently on a wide range of women's health topics. She is also a board member and past president of the Women's StateWide Legislative Network of Massachusetts and a member of the Technical Advisory Committee of the Contraceptive Research and Development Program. In 1989 she received the Public Service Award from the Massachusetts Public Health Association. She is the author of numerous chapters and articles on women and health and sits on the editorial boards of *Women and Health* and *Birth: Issues in Perinatal Care*. Currently her work focuses on promoting women and national health care reform as well as advocating expanded access to midwifery services in the home, birth center, and hospital setting.

Ann Scales received a B.A. from Wellesley College and a law degree from Harvard University and is presently the Weihoffen Professor of Law at the University of New Mexico. She has also taught at the University of Iowa, Boston College, and the University of British Columbia. Ms. Scales writes and lectures widely in the field of feminist legal theory, and is currently finishing a book.

Lauren Schnaper, M.D., is Assistant Professor of Surgery and Oncology at the University of Maryland School of Medicine, where she is also Director of Medical Student Education for the Department of Surgery. Her practice is limited to benign and malignant diseases of the breast, and she is Director of the Breast Evaluation Program of the University of Maryland Cancer Center. She is involved in many national breast cancer activities, most notably as Chairman of the Breast Surgeons Committee of the Cancer and Leukemia Group B, a national clinical research organization. Dr. Schnaper is married to Dr. James M. Carlton, a plastic surgeon. They have three sons.

Susan Stefan is Professor of Law at the University of Miami School of Law. Prior to 1990, she worked as an attorney at the Mental Health Law Project (now the Bazelon Center for Mental Health Law) in Washington, D.C. She received an A.B. from Princeton University in 1980, an M. Phil. from Cambridge University in England, and her J.D. from Stanford Law School. She specializes in issues relating to women in mental health law, and has most recently published "The Protection Racket: Rape Trauma Syndrome, Psychiatric Labeling, and Law," *Northwestern Law Review* 88 (1994), and "Dancing in the Sky Without a Parachute: Sex and Love in Institutional Settings," in Sundram, ed., *Choice and Responsibility: Legal and Ethical Dilemmas in Services for People with Mental Disabilities* (Albany: New York Commission on Quality of Care for the Mentally Disabled, 1994).

Catherine Teare is Project Coordinator of the Adolescent HIV Project and Health Policy Analyst with the National Center for Youth Law in San Francisco. She has worked extensively on policy issues affecting at-risk and HIV-infected children and youth, with particular emphasis on young women, children orphaned by AIDS, and children in foster care. She is the editor of a Special Issue of *Youth Law News* on adolescents in the HIV/AIDS epidemic. Her current work examines access to preventive care and medical treatment for low-income children and adolescents, particularly in managed care.

Library of Congress Cataloging-in-Publication Data

Man-made medicine : women's health, public policy, and reform / edited
  by Kary L. Moss.
        p.   cm.
    Includes index.
    ISBN 0-8223-1811-3 (cloth : alk. paper). — ISBN 0-8223-1816-4 (pbk. : alk. paper)
    1. Women's health services — Government policy — United States.
2. Sexism in medicine — United States.   3. Sex discrimination in
medicine — United States.   4. Women — Health and hygiene — Government
policy — United States.   5. Women — Health and hygiene — United States —
Sociological aspects.   I. Moss, Kary L.
RA564.85.M36   1996
362.1'082 — dc20   96-21855 CIP